Download the Gunner Goggles App Now!

Go to the App Store from your iPhone or iPad and search for Gunner Goggles

T0210200

7:27 PM Mon Jul 23

X

Hi, Welcome to Gunner Goggles

Gunner Goggles is a book and augmented reality app series that allows you to scan AR Targets in our books to access expertly curated content for you, the busy med student.

Up Next: How to Scan

Each Gunner Goggles specialty has its own app; you can purchase other titles at:
ElsevierHealth.com/GunnerGoggles

GUNNER GOGGLES

Medicine

HONORS SHELF REVIEW

EDITORS:

Hao-Hua Wu, MD
Resident, Department of
Orthopaedic Surgery
University of California–San Francisco
San Francisco, California

Leo Wang, MS, PhD
Perelman School of Medicine
University of Pennsylvania
Philadelphia, Pennsylvania

Rebecca Gao, MS
Stanford School of Medicine
Palo Alto, California

FACULTY EDITORS:

Nadia Bennett, MD
Assistant Professor of Clinical Medicine
Perelman School of Medicine
University of Pennsylvania
Philadelphia, Pennsylvania

Eric Goren, MD
Associate Professor of Clinical
Medicine
Perelman School of Medicine
University of Pennsylvania
Philadelphia, Pennsylvania

Temitayo Ogunleye, MD
Assistant Professor of Clinical
Dermatology
Perelman School of Medicine
University of Pennsylvania
Philadelphia, Pennsylvania

Wanda Ronner, MD
Professor of Clinical Obstetrics and
Gynecology
Perelman School of Medicine
University of Pennsylvania
Philadelphia, Pennsylvania

Chuang-Kuo Wu, MD
Professor of Medicine
University of California–Irvine
School of Medicine
Irvine, California

ELSEVIER

ELSEVIER

1600 John F. Kennedy Blvd.
Ste 1800
Philadelphia, PA 19103-2899

Notices

Knowledge and best practice in this field are constantly changing. As new research and experience broaden our understanding, changes in research methods, professional practices, or medical treatment may become necessary.

Practitioners and researchers must always rely on their own experience and knowledge in evaluating and using any information, methods, compounds, or experiments described herein. In using such information or methods they should be mindful of their own safety and the safety of others, including parties for whom they have a professional responsibility.

With respect to any drug or pharmaceutical products identified, readers are advised to check the most current information provided (i) on procedures featured or (ii) by the manufacturer of each product to be administered, to verify the recommended dose or formula, the method and duration of administration, and contraindications. It is the responsibility of practitioners, relying on their own experience and knowledge of their patients, to make diagnoses, to determine dosages and the best treatment for each individual patient, and to take all appropriate safety precautions.

To the fullest extent of the law, neither the Publisher nor the authors, contributors, or editors, assume any liability for any injury and/or damage to persons or property as a matter of products liability, negligence or otherwise, or from any use or operation of any methods, products, instructions, or ideas contained in the material herein.

Library of Congress Cataloging-in-Publication Data
Names: Wu, Hao-Hua, editor.
Title: Gunner goggles medicine : honors shelf review / editors, Hao-Hua Wu, Leo Wang ; faculty editors, Nadia Bennett, Eric Goren, Temitayo Ogunleye, Wanda Ronner, Chuang-Kuo Wu.
Description: Philadelphia, PA : Elsevier, [2019] | Includes bibliographical references.
Identifiers: LCCN 2017048837 | ISBN 9780323510356 (pbk. : alk. paper)
Subjects: | MESH: Clinical Medicine | Test Taking Skills | User-Computer Interface | Study Guide
Classification: LCC RC46 | NLM WB 18.2 | DDC 616--dc23 LC record available at https://lccn.loc.gov/2017048837

Executive Content Strategist: Jim Merritt
Content Development Manager: Lucia Gunzel
Publishing Services Manager: Patricia Tannian
Senior Project Manager: Cindy Thoms
Senior Book Designer: Maggie Reid

Working together
to grow libraries in
developing countries

www.elsevier.com • www.bookaid.org

Printed in China

Last digit is the print number: 9 8 7 6 5 4 3 2 1

Gunner Goggles Honors Shelf Review Series

Gunner Goggles Family Medicine	978-0-323-51034-9
Gunner Goggles Medicine	978-0-323-51035-6
Gunner Goggles Neurology	978-0-323-51036-3
Gunner Goggles Obstetrics and Gynecology	978-0-323-51037-0
Gunner Goggles Pediatrics	978-0-323-51038-7
Gunner Goggles Psychiatry	978-0-323-51039-4
Gunner Goggles Surgery	978-0-323-51040-0

Contributors

SECTION EDITOR

Jacques Greenberg, MD
Resident Physician
Department of Surgery
Cornell University
New York, New York

QUESTIONS EDITOR

Daniel Gromer, MD
Resident Physician
Internal Medicine
Massachusetts General Hospital
Boston, Massachusetts

CONTRIBUTING AUTHORS

Sila Bal, MD, MPH
Resident Physician
Massachusetts Eye and Ear
Boston, Massachusetts
Diseases of the Blood and Blood-Forming Organs

Lauren Briskie, MD
Resident Physician
Emergency Medicine
Christiana Care Health System
Newark, Delaware
Diseases of the Respiratory System

Sierra Centkowski, MD
Resident Physician
Department of Dermatology
Stanford University School of Medicine
Palo Alto, California
Endocrine and Metabolic Disorders

Jacob Charny, MD
Resident Physician
Department of Dermatology
University of Illinois College of Medicine
Chicago, Illinois
Disorders of the Skin and Subcutaneous Tissues

Jacques Greenberg, MD
Resident Physician
Department of Surgery
Cornell University
New York, New York
Cardiovascular Disease
Renal, Urinary, and Male Reproductive System

Daniel Gromer, MD
Resident Physician
Internal Medicine
Massachusetts General Hospital
Boston, Massachusetts

George Hung
Perelman School of Medicine
University of Pennsylvania
Philadelphia, Pennsylvania
Diseases of the Musculoskeletal System and Connective Tissue

Cody Nathan, MD
Resident Physician
Department of Medicine
University of Pennsylvania
Philadelphia, Pennsylvania
Diseases of the Nervous System and Special Senses

William Plum, MD
Resident Physician
Department of Ophthalmology
Columbia University
New York, New York
Diseases of the Respiratory System
Nutritional and Digestive Disorders

Alejandro Suarez-Pierre, MD
Johns Hopkins School of Medicine
Baltimore, Maryland
Nutritional and Digestive Disorders

Junqian Zhang, MD
Resident Physician
Department of Dermatology
University of Pennsylvania
Philadelphia, Pennsylvania
Cardiovascular Disease

Acknowledgments

"If I have seen further than others, it is by standing upon the shoulders of giants."

–Isaac Newton

We would like to thank the many exceptional innovators who helped transform our vision of *Gunner Goggles Medicine* into reality.

To our editorial team at Elsevier, thank you for your unrelenting support throughout the publication process. Jim Merritt believed in *Gunner Goggles* from day one and used his experience as an executive content strategist to point us in the right direction with respect to book proposal, product pitch, and manuscript development. Lucia Gunzel expertly guided us through manuscript submission and revision, no easy feat with two first-time authors. Maggie Reid collaborated with us closely to create the layout design and color schemes. Cindy Thoms and the copy editing team made sure our written content adhered to a high professional standard.

To the editors, authors, and student reviewers of *Gunner Goggles Medicine*, thank you for your scholarship and unwavering enthusiasm. Our outstanding faculty editors — Dr. Nadia Bennett, Dr. Eric Goren, Dr. Temitayo Ogunleye, Dr. Wanda Ronner, and Dr. Chuang-Kuo Wu — took time out of their busy schedules to meticulously edit each chapter and provide numerous invaluable insights on how to improve quality and accuracy. A number of outstanding residents and medical students contributed to the content of this textbook and provided us feedback on high-yield topics for the NBME Medicine Subject Exam, notably Dr. Sila Bal, Dr. Lauren Briskie, Dr. Sierra Centkowski, Dr. Jacob Charny, Dr. Jacques Greenberg, Dr. Daniel Gromer, George Hung, Dr. William Plum, Dr. Alejandro Suarez-Pierre, and Dr. Junqian Zhang.

To our augmented reality (AR) team, thank you for your creativity and dedication during the development of the *Gunner Goggles* AR application. Nadir Bilici, Brian Mayo, Vlad Obsekov, Clare Teng, and Yinka Orafidiya helped us develop and test the initial *Gunner Goggles* AR prototype. Tammy Bui designed the *Gunner Goggles* logo and AR app icon.

We would also like to thank the Wharton Innovation Fund for awarding us seed money to help pursue development of *Gunner Goggles* AR.

You all continue to inspire us, and we are incredibly grateful and deeply appreciative for your support.

–Hao-Hua, Leo, and Rebecca

Contents

Introduction

Hao-Hua Wu and Leo Wang

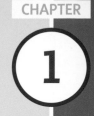
I. The Gunner's Guide to a Better Test Score

Curious why certain classmates perform well on every exam? Frustrated by how few of these "gunner" peers share study secrets?

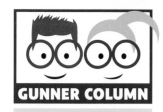

At *Gunner Goggles*, our goal is to reveal and demystify. By integrating *augmented reality (AR)* into this review book, we **reveal** how the best students approach topics, conceptualize complex disease, and allocate study time efficiently. By organizing each topic according to the National Board of Medical Examiners (NBME) format, we **demystify** exam content and the types of questions one can expect on test day.

Of the tests medical students strive to conquer, shelf exams boast the highest ratio of importance to study resource quality. For instance, performance on shelf exams typically informs final clerkship grades, which are the most important criteria on the medical school transcript for residency application. Yet, there is no single authoritative study resource for the shelf across all disciplines. Most importantly, no current book specifically targets shelf exam prep. So students must rely on miscellaneous resources and anecdotal advice to get the job done.

In light of this void in authoritative test prep, we have created the *Gunner Goggles* series to provide you with the most effective shelf exam testing resource. *GG* stands out for three important reasons:

First, readers have the opportunity to enhance understanding of important shelf topics by using the **AR** features on each page. With an iPhone or iPad, users can download the *Gunner Goggles* AR iOS app and use it to turn book figures into three-dimensional (3D) images, access high-yield videos and view pertinent digital media. More on how AR technology works can be found on page 2.

Second, *Gunner Goggles* provides a plethora of tips on how to manage time efficiently when studying for the shelf. Mnemonics and strategies for how to approach difficult concepts can be found in the blue "Gunner Column" to the right or left of each page. We also tell you how to *think* about these concepts so that the study of medicine never feels like a laundry list of items you simply have to memorize.

Third, this review book is written and organized optimally for shelf exam test prep. Each chapter is organized according to the NBME Clinical Science Subject Examination and USMLE Course Content outlines. In addition, a concise summary of how topics are tested prefaces each chapter.

As experts on the shelf exam, we understand how difficult it is to carve out time to study while juggling clinical responsibilities during your clerkship rotation. We also know that each student's learning curve is different based on the timing of the rotation (first block vs. last block), year in medical school (MS3 vs. MD/PhD returning after graduate school), and future career interests (e.g., an aspiring orthopedic surgeon learning about obstetrics and gynecology). However, we believe that any student can perform well on the shelf with the right strategy and study resources.

We created this book anticipating the needs of all types of students, and hope that *Gunner Goggles* will be the most comprehensive, authoritative shelf exam review book that you ever use. We are confident that *Gunner Goggles* will enable you to achieve your test performance goals and stick it to your "gunner" classmates, whose advice, or lack thereof, you won't be needing after all.

II. Augmented Reality: A New Paradigm for Shelf Exam Test Prep

Think of AR as your best friend.

To use it, download the free *Gunner Goggles Medicine* application on your iPad or iPhone and create your own optional profile. Now with the application open, point your smart mobile camera at this page.

Notice how on your camera, there are now links you can click on, 3D figures you can rotate, and a video you can watch. You have just unlocked the AR features for this page!

Take a moment to play around with these AR features on your smart mobile device. The way this works is anytime you see the *Gunner Goggles* icon 🔵🔵 in the blue Gunner Column, there is an AR feature accompanying the text which you have the opportunity to interact with.

Still not convinced? Here are three reasons why AR is your ideal study companion.

99 AR
Gunner Goggles Introduction Video

99 AR
Gunner Goggles Contact

Presentation

AR breaks the boundaries of how information can be presented in this textbook.

Traditionally, if you wanted to learn about a disease in a review book, you would be expected to read and memorize a block of text similar to the following:

"Huntington disease (HD) is a GABAergic neurodegenerative disorder that is caused by an autosomal dominant mutation leading to CAG repeats on chromosome 4. Patients typically present in the fourth and fifth decade of life with chorea, memory loss, caudate atrophy on neuroimaging, and motor impairment, depending on the variant. Although there is no cure for Huntington's, the movement disorders associated with the disease, such as chorea, can be treated with drugs like tetrabenazine and reserpine to decrease dopamine release."

Having read (or most likely glazed) through that last paragraph, do you feel comfortable enough to answer questions about the genetics, presentation, and treatment of Huntington's right now? A week from now? Three weeks from now when you have to take your shelf exam?

Here's where AR comes in. Use your *Gunner Goggles* app to check out how we're able to present HD in different, memorable ways.

For visual learners, here's a video of an effective HD mnemonic →

If you are an audio learner, here's a link to key points about Huntington's for the shelf →

Forgot your neuroanatomy? Here's where the caudate is →

What's the difference between chorea, athetosis and ballismus again? Chorea looks like this →

Now write a one-line description of Huntington's in your own words in the margins of this page for future reference. It's much easier with AR, right? Like we said, your best friend.

99 AR
Huntington Disease Mnemonic

99 AR
Huntington's Podcast

99 AR
The caudate nucleus is part of the basal ganglia.

99 AR
Chorea Patient Example

Evaluation

The GG Medicine app has the potential to exponentially enhance how you can evaluate your own understanding of the material. Although not available with the first edition, we are in the process of developing a personalized question bank as well as a flashcards feature. Our vision is to allow you to scan a topic on the page for immediate access to relevant practice questions and flashcards. In future versions, you will also be able to create your own flashcard deck and track your mastery.

gg AR

In addition the GG app can keep track of the AR Targets scanned and the Learning links viewed. These links are saved to a Link Library which you can view at any time. You can also like or dislike a Learning Link with an opportunity to provide us feedback for better resources available.

As development of the GG Medicine app is an ongoing process, we encourage and welcome your feedback. If you like the idea of having a personalized question bank and flashcard feature or have an idea for how we can improve the GG app to better serve your studying needs, please provide us feedback through an in-app message. You can also email us at GunnerGoggles@gmail.com.

Community Engagement

Studying for the shelf can be isolating. Our vision is to develop a feature in the GG Medicine that would allow you to connect with chapter authors and fellow readers. We are in the process of developing a medium in which shelf-related inquiries can be discussed among authors and readers through an optional short message system (SMS) feature.

Given that the community engagement feature is in development and unavailable for the first edition, we welcome your input on how we can connect you with the people who will enable your test day success.

To provide feedback, please scan the page and vote. You can also email us GunnerGoggles@gmail.com for any comments or suggestions.

Augmented Reality Frequently Asked Questions

"Since AR is integrated into _Gunner Goggles Medicine_, does this mean I have to pull out my iPad of iPhone for every page of the book?"

No, only if you need it. Some may use AR more than others, depending on background and level of comfort with medicine. For instance, you may already have a solid understanding of Huntington's and only need to read the text as a refresher. On the other hand, if you are less comfortable with Huntington's, the AR features are there just in case.

"Can't I just look up everything I don't know on my own? Why do I have to use the _Gunner Goggles_ app?"

You can absolutely look things up on your own. But that takes time. And sometimes you can't find the best reference or mnemonic. Our team of experts has already gone through the trouble of identifying potential sources of confusion for you and found the perfect resources. In the *Gunner Goggles* app, we have compiled the slickest and most concise resources one can use to better understand a topic. Videos, audio files, and images are first vetted by subject experts for accuracy of content. They are then evaluated by students like yourself for utility of content to enhance test performance. Only resources with the most Gunner votes are embedded into each page.

"What if a link doesn't work or I want something on the page to change?"

Please tell us! Another advantage of AR is that we can immediately receive and implement your feedback. Just use the *Gunner Goggles* app to text us your concerns and our tech support team will respond ASAP!

III. Study Smart: Mnemonics and Gunner Study Tips

Even with incredible AR features at your disposal, you won't be able to optimize exam performance unless you know how to study. Below are the four most important things one can do to study for the Medicine shelf under the time restraints imposed by clerkships.

Understand the Organizing Principle

The easiest way to both save time and perform well on the shelf is to understand how a specific disease or concept fits into the big picture. For instance, knowing the buzz words, diagnostic steps, and treatment plan for histoplasmosis will likely lead to only one correct answer on the test. However, understanding that histoplasmosis exists on a spectrum of fungal infections (blastomycosis, coccidioidomycosis) differentiated by geographic region can help you answer any question when the otherwise healthy adult patient presents with a respiratory fungal infection.

Create Effective Mnemonics

If you have photographic memory, skip this section. For the rest of us mere mortals, the following outlines the organizing principles of what constitutes a Gunner mnemonic.

Mnemonics are important when

1. You have to learn a lot of material.
2. You want to teach something to your colleagues during morning rounds. Attendings and residents are always impressed when they can learn something from a medical student.
3. You want to remember something 15 years from now when you are working the 30th hour of a busy call day.

Organizing principles (OP) for mnemonics are as follows:

1. Use the spelling of a name to your benefit (**Spell**)
   Example:
   a. "8urk14tt's" lymphoma (Burkitt lymphoma), lep"thin" (leptin), "supraoptiuretic" nuclei (supraoptic nuclei that produces antidiuretic hormone)
   b. Tenofovir is the only NRTI nucleoTide
   c. We"C"ener's granulomatosis (GPA) for C-ANCA and Cyclophosphamide tx

Trisomy 13 mnemonic

2. Create an acronym that contains distinguishing syllables or letters of names (**Distinguish**).
   Example:
   a. Chronic Alcoholics Steal PhenPhen and Nevar Rifuse Grisee Carbs (Chronic alcohol abuse + St John's wort + phenytoin + phenobarb + nevaripine + rifampin + griseofulvin + carbamazepine)
      • Reinforce the mnemonic by spelling the name of the item to be memorized accordingly.
      • For example, "Refus"ampin, "Never"apine, "Greasy"ofulvin, "Carb"amazepine, etc.
      • This ties mnemonic OP 1 with mnemonic OP 2.
3. Drawings help (**Draw**)
   Example: Trisomy 13 looks like polydactyly + cleft lip when the number 13 is rotated 90 degrees clockwise (the horizontal 1 is the extra digit, and the cleft of the horizontal 3 is the cleft lip).
4. Counting the letters of a word (**Count**)
   Example: Patau syndrome = 13 letters = Trisomy 13
5. Arrange acronym in alphabetical order (**Arrange**)
   Example: ABCDEF for diphtheria (ADP ribosylation, beta prophage, C Diphtheria, elongation factor 2)
   Examples of instructors who practice this concept well are Dr. John Barone of Kaplan and Dr. Husain Sattar of Pathoma.

On the flip side, here are examples of poor mnemonics (although you may remember them now, given how they were highlighted in this text).

a. Blind as a bat, mad as a hatter, red as a beet, hot as Hades, dry as a bone, the bowel and bladder lose their tone, and the heart runs alone = poor mnemonic for anticholinergic syndrome
   • This mnemonic forces you to memorize extra and extraneous things (like bat, beet, hare, and desert), which have nothing to do with anticholinergic syndrome.
b. WWHHHHIMP (withdrawal + Wernicke + hypertensive crisis + hypoxia + hypoglycemia + hypoperfusion + intracranial bleed + meningitis/encephalopathy + poisoning) = poor mnemonic for causes of delirium
   • Wait, how many *H's* does this mnemonic have again?

A good rule of thumb: if you can still remember a mnemonic under a high-pressure situation (attending pimps you) or after a 7-day period, then you have a winner.

Ultimately, the best mnemonics are the ones you invent and apply repeatedly. So use these mnemonic principles to give yourself a solid head start.

Devise a Study Schedule and Stick to It

The third most important piece of advice for the shelf is to create a study schedule at the beginning of the rotation and follow it. Rotations are draining, and oftentimes you may find yourself coming home after a 12-hour shift not wanting to study. However, if you are mentally committed to following a schedule, you will find creative ways to get studying done. For example, some students wake up an hour early to read before pre-rounds. Other students fit study material into their white coat and read during downtime.

Distinguish Rotation-Knowledge From Shelf-Knowledge

Most things you learn on rotation do not apply to the shelf exam and vice versa. For example, you may be able to impress your medicine attending by committing the prevalence of type 2 diabetes in the US adult population to memory. However, with only 150 minutes to answer 100 lengthy questions on the shelf, details like that have no real utility.

Thus, be able to compartmentalize. Know exactly what is needed for clinics and what is expected on the shelf to save yourself precious study time.

99 AR

NBME Shelf Exam Website

IV. Intro to the National Board of Medical Examiners Clinical Science Medicine Subject Exam

The Clinical Science Medicine NBME Shelf Exam is a 110-question computerized exam administered over a recommended course of 2 hours and 45 minutes, typically at the conclusion of one's medicine clerkship rotation. The test questions come from either retired Step 2 clinical knowledge (CK) questions or are written by a committee of faculty across the country. Thus it is important to master shelf exam style questions to set yourself up nicely for Step 2 CK.

Unlike Step 1, shelf exam questions focus almost exclusively on disease processes rather than normal processes. That being said, the most high-yield principles to know for the medicine shelf are normal lab values. Knowing what values to expect for the basic metabolic panel will help you quickly identify abnormal processes, such as hyper/hyponatremia, anion gap metabolic acidosis, or acute kidney injury.

According to the NBME, the exams are curved to a mean of 70 with a standard deviation of 8. The curve does not take into account timing of rotation. For instance, students who take the exam during their first block will be held to the same statistical standard as students who take the exam during their fourth clerkship block. However, the NBME does release "quarterly norm information" to medical schools in order to make clerkship directors aware of the relationship between exam score and rotation timing. Importantly, as of now, shelf exam scores are sent to the school directly; students cannot request their shelf exam score independent of their school.

99 AR

Medicine Outline

Although different medicine clerkships have different standards for determining grades, in general, each program has its own internally generated shelf exam cutoff score one needs to achieve in order to be eligible for the highest clerkship grade (e.g., honors). If this is the case, confirm the cutoff score with your clerkship director so that you have a reasonable performance goal to shoot for.

Students are expected to master content organized into these following categories:

General Principles, Including Normal Age-Related Findings and Care of the Well Patient	1%–5%
Immune System	1%-5%
Blood and Lymphoreticular System	5%-10%

Nervous System and Special Senses	5%-10%
Skin and Subcutaneous Tissue	5%-10%
Musculoskeletal System	5%-10%
Cardiovascular System	10%-15%
Respiratory System	10%-15%
Gastrointestinal System	8%-12%
Renal and Urinary System	8%-12%
Female Reproductive System and Breast	1%-5%
Male Reproductive System	1%-5%
Endocrine System	5%-10%
Multisystem Processes and Disorders	3%-7%
Biostatistics, Epidemiolgoy/Population Health, and Interpretation of the Medical Literature	1%-5%
Social Science, Including Medical Ethics and Jurisprudence	1%-5%

Currently, the NBME Medicine Content Outline breaks down question types into three categories:

Physician Tasks

Applying Foundational Science Concepts	10%-15%
Diagnosis: Knowledge Pertaining to History, Exam, Diagnostic Studies, and Patient Outcomes	50%-55%
Health Maintenance, Pharmacotherapy, Intervention, and Management	30%-35%

However, devising a study plan from these three categories can be confusing. "Applying Foundational Science Concepts," for instance, is vague and difficult to prepare for. Instead, many students prefer to study according to Physician Tasks provided in older content outlines. Since every subject exam question asks about one of four things -- 1) protocol for promoting health maintenance (Prophylaxis [**PPx**]), 2) the mechanism of disease (**MoD**), 3) steps to establishing a diagnosis (**Dx**), and 4) steps of disease management (**Tx/Mgmt**) – we recommend studying according to Physician Tasks from the 2016 Content Outline.

In addition, the NBME breaks down questions by Site of Care, including

- Ambulatory (55%-65%)
- Emergency Department (50%-55%)
- Inpatient (30%-35%)

Our recommendation is to not worry about site of care and focus on studying content related to Physician Tasks.

Gunner Goggles Medicine presents material to reflect how the NBME structures its shelf exams. Each chapter that follows falls into the main testable categories of general principles (Chapter 2) or organ systems (Chapters 3–13). Each disease will also be presented in a "PPx, MoD, Dx, and Tx/Mgmt" format, which represents the four physician tasks the NBME can test you on. Since establishing a diagnosis is weighted especially heavily (40%–45%), a "Buzz Words" category has been added to show readers how to quickly identify the disease process from just a few key words. A "Clinical Presentation" section has also been added to more thoroughly describe the disease. However, it is important to note that Buzz Words are sufficient in correctly identifying the corresponding disease on the shelf. The detail provided in the Clinical Presentation section is only meant to augment your understanding, particularly if it is your first pass and you are unfamiliar with the material. However, by the end of studying, the focus should primarily be on Buzz Words.

Finally, here are four things to keep in mind when studying for the medicine shelf.

1. If pressed for time, practice identifying disease processes only through "Buzz Words." For instance, a patient with atrophy of the caudate nucleus and progressive memory loss should immediately evoke HD. Patients with sclerosing cholangitis on the shelf exam always have underlying ulcerative colitis.

2. Many tested disease processes can also appear on other shelf exams, and these are most often the most high-yield topics. Examples of these multidisciplinary diseases include lupus, syphilis, and HIV.

3. Make sure to begin doing questions early (e.g., 10 questions a day starting from day 1). Ideally you should make a second pass of the most high-yield questions.

4. For each question, write a one-line take-home point in an Excel spreadsheet. This makes for quick and easy review in the days leading up to the exam.

If any questions arise while studying, use the *Gunner Goggles* app to access the AR features embedded on each page.

Good luck and happy hunting.

—The *Gunner Goggles* Team

General Principles for the Internal Medicine Shelf

Leo Wang, Daniel Gromer, Hao-Hua Wu, and Rebecca Gao

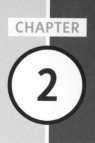

Introduction

Up to 5% of the test will be on General Principles. Although this chapter may seem long relative to the number of questions you will get, you should already be familiar with many of these concepts from your first few years of medical school. This chapter should serve as a refresher only.

This chapter also contains many organizing principles that can be applied to other chapters and to other shelf exams; for example, being able to read vital signs and the metabolic panel is just as important in surgery as it is in medicine.

This chapter is divided into (1) How to Read the Vital Signs and Metabolic Panel, (2) How to Read an Electrocardiography, (3) How to Deal with Bacteria and Antibiotics, (4) How to Look at a Chest X-Ray, (5) Biostatistics and Epidemiology for the Medicine Shelf, (6) Medical Ethics for the Medicine Shelf, (7) Vitamin Deficiencies, (8) Chemical Poisoning, (9) Shock, and (10) Paraneoplastic Syndromes. The final section is Gunner Practice. Anticipate spending approximately 10 hours on this chapter and referencing it repeatedly over the course of your shelf review.

How to Read the Vital Signs and Metabolic Panel

The vital signs you will most frequently encounter on the shelf are blood pressure (BP), heart rate (HR), respiratory rate (RR), temperature, and occasionally O_2 sat.

- **Blood pressure:** BP is a measure of volume status for the purposes of the shelf. It tells you if someone needs fluids (or may be actively bleeding) if too low. If too high, worry about hypertensive urgency/emergency, which increases risk for hemorrhages.
- **Heart rate:** HR is the first thing that changes in response to disease but is super nonspecific. There isn't too much to know regarding an HR, but recognize both brady (<60) and tachy (>100) arrhythmias. The most important thing to be able to recognize here is to

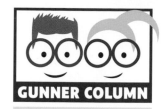

GUNNER COLUMN

order an electrocardiography (EKG) and correlate HR with EKG abnormalities.

- **Respiratory rate:** RR is important as a marker for acid base status on the shelf exam. Patients who are hyperventilating (>20) may be acidotic, and patients who are hypoventilating (<10) may be alkalotic. Extremely low RRs should be indicative of opiate overdose.
- **Temperature:** Temperature greater than 100.4°F is a fever and should raise suspicion for infection or inflammation. Extremely high temperatures greater than 104°F should raise suspicion of malignant hyperthermia or neuroleptic malignant syndrome.
- **O_2 sat:** Most people's O_2 sat should be 100, but in the hospital as long as greater than 90 they are in the clear. If below 90, suspect respiratory pathology, further delineated in Chapter 7.

One of the most important lab tests that every medical student should understand is the basic metabolic panel. It consists of the following measurements: Na, K, Cl, HCO_3, BUN, Cr, Glu, Ca, Mg, and Phos. A more extensive version of this consists of the following additional measurements: Alk Phos, total bilirubin, total protein, and occasionally AST/ALT. This is called the complete metabolic panel. The combination of protein, albumin, bilirubin, AST/ALT, and Alk Phos is often referred to as liver function tests.

Understanding contexts when these measurements are used and when they are abnormal will therefore be **imperative** to the medicine shelf.

From the BMP, the two most important electrolytes routinely tested on the medicine shelf are Na and K. Calcium is lower yield but fair game. Changes in chloride or magnesium are rarely ever tested. Thus, on every BMP you see, the first two things you look at should be Na and K. Memorize their normal values (135–145 mEq/L for Na, 3.5–5 mEq/L for K). Remember, sodium levels are really high in the blood but low in the cell. Conversely, potassium levels are really low in the blood but really high in the cell. This seems obvious, but you can get a lot of questions right by fleshing out this concept. If sodium levels have gone down and you are unclear as to where they're going, they might still be in the cell (Na/K ATPase pumps Na out).

There are two salient points to the medicine shelf—first, electrolyte abnormalities should be assessed in the context of changes. If an abnormal sodium level appears out of nowhere, one of the first things you should do is get another BMP. Second, understand that electrolyte levels are dependent on volume status and kidney status. Always think about volume status first when assessing a change in an electrolyte. Most of the time, this can help provide an easy explanation. Finally, recognize the function of the kidneys in promoting electrolyte balance. A patient in renal failure will have electrolyte disturbances.

Hyponatremia

Buzz Words: Low sodium + headaches + nausea progressing to seizures/coma

Clinical Presentation: Hyponatremia is a common clinical finding that can be caused by a variety of causes. There are three kinds of hyponatremia: isotonic hyponatremia, hypotonic hyponatremia and hypertonic hyponatremia. Isotonic hyponatremia is also known as pseudohyponatremia.

The easiest to understand is isotonic hyponatremia and can be determined by looking at serum osmolality. If serum osmolality is NORMAL (280–295 mOsm/kg), it is most likely pseudohyponatremia caused by extraordinary levels of lipid/protein which interfere with sodium detection. This is the least high yield of all the three types.

Hypotonic hyponatremia is caused by several different things. This occurs in the setting of a low serum osmolality (<280 mOsm/kg). The next most important thing to do here is to look at volume status.

- **Euvolemic** = most likely SIADH, diuretic use, or some endocrinopathy such adrenal insufficiency.
- **Hypovolemic** = look at urine sodium next.
  - If >20 mEq/L, sodium is being lost through the urine.
  - If <20 mEq/L, sodium is being lost from elsewhere.
- **Hypervolemic** = look at urine sodium as well.
  - If >20 mEq/L, think of renal failure.
  - If <20 mEq/L, think of problems such as such as cirrhosis and nephrotic syndrome.

Finally, hypertonic hyponatremia is really caused only by hyperglycemia in the context of the medicine shelf. Hypertonic hyponatremia is a finding of serum osmolality greater than 295 mOsm/kg.

PPx: Manage risk factors/causative etiologies described previously.

MoD: See previous.

Dx:

1. BMP

Hypoantremia video

2. Physical exam (PE)/BP/vitals to determine volume status
3. Urinalysis/urine output

Tx/Mgmt:
1. Normal saline
2. Water restriction
3. Monitor Na with BMP every 2 hours

Hypernatremia

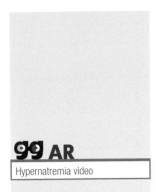

Hypernatremia video

Buzz Words: Serum sodium >145 mmol/L + altered mental status + seizures + coma + dry membranes and decreased salivation

Clinical Presentation: Like hyponatremia, there are three types of hypernatremia: euvolemic, hypovolemic, and hypervolemic. These also all depend on volume status, so measurements of things like BP will be vital to understanding this patient's presentation.

    Euvolemic hypernatremia is caused by pure water loss. Total body sodium is unchanged. Such causes include both central and nephrogenic diabetes insipidus, dehydration, or insensible losses (such as rigorous exercise).

    Hypovolemic hypernatremia is caused by loss of both water and sodium. The most important thing to look at here is urine sodium to determine if the sodium is being lost through the urine. If urine sodium is greater than 20 mEq/L, suspect a diuresis. This can be caused by loop diuretics but can also be caused by things like mannitol or glucose, which can concentrate sodium in the nephron tubules.

    Hypervolemic hypernatremia is actually caused by a primary sodium gain with a decrease in total body water. There are a few causes—the most important and high yield for the medicine shelf is increases in aldosterone, which stimulates sodium reuptake. Other causes include sodium bicarbonate infusion, hypertonic injections/dialysis, or salt tablets.

PPx: Manage risk factors described previously, hydration.

MoD: See earlier.

Dx:
1. BMP
2. PE/vitals for volume status
3. Urine sodium

Tx/Mgmt:
1. Hypovolemic
   - Treat with oral fluids
   - If symptomatic, give 0.9% saline
   - Once euvolemic, give 5% dextrose

- Endocrinology consult for diabetes insipidus
2. Euvolemic
   - Hypertonic saline
3. Hypervolemic
   - Diuretics to remove excess sodium; if end stage renal disease (ESRD), dialysis to remove excess sodium

Hypokalemia

Buzz Words: Flattened T waves/presence of U waves on EKG + arrhythmias + muscle weakness/cramps/fatigue + decreased DTRs

Hypokalemia ECG

Clinical Presentation: Low potassium is a dangerous medical emergency. Hypokalemia should be categorized based on urinary potassium secretion.
- **If urine potassium secretion is low (<20 mEq/L):** potassium losses are occurring from extrarenal sources, such as through diarrhea or vomiting.
- **If urine potassium secretion is high (>20 mEq/L):** there are a plethora of causes. One of the major causes is metabolic acidosis, and two important causes on the medical shelf will include renal tubular acidosis or diabetic ketoacidosis. The most important sign to recognize either of these will be low serum bicarbonate. In the setting of normal serum bicarbonate, one should look at volume status and BP. In hypervolemic states or in the setting of high BP, causes include excess of glucocorticoids/mineralocorticoids. In the setting of low volume or BP, causes include loop diuretics and some congenital diseases.

PPx: N/A
MoD: See earlier.
Dx:
1. BMP
2. EKG for arrhythmias and flattened T waves
3. Urine K
4. PE/vitals for volume status
Tx/Mgmt:
1. Slowly replace K (rapid replacement → arrhythmia)
2. Potassium sparing diuretics (amiloride, triamterene, spironolactone, eplerenone)
3. Correct acid-base status

Hyperkalemia

Buzz Words: Peaked T waves on EKG + muscle weakness + decreased DTRs + respiratory distress

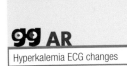

AR

Hyperkalemia ECG changes

Clinical Presentation: Hyperkalemia is an elevation of potassium in serum. The most common abnormality is arrhythmia, although this will depend on the level of elevation. Patients may also have nausea, vomiting, diarrhea, and if severe, flaccid paralysis.

PPx: Reduce dietary K.

MoD: Can occur secondary to potassium sparing diuretics (spironolactone, eplerenone, amiloride, triamterene) or ACEIs. Can also be secondary to decreased kidney function, rhabdomyolysis, and aldosterone deficiency.

Dx:
1. BMP (K > 5.0 mEq/L)
2. EKG for peaked T waves, prolonged PR

Tx/Mgmt:
1. Calcium gluconate (restores threshold potential)
2. Dextrose/insulin
3. Salbutamol
4. Sodium bicarbonate
5. Dialysis
6. Loop diuretics
    Other tests to understand include thyroid studies, which include TSH, T3, T4, FT3, and FT4. Coagulation studies include PT, PTT, INR, and bleeding time. Lipid panel includes TC, HDL, LDL, and TGs. The urinalysis includes urine creatinine, protein, and tests the specific gravity, pH, leukocyte esterase, nitrites, protein, blood, glucose, ketone, bilirubin, and urobilinogen. These tests will be described in later chapters as they come up.

How to Read an Electrocardiography

It is imperative for students to be able to interpret an EKG. An EKG (sometimes ECG) is a record of how the electrical activity *changes over time* across various axes in the heart. Changes in electrical activity are essentially measures of what is happening on the level of the cardiomyocytes in terms of action potential conduction. Let's start with the basics, the waveforms. The waveforms are P, Q, R, S, and T (Fig. 2.1).

    The P wave represents the depolarization of the atrium which leads to atrial contraction and blood pumping into the ventricles. The QRS waves join to form a complex that normally starts with an inverted peak (Q) followed by an upright peak (R) followed by an inverted peak (S). The

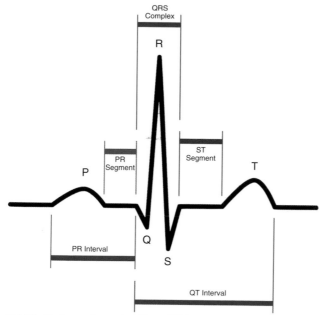

FIG. 2.1 Electrocardiography. (From Wikimedia Commons: https://commons.wikimedia.org/wiki/File:SinusRhythmLabels.svg. Created by Anthony Atkielski. In the public domain.)

summation of the QRS complex represents depolarization of the ventricle and ventricular contraction. Note that not all QRS complexes must show all three waveforms of the Q, R, and S. The T wave represents ventricular repolarization—remember, any time a muscle contracts and depolarizes, it must repolarize!

Now that you know what all the peaks are, let's go through the EKG the way Gunner Jim approaches it. Start with the rate:

1. Find any two consecutive R waves or any two consecutive P waves
2. Count the number of big boxes between these two R waves or P waves
   - 1 big box = 300 BPM
   - 2 big boxes = 150 BPM
   - 3 big boxes = 100 BPM
   - 4 big boxes = 75 BPM
   - 5 big boxes = 60 BPM
3. Notice that the previous calculation is just 300/(# of squares between P-P or R-R). So if you count 2.5 big boxes, that is 300/2.5 or 120 beats/min.
4. Report the rate as normal (60–100), tachycardic (>100), or bradycardic (<60). In our example, there

QUICK TIPS

If you're wondering where atrial repolarization is, it's because it's hidden in the QRS complex. This is called the Ta Wave and is recognized only by the best of electrophysiologists and only during AV blocks.

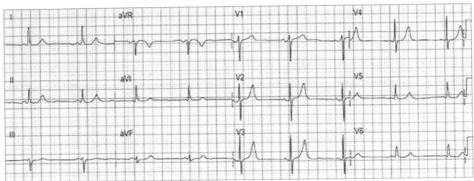

FIG. 2.2 Electrocardiography. (From Timmis AD, Archbold A: Cardiovascular system. In Glynn M, Drake W, editors: *Hutchison's clinical methods: an integrated approach to clinical practice*, ed 23, London, 2012, Elsevier Ltd., figure 11.11.)

are approximately 5 boxes between the two Q waves shown. Therefore this patient has a regular HR of 60 BPM (Fig. 2.2).

Next, determine the rhythm. This is Gunner Jim's favorite and the easiest to understand. Look at all the QRS complexes. Is the distance between them all the same? Or are they different? The rhythm is described as either:

1. Regular: distance between QRS complexes is the same throughout the EKG
2. Irregularly irregular: distance between QRS complexes varies throughout the EKG
3. Regularly irregular: distance between QRX complexes varies throughout the EKG but there is a pattern:
   - For example, if there were 2 boxes between the first two QRS complexes, 3 boxes between the second two, and 4 boxes between the fourth two, and then repeated 2, 3, 4, 2, 3, 4, 2, 3, 4, this would be a regularly irregular pattern. This can be tough to spot!

Finally, determine the axis. We will not go into detail over how an axis should be determined. The general principle to remember here is that the waveforms will point upward and be positive when measured in an axis that runs parallel to the direction of electricity. In general, the electrical signal from the heart starts from the **right hand** side and runs to the **left leg** in a diagonal down the body (Fig. 2.3). Thus measurements that measure in that general axis should be **positive**, whereas measurements in the opposite direction to that axis are negative.

The overall point of the axis is to determine in which direction the electrical activity is going. Remember, the axis of positive electrical activity in the heart should be

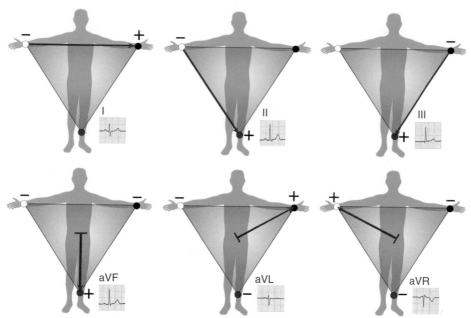

FIG. 2.3 Electrocardiography axes. (From Wikimedia Commons: https://commons.wikimedia.org/wiki/File:Limb_leads_of_EKG.png. Created by Npatchett. Used under Creative Commons Attribution License Share Alike 4.0 International License.)

heading from the right hand to the left leg, which is also the equivalent of 0–90 degrees (Figs. 2.4 and 2.5).

Gunner Jim and Jess use the following, efficient algorithm.

1. Look at Lead I and determine if the QRS inflection is overall upright (positive) or inverted (negative).
   a. If Lead I is **negative** that is NEVER normal. Then you look at lead AVF:
      i. If AVF is positive, you have right axis deviation and your axis is between 90 and 180 degrees.
      ii. If AVF is negative, you have extreme far left or far right axis deviation and your axis is between −90 and 180 degrees.
   b. If Lead I is positive, you most likely have a normal axis.
      i. Confirm you have a normal axis (−30 to 90 degrees) by looking at AVF. It should also be positive.
      ii. If AVF is negative, you most likely have left axis deviation. Confirm by looking at Lead II:
2. If Lead II is negative, you have left axis deviation (−30 to −90 degrees).

Next, look at the PR interval. This is the distance from the beginning of the P wave to the beginning of the Q wave.

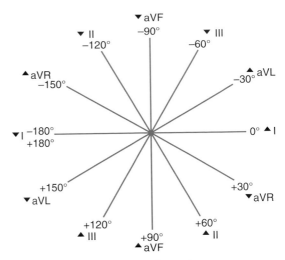

FIG. 2.4 Electrocardiography axes.

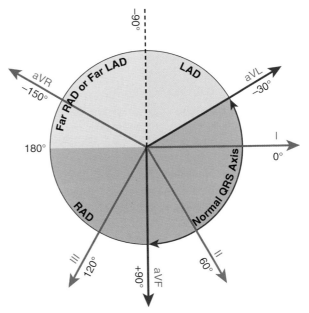

FIG. 2.5 Electrocardiography axes.

The maximum distance between these two points should be 1 big box, or five small boxes (200 ms). Anything longer indicates pathology between atrial depolarization and ventricular depolarization.

Next, look at the QRS interval. This is the distance from the beginning of the Q wave to the end of the S wave. The entire duration of the QRS complex should correspond to three small boxes (120 ms) or 3/5 of a large box.

Anything longer than that indicates pathology in ventricular depolarization.

Next, look at the ST interval. This is where the S wave ends and T wave begins. The duration of the ST segment should be no longer than 120 ms or three small boxes. Anything longer indicates a disconnect between ventricular depolarization and ventricular repolarization.

Next, measure the QT interval. This is the distance between the beginning of the Q wave and end of the T wave. This corresponds to the actual length of action potential. To calculate a QT interval, you will need to correct for the HR (since HR will change the AP length). The calculation for this is QTC = QT/(sqrt[RR]). A normal QTC will be less than 460 ms. Remember, each small box is 40 ms and each large box is 200 ms. A disconnect here indicates problems in action potential propagation.

These are the basics for interpreting an EKG. These skills should translate both on the medicine shelf and in the clinics. You should be able to recognize pathologic causes that distort specific aspects of the EKG. Although these are not covered here, you should be able to recognize specific changes such as ST segment elevation (myocardial infarction [MI]) or elevated T waves (hyperkalemia).

Some common EKG findings with their clinical correlates:
- ST elevation—MI
- ST depression—myocardial ischemia, subendocardial infarction
- Peaked T waves—hyperkalemia (usually preceding MI)
- ST elevation in all lead—pericarditis (note MI does not elevate in all leads)
- Absent P waves, irregular QRS—atrial fibrillation
- Regular P waves, multiple P waves for every QRS—atrial flutter
- Rapid irregular QRS complexes, no P waves—ventricular fibrillation
- PR > 200 ms, 1 P wave for every QRS—1st degree AV block
- PR lengthening per contraction with eventual disappearance of QRS—2nd degree AV block
- No connect between P wave and QRS—3rd degree AV block
- QRS > 120 ms—LBBB, RBBB
- Early upstroke in QRS complex (delta wave)—Wolf Parkinson White
- Low voltage (amplitude of QRS)—obesity

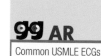

99 AR
Common USMLE ECGs

99 AR

Antibiotic Treatment Ladder

How to Deal With Bacteria and Antibiotics

The medicine shelf will test your ability to understand usage of different antiinfectious agents and their implications. Here we will discuss an approach to learning bacteria, antibiotics, and go through common antibiotic, antiviral, and antifungal drugs.

Bacterial infections are among concepts medical students struggle most with—specifically, which kinds of bacteria like to cause infections where. An organizing principle in this section is to organize bacteria based on where they like to live. If you understand this, you will understand where they like to cause infection.

Let's start with the largest organ in the body: the skin.

What kinds of bacteria like to live on the skin? Most bacteria which live on the skin flora are commensal or mutualistic but will cause disease during specific pathologies like trauma or immunosuppression. The most common bacteria on the skin include *Staphylococcus epidermidis*, *Staphylococcus aureus*, *Streptococcus pyogenes,* and *Propionibacterium acnes*. Thus associate these bacteria with common infections of the skin, including atopic dermatitis, psoriasis, acne vulgaris, folliculitis, and impetigo. These infections are better expounded upon in the dermatology section. Common antibiotics used are the β-lactams, such as: cefazolin (first-generation cephalosporin), nafcillin, methicillin.

Next, let's move to the nasopharynx and oropharynx, which are directly connected to the skin via the nasal and oral orifices. Remember—the flora of these areas cannot differ too much from the skin because there is no physical barrier between them. Think about *S. aureus*, *S. pyogenes*, *S. epidermidis*, *Haemophilus influenzae* and *Streptococcus pneumoniae*, and *Neisseria meningitidis* as natural colonizers of the nasopharynx. Notice this doesn't differ too much from skin mucosa, does it? The natural colonizers of the nasopharynx and oropharynx will cause pharyngitis and sinusitis. The most common causes of pharyngitis include *S. pyogenes* and *H. influenzae*. The most common causes of sinusitis include *S. pneumoniae*, *H. influenzae*, and *Moraxella catarrhalis*, with occasional *S. aureus* and *S. pyogenes*. Notice the huge amount of overlap between infectious etiologies of these different conditions! Common antibiotics used are the β-lactams, specifically amoxicillin, one of the most commonly used antibiotics for Strep pharyngitis or sinusitis.

Another organ directly connected to the sinuses is the brain. Thus most bacterial causes of meningitis come from the sinuses, and the most common causes of bacterial meningitis include *S. pneumoniae*, *N. meningitidis*, and *H. influenzae*. Common antibiotics used are directed against the aforementioned three organisms. Ceftriaxone is the prime example. Ampicillin is often added for protection against Listeria in the elderly or immunocompromised.

Let's move next to the lower respiratory tract. There are no natural colonizers here, so bacteria get here through colonizers of either (1) the upper respiratory tract or (2) the gastrointestinal (GI) tract (from vomiting). It should come as no surprise then that the most common causes of pneumonia are *S. pneumoniae* or atypical organisms such as *H. influenzae* and *Mycoplasma pneumoniae*. The most common bacteria that form lung abscesses are anaerobes from the GI tract—more on this to follow. Common antibiotics used are directed against atypical organisms: clindamycin, azithromycin.

In the GI tract, oxygen is low. Thus bacteria that survive in the low oxygen content of the GI tract tend to be anaerobes and gram negatives. The intestinal microflora consists of a TON of different bacteria, most which you will not be responsible for. Recognize some of the most common bacteria: *Bacteroides* species, *Enterococcus* species, *Escherichia coli*, *Enterobacteriae*, *Klebsiella*, *Clostridium perfringens*. One thing these all have in common is that they are anaerobes. These bacteria normally do not cause any harm unless in the body is immunocompromised OR if the bacteria get into a place they do not belong. Unfortunately, it is very easy for these bacteria to get to undesirable places. Aspiration of gastric contents can lead to aspiration pneumonia caused by anaerobic gut flora. These bacteria are also some of the most important causes of urinary tract infections and other infections of the genitourinary tract due to the proximity of the GI tract to the urethra. They also are frequent causes of cholecystitis and appendicitis. Common antibiotics used have properties against anaerobes, including piperacillin/tazobactam (Zosyn), cefepime, meropenem, and metronidazole. A few organizing principles begin here—meropenem and cefepime are really only prescribed to include pseudomonas coverage and are not frequently used. For coverage of genitourinary tract infections, including UTIs, physicians like to begin with TMP/SMX, levofloxacin, or nitrofurantoin.

In the reproductive tract, most organisms are gram negative and require different types of treatment. However, there are some exceptions that defy the organizing principles (e.g., syphilis treated with penicillin). Thus it is more useful to think of treatment of STIs in a case by case basis. The types of sexually transmitted infections and the treatment needed are covered in Chapter 9.

Problem organisms are organisms that defy the organizing principles laid out due to developed resistance and difficulty with antibiotic penetrance. Just know how to recognize these symptoms and the corresponding antibiotics used.

Methicillin-Resistant Staphylococcus aureus

Buzz Words: Dialysis + long inpatient stay
Tx/Mgmt:
1. Vancomycin
2. Daptomycin
3. Linezolid

Pseudomonas

Buzz Words: Cystic fibrosis + human immunodeficiency virus (HIV) + clindamycin
Tx/Mgmt:
1. Cefepime
2. Levofloxacin
3. Piperacillin-tazobactam

Enterococcus

Buzz Words: UTI + abdominal infection
Tx/Mgmt:
1. Amoxicillin
2. Ampicillin

Bacteroides fragilis

Buzz Words: GI + rotten teeth + vaginal tract infection
Tx/Mgmt:
1. Amoxicillin-clavulanate
2. Metronidazole

So now that you know all of these things, how do you prescribe antibiotics?
1. First, when someone presents with a serious infection, order a blood culture immediately. Blood cultures must ALWAYS be ordered before antibiotics are started because antibiotic administration can mask infection.
2. Use whatever diagnostic means needed to help better elucidate a bacterial source of infection. For UTI or pyelonephritis, this may be a urinalysis or urine culture. For pneumoniae, this may be a chest x-ray (CXR). For meningitis, this may be a lumbar puncture.
3. Next, use your HPI to start a patient on a broad-spectrum antibiotic that will cover your suspected bacterial

etiologies—you may not receive the results from the blood culture or imaging from a while. What does this mean? If a patient comes in with meningitis, you should recognize the most common etiologies include *S. pneumoniae*, *N. meningitidis*, and *H. influenzae*. Ceftriaxone will cover all of these (vancomycin is often prescribed because methicillin-resistant *Staphylococcus aureus* is a problem and is nosocomially spread). As a rule, always use the weakest antibiotic you can use to save your big guns for the bigger bugs. This helps to prevent antibiotic-resistant bacteria.

4. When you have identified an infectious agent, place them on the narrowest, weakest antibiotic that will cover their infectious agent. Most hospitals have charts for what works and what doesn't, based on local resistance patterns, and every bacteria is different. The key here is that once you know what's causing an infection, you don't need them to be on broad spectrum antibiotics!

Common Antibiotic Toxicities Tested on the Medicine Shelf

Don't worry, you won't have to memorize all those drug side effects from Step 1 to do well. Next is a list of the most commonly tested side effects seen on the medicine shelf.

- Difficulty hearing (ototoxicity) → Aminoglycosides
- Teeth discoloration → Tetracycline
- Pseudomembranous colitis → Clindamycin
- Orange urine → Rifampin
- Aplastic anemia → Chloramphenicol
- Renal toxicity → Aminoglycosides
- Red man syndrome → Vancomycin

How to Read a Chest X-Ray

There is no perfect way to read a CXR, but we recommend one thing: do it the same way every time (Fig. 2.6). The only way you catch things is by taking the exact same, thorough approach to every CXR you see. Although this is less relevant for the medicine shelf, you should be able to apply these principles to be able to rule in or rule out the most common thoracic pathologies. The strategy we like to follow is the ABCDEFGH steps of reading a CXR: Airway, Bone, Cardiac, Diaphragm, Effusion, Fields, Gastric, Hilum.

1. First, ensure you understand the orientation and position of the patient. Are they on their side? Upright? Supine? This affects where different organs will sit in the thoracic cavity.

99 AR
Johns Hopkins Antibiotics Guide

99 AR
Stanford antibiotics review

99 AR
How to read chest x-ray series

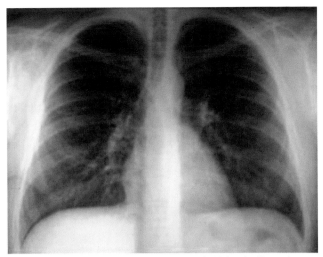

FIG. 2.6 Normal x-ray. (From Hamad HM, Galrinho A, Abreu J, Valente B, Bakero L, Ferreira RC: Giant pericardial cyst mimicking dextrocardia on chest x-ray. *Rev Port Cardiol* 32(1):49–52, 2013.)

2. Check for inspiratory quality—a good CXR should illuminate 9 pairs of ribs posteriorly.
3. Airway
   - Ensure trachea is midline
     - If not, suspect, atelectasis, pneumothorax, effusions
   - Ensure carina angle is 60–100 degrees. The carina is where the trachea divides into two bronchi.
     - Carina greater than 100 degrees in atelectasis, cardiac hypertrophy, lymphadenopathy
   - Check the mediastinum.
     - If widened, suspect tumors, lymphadenopathy, and vascular problems (hematomas, aneurysms).
   - Look for pacemakers, tubes, foreign bodies, etc.
4. Bones
   - Look at the clavicles, ribs, spine and humerus for signs of fracture, dislocation, subluxation or lytic lesions; assess for osteoarthritis changes.
5. Cardiac
   - Check heart size, aortic size
     - If larger, suspect cardiac hypertrophy, aortic aneurysms/dissection
6. Diaphragm
   - If diaphragm cannot be seen, suspect pleural effusion
   - Right side of diaphragm should be slightly higher than left but may be significantly higher than left in effusion, diaphragmatic collapse, or paralysis

- Flattened diaphragm in chronic obstructive pulmonary disease (COPD) and other obstructive lung problems
7. Effusion
   - Look at costophrenic angle for "blunting"
   - Look for pleural thickening or calcifications.
8. Fields
   - Identify infiltrates and their location.
   - Identify pattern of infiltration (reticular or nodular/alveolar)
   - Assess Kerley B lines, air bronchograms, pulmonary nodules
   - Assess hyperlucency (too much air) or hypolucency (too much parenchyma/fluid).
9. Gastric
   - Look for free air in the gastric bubble and position below diaphragm
10. Hilum
   - Assess for position, size, lymph nodes, calcifications or mass lesions.

Biostatics and Epidemiology for the Medicine Shelf

For the Medicine shelf, there are times when you are tested on sensitivity and specificity of tests. This is the same material that you learned for Step 1. If you remember your stats from Step 1 (e.g., sensitivity, specificity, NPV, PPV, OR, RR, ARR, type 1 and 2 error, null hypothesis), feel free to skip this section. Otherwise spend no more than 30 minutes reviewing the material below (Table 2.1).

Sensitivity—how many people who have the disease will test positive?
- True positives/(total who test positive for disease)
  - Total who test positive for disease = false positive (people who don't have disease but actually test positive falsely) and true positive (people who have disease and test positive)
- True positives/(false positives + true positives)

Specificity—how many people who don't have the disease will test negative?
- True negatives/(total who test negative for disease)
  - People who test negative for disease—false negative (people who actually have the disease and test falsely negative) and true negative (people who don't have the disease and test negative)
- True negatives/(false negatives + true negatives)

99 AR

UVA Chest XR Tutorial

TABLE 2.1 Diagnostic Tests

		DISEASE		
		+	−	
Test	+	TP (patients with disease, test positive)	FP (patients without disease, test positive)	PPV = TP(/ TP+FP)
	−	FN (patients with disease, test negative)	TN (patients without disease, test negative)	NPV = TN/ (TN+FN)
		Sensitivity = TP/ (TP+FN)	Specificity = TN/ (TN+FP)	

FN, False negative; *FP*, false positive; *TN*, true negative; *TP*, true positive; *NPV*, negative predictive value; *PPV*, positive predictive value.

TABLE 2.2 Risk Factor Versus Disease

		DISEASE	
		+	−
Risk factor	+	A	B
OR	−	C	D
Intervention			

Positive Predictive Value—how many people who test positive actually have the disease?
- True positives/(total people who have the disease)
  - Total people who have the disease = true positives (have disease, test positive) and false negatives (have disease, test falsely negative)
- True positives/ (true positive + false negative)

Negative Predictive Value—how many people who test negative actually don't have the disease?
- True negatives/(total people who don't have the disease)
  - Total people who don't have disease = true negatives (don't have disease, test negative) and false positives (don't have disease, test falsely positive)
- True negatives/(true negatives + false positives) (Table 2.2)

This is the only thing used in case control studies:

Odds Ratio (OR): Only used in case control studies; odds of being exposed to risk factor in patients with disease divided by odds of being exposed to risk factor in patients without disease

$$OR = (a/c)/(b/d)$$

Everything else is used in cohort studies:

Relative Risk (RR): Only used in cohort studies, risk of getting disease in patients with risk factor divided by risk of getting disease in patients without risk factor

$$RR = [a/(a+b)]/[c/(c+d)]; \text{ relative risk}$$
$$\text{reduction} = 1 - RR$$

Attributable Risk (AR; risk gain): Only used in cohort studies looking at a negative exposure (i.e., smoking for lung cancer), risk of getting disease in patients with risk factor minus risk of getting disease in patients without risk factor

$$AR = a/(a+b) - c/(c+d); \text{ number needed}$$
$$\text{to harm} = 1/AR$$

Absolute Risk Reduction (ARR; risk loss): Only used in cohort studies looking at a positive exposure or preventative measure (i.e., exercise for MI), risk of getting disease in patients without preventative measure minus risk of getting disease in patients with preventative measure

$$ARR = c/(c+d) - a/(a+b); \text{ number}$$
$$\text{needed to treat} = 1/ARR$$

Finally, understand the basics behind statistical testing. Anytime you run a statistical test, you are determining if there is or is not a relationship between two variables. For example, is there a relationship between smoking and lung cancer? Yes. Is there a relationship between a positive pregnancy test and lung cancer? No. Is there a relationship between a positive pregnancy test and pregnancy? Yes. Do men weigh more than women? Yes. Statistical testing is the way we are able to say yes, no, yes, and yes to the previous questions with some amount of certainty, although any real statistician will tell you that you cannot say anything with absolute certainty in statistics.

The null hypothesis is the assumption that there is no relationship between two variables you are testing. For example, your null hypothesis could be that smoking does not cause lung cancer, or that sex does not influence weight. You then run a statistical test that will assess that relationship. You will only need to know two for the medicine shelf.

1. T-tests test whether two variables are from the same group or from different groups. Imagine that the average weight of men is 150 and average weight of women is 100. The t-test would find these two averages come from different groups; another way of rephrasing this is that your sex influences your weight

and the two variables are related. Here, you would reject the null hypothesis if and only if $P < .05$. We discuss this later.

2. An ANOVA tests whether several variables are from the same group or from different groups. Imagine that the average BP of construction workers is 140, doctors is 120, nurses is 130, lawyers is 110 and that astronauts is 210 (this is absolutely not true, by the way). The ANOVA would find that astronauts have a much higher BP than the other groups. Another way of saying this would be that your occupation influences your BP.

Here you would again reject the null hypothesis under specific conditions (Bonferroni correction) that are not relevant to the medicine shelf.

Every statistical test requires you pick an alpha threshold that you are comfortable with. Most people pick 0.05, or 5%. Alpha is your chance of making a type I error, (stating there is a difference when one does not really exist, or erroneously rejecting the null)—put simply, it's your odds of finding a relationship and not being wrong about it, or your odds of getting a false-positive result.

The P-value your statistical test gives you is the odds of a type I error. The lower the better, and the more likely it is you can actually reject your null hypothesis without committing a type I error. For example, if I were to receive a P-value of .01 from a statistical test between the weights of men and women, I would conclude there is only a 1% chance that we committed a type I error if I reject the mean. That means if we run this test 99 times, we would get the same result 99 times and only 1 of those times would we actually have incorrectly rejected the null. Put simply, it means that we have a 99% chance of finding this same relationship (sex influences weight) if we did the test again. Conversely, if we got a P-value of 0.5 or 50%, this means that there is a 50% chance that if we did this test again that we would get a different relationship—thus half the time sex influences weight, the other half of the time it doesn't. We wouldn't be able to conclude that sex influences weight here!

The other concept that relates closely to alpha is beta. Beta is the opposite of the alpha, and is the likelihood of accepting the null when there is a real relationship. This is a type II error, the odds of you actually concluding that positive pregnancy tests have no relationship with pregnancy, when in reality there is an obvious relationship. While alpha is set at very low thresholds like 0.05, beta is usually set around 0.2. This means that we are okay with as high of a 20% chance of making a type II error, whereas we set alpha

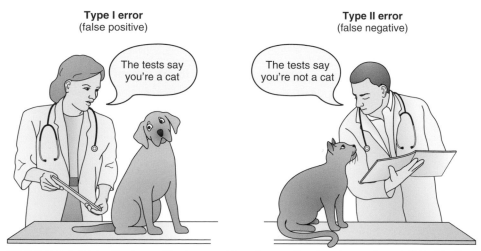

FIG. 2.7 Remember, we're more willing to accept type II errors than type I errors from statistical testing, but we really shouldn't be making either!

at much lower. Why? It's because false negatives are bad, but false positives are even worse. We want to be able to trust the results of a positive statistical test more than we want to be able to trust the results of a negative one; if our positive tests were getting a bunch of false-positive measurements, they'd be meaningless. Remember beta is influenced by three things: sample size, effect size, and precision of measurement. Increasing all of the aforementioned will decrease beta, and decrease odds of a type II error (Fig. 2.7).

Medical Ethics for the Medicine Shelf

Patient characteristics associated with adherence can appear on any shelf exam, and medicine is fair game. Learn what to do and not to do in the following ethical scenarios. These concepts test your mastery of building the patient-doctor relationship, the strength of which is most closely related to patient adherence. In general, think how your doctoring or doctor-patient preceptor/mentor would respond and answer accordingly. The safest answer is usually correct. When in doubt, prioritize the patient's autonomy and comfort first and foremost.

Patient With Suicidal Ideation

Action

Assess threat (e.g., detailed plan vs. passing thought); if threat is serious (e.g., detailed plan, consistent suicidal ideation [SI]), make sure patient is admitted to hospital voluntarily or involuntarily. Patients may be held involuntarily if threat to self or others.

Avoid

Assuming threat is not serious, question stem may contain fillers to obfuscate severity of SI admission.

Patient Nonadherent to Treatment or Test

Action

Ask why patient is nonadherent and be respectful.

Avoid

Referring patient to another physician.

Patient Nonadherent to Total Lifestyle Change, Behavior

Action

Ask about patient's willingness to change behavior. If patient is not willing, then provider cannot move on to the next step and why the issue needs to be addressed.

Avoid

Forcing patient to change if not willing to or scaring patient. Remember, D.A.R.E. does not work.

Patient Who Acts Seductively

Action

Set limits, define tolerable behavior, see patient with chaperone.

Avoid

Refusing to care for patient, asking open-ended questions, referring patient to another physician, entering into relationship with patient (never the right answer).

Patient Who Is Angry

Action

NURSE: Name the emotion (e.g., "You appear angry."). Understand why and thank patient for sharing. Recognize what patient is doing right. Show support for the patient. Explore emotion.

Avoid

Taking patient's anger personally.

Patient Who Is Sad and Tearful

Action

NURSE: Name the emotion (e.g., "You appear angry."). Understand why and thank patient for sharing. Recognize what patient is doing right. Show support for the patient. Explore emotion.

Avoid

Using patronizing statements such as "do not worry," rushing patient, and stating "I understand"; instead, further explore emotion to better understand where patient is coming from.

Patient Who Complains About Another Doctor

Action

Recommend patient speak to the other doctor directly.

Avoid

Saying anything to disparage the other doctor, intervening with care unless emergent need.

Patient Who Complains About You or Your Staff

Action

Verify complaint, speak to staff member who was named in complaint.

Avoid

Blaming patient, being defensive.

Patient to Whom You Must Break Bad News

Action

SPIKES: Set-up patient encounter by making sure patient is sitting in a chair with social support nearby. Ask about patient perception of what is going on. Ask patient for an invitation or permission to share the bad news. Explain your own knowledge of the bad news; make sure to preface by statements that convey the gravity of the situation (e.g., "I'm worried" or "I have bad news"). Manage patient's emotion after bad news is shared. Summarize situation and suggest concrete next steps.

Avoid

Sharing bad news when patient is in a vulnerable position (e.g., standing up while on the phone), breaking bad news without warning.

Patient Being Evaluated for Decision-Making Capacity

Action

Determine if patient meets criteria for being a legally competent decision maker, including the following criteria:
- Patients ≥18 or legally emancipated through marriage, military, or financial independence
- Patient makes and communicates a choice.
- Patient knows and understands benefit and risks.
- Patient's decision is stable over time.

- Decision is congruent to patient value system
- Decision is not a result of mood disorder, hallucinations, or delusions

Patients with adequate decision-making capacity can refuse labs, imaging (e.g., computed tomography [CT] scans), and medical treatment.

Avoid

Assuming patient lacks decision-making capacity if less than 18 (remember marriage, military, and financial independence from parents).

Patient Who Is a Jehovah's Witness and Needs Blood Transfusion

Action

Determine if patient meets criteria for not needing informed consent (e.g., legally incompetent, implied consent in emergency with no ability for communication, patient waived right to informed consent).

Avoid

Giving blood if patient does not give consent and also does not meet any of the exceptions.

Patient With Meningitis Refusing Treatment

Action

Determine if patient has right to refuse treatment; in this case, patient does not have a right because doing so would pose a threat to the health and welfare of others.

Avoid

Consulting hospital ethics committee unless there is a dilemma with no clear way to proceed.

Pediatric Patient With Nonemergent, Potentially Fatal Medical Condition and Parents Refuse Treatment

Action

Seek a court order mandating treatment.

Avoid

Complying with parents' demand.

Patient With Human Immunodeficiency Virus Diagnosis Refuses to Share With Significant Other

Action

Assess confidentiality rules; in this case, significant other needs to be legally notified to prevent harm

QUICK TIPS

- Pediatric patient + emergent condition + no parental approval → proceed with treatment anyway
- Pediatric patient + non-emergent condition + no parental approval → proceed with treatment only after legal approval granted

from transmission. Encourage patient to discuss health and medical conditions with loved ones. Share patient results with local health department.

Avoid
Allowing patient to avoid disclosing potentially fatal communicable disease.

Vitamin Deficiencies

Vitamin deficiencies are frequently tested on the medicine shelf. Be able to identify vitamin deficiencies based on the buzz words, and recognize the diagnostic steps in differentiating between them. All vitamin deficiencies occur through supplementation of the missing vitamin, so this basic principle is not frequently tested.

Vitamin A (Retinol) Deficiency

Buzz Words: Night blindness + dry skin + alopecia + corneal degeneration
PPx: Vitamin A supplementation
MoD: Vitamin A is needed to bind a protein in retina. Lack thereof can cause inability to see through dim light at night (night-blindness).
  • Deficiency occurs rarely in fat malabsorption syndromes that are caused by cystic fibrosis, biliary atresia, and sprue.
Dx:
1. Clinical symptoms
Tx/Mgmt:
1. Vitamin A supplementation

Vitamin B1 (Thiamine) Deficiency

Buzz Words:
  • Peripheral neuropathy w/ symmetric impairment of sensory, motor, and reflex functions → distal > proximal limb segments with calf muscle tenderness → dry beriberi
  • Confusion, muscular atrophy, "edema," tachycardia, cardiomegaly, CHF with peripheral neuropathy → **wet beriberi**
  • Alcoholic with retrograde and anterograde amnesia and confabulation (altered mental status, ophthalmoplegia, ataxia [AOA]) → Wernicke-Korsakoff syndrome
PPx: None; avoid abusing alcohol

QUICK TIPS
Beriberi means extreme weakness. The difference between dry and wet beriberi is whether or not there is edema of the lower extremities. In wet beriberi the legs are edematous and "wet."

QUICK TIPS
Wernicke vs. Korsakoff: Wernicke = AOA, Korsakoff = confabulation

MoD: Thiamine deficiency → catabolism of sugars and amino acids in neurons

Dx:
1. History and physical

Tx/Mgmt:
1. Intravenous (IV) infusion of Vitamin B1 in the acute stage (Wernicke encephalopathy)
2. In the chronic stage (Korsakoff syndrome), only supportive care can be provided

Vitamin B3 (Niacin; Nicotinic Acid) Deficiency

Buzz Words: Diarrhea + dementia + dermatitis→ pellagra

PPx: None

MoD: Decreased NAD production (NAD and its phosphorylated NADP form are cofactors required in many body processes); often from deficiency in tryptophan—occurring in people who consume only corn—lacking nicotinic acid and tryptophan that can be converted into nicotinic acid. Primarily causes symptoms of three organs (GI, nervous system, and skin).

Dx:
1. Clinical syndrome—diarrhea, skin changes, and neuro (memory problems, inattention, confusion, spasticity)

Tx/Mgmt:
1. Nicotinamide (same structure but lower toxicity)

Vitamin B6 (Pyridoxine) Deficiency

Buzz Words:
- Skin rash, atrophic glossitis with ulceration, angular cheilitis, conjunctivitis, intertrigo, and neurologic symptoms of somnolence, confusion with sideroblastic anemia in patient with tuberculosis taking isoniazid therapy → B6 (pyridoxine) deficiency
- Seizures in infants (pyridoxine-responsive seizure)

PPx: Vitamin supplementation with isoniazid for patients receiving tuberculosis treatment

MoD: Cofactor in reactions of amino acid, glucose, lipid metabolism → Neuropathy from impaired sphingosine synthesis

Dx:
- Seizures in infants
- Neuropathy in adults

Tx/Mgmt:
1. Pyridoxine hydrochloride to replace vitamin B6

History of Pellagra

Vitamin B12 (Cobalamin) Deficiency

Buzz Words: Bone marrow promegaloblastosis (megaloblastic anemia from inhibition of purine synthesis) + GI symptoms + weakness + spasticity + absent reflexes + diminished vibration and position sensation + subacute degeneration of spinal cord + memory loss + depression

PPx: B12 supplementation, diet including animal products

MoD: Decreased B12 → Impaired DNA synthesis and regulation, fatty acid, and amino acid metabolism. Also known as subacute combined degeneration of the spinal cord that presents with posterior and lateral column signs.

Dx:

1. Labs → low vitamin B12 levels with elevated methylmalonic acid
2. Antiintrinsic factor antibodies to rule out (r/o) pernicious anemia

Tx/Mgmt:

1. Vitamin B12 supplementation

QUICK TIPS
B12 vs. folate deficiency: There are no neurologic symptoms and methylmalonic acid levels are normal in folate deficiency.

Vitamin D Deficiency

Buzz Words:

- Adult + bone pain + weakness + poor fracture healing + hypocalcemic tetany

Clinical Presentation: Prolonged vitamin D deficiency can cause myelopathy (weakness in legs) as well. An adult with poor nutrition will present with bone pains, weakness, and fractures.

PPx: Consumption of dairy products and sun exposure

MoD: Decreased vitamin D → decreased intestinal absorption of calcium and phosphate → decreased bone mineralization

Dx:

1. Serum level of 25-hydroxyvitamin D
2. PTH levels to r/o endocrine disorder

Tx/Mgmt:

1. Vitamin D supplementation

QUICK TIPS
Calcitriol = active form of vitamin D

Vitamin E Deficiency

Buzz Words: Hemolytic anemia + muscle weakness + acanthocytosis + spinocerebellar ataxia + loss of vibratory sensation and proprioception

PPx: None

MoD: Vitamin E protects cellular membranes and is an antioxidant.

QUICK TIPS
Cystic fibrosis patients = vitamin E deficiency 2/2 pancreatic dysfunction

Dx:
1. H&P—ataxic gait and weakness in legs
Tx/Mgmt:
1. Vitamin E supplementation

Vitamin C Deficiency

Buzz Words: Weakness, fatigue + curly hair + dry mouth + gum bleeding + poor wound healing
PPx: Vitamin C in diet from citrus fruits and vegetables
MoD: Vitamin C or ascorbic acid accelerates many biochemical processes, especially in the synthesis of collagen.
Dx: PE
Tx/Mgmt:
1. Vitamin C supplementation

Vitamin K Deficiency

Buzz Words: Abnormal bleeding

Zinc Deficiency

Buzz Words: Hypogonadism + delayed wound healing + developmental problems + unable to taste, unable to smell + hair loss + skin rash

Chemical Poisoning

There are four chemical agents that frequently appear on the medicine shelf: ethylene glycol, CCL4, aspirin, and acetaminophen. Understanding the Buzz Words that describe their toxicities, as well as how to treat them, is key and will be sure to yield you a few points on the test.

Ethylene Glycol Poisoning

Buzz Words:
- Acute back pain + hematuria + oliguria in s/o high anion gap metabolic acidosis
- Oxalate crystals in urine + homeless alcoholic man
- Intermittent flashing spots + blurred vision + paint thinner spill + mydriasis + hyperemia of optic disc + Anion gap metabolic acidosis → alcohol (e.g., ethylene or methylene glycol) toxicity

Clinical Presentation: Ethylene glycol toxicity can be seen in patients who suffer from alcohol abuse looking for an alternative to feed the addiction. Patients (typically homeless) will present with oxalate crystals in urine.

MoD: Ethylene glycol is metabolized to glycolic acid = toxic to renal tubules (nephropathy) + induces oxalic acid to precipitate to calcium oxalate crystals

Dx:
1. UA (dumbbell shaped calcium oxalate crystals)

Tx/Mgmt:
1. Fomepizole (alcohol dehydrogenase inhibitor)
2. Dialysis

Carbon Tetrachloride Toxicity

Buzz Words: Dry cleaning industry exposure + liver damage → CCl4 toxicity

Clinical Presentation: Patients who experience CCl4 toxicity will have hepatic dysfunction and often have had some exposure to the dry cleaning industry.

PPx: Avoid dry cleaning industry

MoD:
- CCl4 oxidized by liver P450 → free radical generation → leads to reversible injury (cell swelling) of the hepatocyte → hepatocyte can no longer synthesize proteins 2/2 RER swelling → no proteins, including apolipoproteins synthesized → fat in the hepatocytes cannot be transported out → fatty change of liver
- Free radical generation also reacts with lipids of cell membrane → lipids are degraded and produce H_2O_2 (process of lipid peroxidation) → vicious cycle of ROS generation

Dx:
1. Liver panel

Tx/Mgmt:
1. Supportive

Aspirin Toxicity

Buzz Words:
- Tinnitus + respiratory alkalosis → early stage aspirin toxicity
- Microvesicular fatty infiltration + death 2/2 increased ICP and herniation → Reye syndrome (aspirin-mediated)
- Viral infection (e.g., influenza B, varicella-zoster virus [VZV]) + aspirin use in child + acute liver failure (elevated AST/ALT) + normal alkphos/bili + encephalopathy + hyperammonemia → Reye syndrome

Clinical Presentation: Reye syndrome is a dangerous complication in children who receive aspirin for virus-induced fever. This is because aspirin is mitochondrial toxin that can cause acute hepatic dysfunction in young individuals. Can lead to microvesicular fatty infiltration

PPx: Avoid giving aspirin to child with viral infection

MoD: Aspirin irreversibly inhibits COX → leads arachidonic acid down leukotriene pathway instead producing a lot of broncho-constricting prostaglandins. Can also induce G6PD hemolysis.

Dx:

1. Liver panels

Tx/Mgmt:

1. Sodium bicarbonate to alkalinize the urine

Acetaminophen Toxicity

Buzz Words: AST:ALT in 1000s + Centrilobular necrosis 2/2 increased oxidative stress (since glutathione depleted by acetaminophen-metabolite N-acetyl-p-benzoquinoneimine [NAPQI])

Clinical Presentation: Patients with acute acetaminophen toxicity classically present with AST:ALT ratio greater than 1000, one of only a few conditions to have such a ratio on the shelf exam. Tylenol toxicity occurs in phases. At less than 24 hours, patients may be asymptomatic or may report nausea/vomiting and diaphoresis. From 18 to 72 hours after digestion, patients can complain of RUQ abdominal pain. From 72 to 96 hours, patients may experience jaundice, acute renal failure, and hepatic encephalopathy 2/2 hepatic necrosis and dysfunction. After 96 hours from ingestion, patients who survive and are treated with N-acetylcysteine (NAC) can make a full recovery.

Phases of acetaminophen toxicity

PPx:

- Take less than 3 g of acetaminophen per 24 hours.
- Avoid mixing alcohol and acetaminophen.

MoD: Acetaminophen activates P450 and uses up glutathione, leaving liver susceptible to free radical injury. Alcohol also activates P450 system and can exacerbate symptoms.

Dx:

1. Liver panels
2. UDS

Tx/Mgmt:

1. NAC: Acts as glutathione substitute to bind to NAPQI from acetaminophen and to provide sulfhydryl groups to enhance nontoxic sulfation of acetaminophen

Types of Shock

Septic shock is an important concept to know for clerkships but is not as frequently tested on the shelf. The body is in shock when there is inadequate tissue perfusion. There are four types of shock according to the NBME: cardiogenic, hypovolemic, septic, and neurogenic. Although you may here of other types of shock (e.g., distributive and obstructive) during your rotations, these are the four the NBME have designated for you to learn for the shelf as outlined on the USMLE content outline. The initial management of all types of shock include ABCs, fluids, stat labs (e.g., CBC/BMP/coags/lactate), and labs to look for etiology (e.g., EKG, UA/UCx, CXR). Make sure to differentiate types of shock as well as diagnostic and treatment steps.

99 AR
Types of shock

Cardiogenic Shock

Buzz Words: Cardiac dysfunction + decreased BP/HR + abnormal EKG + evidence of inadequate tissue perfusion (e.g., elevated lactate)

Clinical Presentation: Cardiogenic shock is shock caused by cardiogenic dysfunction leading to decreased absolute cardiac output. Treat with drugs or interventions that get the heart beating properly again. Fluids may help but will not correct underlying etiology.

PPx: Avoid coronary artery disease.

MoD: Inadequate tissue perfusion 2/2 inadequate supply of blood from heart. Could be from MI, tension PTX, tamponade.

Dx:

1. EKG
2. Troponins/CPK
3. CXR
4. ABGs
5. Helical CT to r/o PE
6. Echo

Tx/Mgmt:

1. Treat according to underlying cause of cardiac dysfunction
2. Inotropic or vasopressor agents

99 AR
Guide on how to treat cardiogenic shock from Merck Manual

Hypovolemic Shock

Buzz Words:

- Pulsatile midline abdominal mass + hypovolemic shock (increased HR, decreased BP) → ruptured abdominal aortic aneurysm

- Tender adnexal mass + hypovolemic shock (increased HR, decreased BP) → ectopic pregnancy

Clinical Presentation: Hypovolemic shock is inadequate tissue perfusion due to inadequate volume. Again, for the purposes of the shelf, just be familiar with this concept and focus instead on the types of disease processes (e.g., AAA rupture, ectopic pregnancy, pancreatitis) that can lead to this type of shock.

PPx: Avoid rupture of aneurysm, ectopic pregnancy, etc.

MoD: Inadequate tissue perfusion 2/2 inadequate volume; hemorrhagic versus nonhemorrhagic

Dx:
1. Trend HR and BP (tachycardia earliest sign of hypovolemia; hypotension late stage sign)
2. Measure urine output
3. Identify sources of bleeding if hemorrhagic (e.g., FAST exam for abdominal trauma, abdominal CT, hCG to r/o pregnancy)

Tx/Mgmt:
1. Stop bleeding if hemorrhagic (through surgery or otherwise)
2. Administer resuscitative fluids
3. pRBCs and plasma

Septic Shock

Buzz Words: Fever, chills + signs of infection + immunocompromised patient + increased HR (early) + decreased BP (late) + altered mental status → septic shock

Clinical Presentation: Septic shock is inadequate tissue perfusion from vessel vasodilation and subsequent hypotension 2/2 release of inflammatory markers in response to infection. The key in septic shock is to isolate the source of infection and treat the underlying cause. Common etiologies include UTI and pneumonia.

- **Sepsis** = SIRS + infection source
- **Severe sepsis** = End-organ damage from hypoperfusion
- **Septic shock** = Severe sepsis unresponsive to fluid resuscitation

PPx: Sterile technique when performing invasive procedures

MoD: Inadequate tissue perfusion 2/2 vasodilation from inflammatory markers

Dx:
1. Monitor vital signs
2. CBC with differential, BMP, lactate
3. CVP, PaO_2 readings

4. Blood cultures
5. Search for source: CXR, UA/UCx, culture wounds

Tx/Mgmt:
1. Aggressive IV fluid resuscitation
2. O_2
3. **Broad-spectrum antibiotics**

Neurogenic Shock

Buzz Words: Warm skin + sympathetic denervation + increased HR but decreased BP + spinal cord injury

Clinical Presentation: Neurogenic shock is inadequate tissue perfusion 2/2 sympathetic nerve denervation. Most commonly occurs in patients who are undergoing spine surgery.

PPx: Avoid injury of spinal cord during surgery.

MoD: Lesion of sympathetic chain or sympathetic nerves → loss of vascular tone
1. Monitor vital signs
2. CBC with differential, BMP, lactate
3. CVP, PaO_2 readings

Tx/Mgmt:
1. Fluids

Paraneoplastic Syndromes

Paraneoplastic syndromes are disorders caused by a central neoplastic process. These traditionally do not fit into any specific organ system and can affect multiple organ systems at once. As such, they are fair game for the medicine shelf. For instance, patients with small cell carcinoma may present with Cushing features because the neoplasm itself upregulates ACTH. These are important because they lend important clues to what type of cancer ails the patient. The principle here is to recognize the buzz words only. Treating the primary cancer will treat the paraneoplastic syndrome.

Proximal muscle weakness + improvement with use + lung mass	Lambert-Eaton syndrome 2/2
2 atrophic adrenal glands + Cushing syndrome	Exogenous steroids
1 atrophic adrenal gland + Cushing syndrome	Unilateral adrenal adenoma
0 atrophic adrenal glands + Cushing syndrome	Paraneoplastic ACTH secretion and ACTH pituitary adenoma

99 AR

Make sure to use the qSOFA score for sepsis identification. Look to see if patient is (1) has new or worsened alterened mentation, (2) respiratory rate ≥22, (3) systolic BP ≤ 100. If yes to all three, test full SOFA score, assess for evidence of organ dysfunction with serum lactate, and search for source of infection.

QUICK TIPS

SOFA and qSOFA scores will NOT be on the medicine shelf but will be useful for you while taking care of patients during clerkships

99 AR

Example of how to select antibiotics for coverage, Merck Manual

- SIADH + Lambert Eaton + paraneoplastic encephalitis → small cell carcinoma
- Hyperthyroidism + scrotal mass → testicular malignancy which secretes beta-hCG (mimicking TSH)
- Elevated EPO, renin, PTHrP and aCTH → paraneoplastic syndrome of RCC
- Paraneoplastic EPO production → HCC, RCC, hemangioblastoma, pheochromocytoma
- Opsoclonus-myoclonus → neuroblastoma

GUNNER PRACTICE

1. A 77-year-old female is brought to the Emergency Department by her grandson, with pain in her arm after a fall. She had been exiting her apartment so that he could take her on some errands after a Saturday afternoon nap when she lost her balance and fell onto the sidewalk. Her past medical history is significant for hypertension, asthma, spinal stenosis, and type 2 diabetes mellitus, and her medications include lisinopril, hydrochlorothiazide, amlodipine, acetaminophen, tramadol, metformin, glyburide, zolpidem, albuterol, and fluticasone-salmeterol. Her vital signs are T 97.6 HR 89 BP 130/78 RR 16 SpO$_2$ 98% on room air. Finger stick blood glucose is 106. Radiographs of the right upper extremity show a simple, nondisplaced fracture of the humerus. Vascular and neurologic exams of the right arm, forearm, and hand reveal no abnormalities. Head CT is also negative. She is to be discharged home with close follow-up with orthopedics. To prevent future falls, which of the following medications should be discontinued most?
   A. Metformin
   B. Lisinopril
   C. Glyburide
   D. Zolpidem
   E. Albuterol
2. A 64-year-old male comes to your office for a follow-up appointment. You were the attending on the General Internal Medicine service that cared for him in the hospital 2 months ago. He was initially admitted for hypercarbic respiratory failure in the setting of a COPD exacerbation, which resulted in intubation. Unfortunately, he subsequently caught a ventilator-associated pneumonia, and respiratory cultures grew *Pseudomonas aeruginosa*. After a prolonged hospital stay and multimodal treatment, he was discharged to a skilled nursing facility,

where he remained until this past week. In the office, he appears well. His vital signs are T 98.4 HR 84 BP 134/80 RR 20 SpO$_2$ 94% on his home 2 L of oxygen by nasal cannula. He complains of difficulty hearing since his hospitalization, and, indeed, he displays a significant auditory deficit bilaterally. He denies vertigo, otalgia, tinnitus, nausea, and sinus pain and congestion. Which of the following medications given to him in the hospital most likely caused his new hearing deficit?

A. Cefepime

B. Gentamicin

C. Methylprednisolone

D. Acetaminophen

E. Ipratropium bromide

3. A 63-year-old female comes to your office for a follow-up appointment in February. You were the attending on the General Internal Medicine service that cared for her in the hospital last week. She had been admitted for a COPD exacerbation. She also has a history of hypertension and type 2 diabetes mellitus and actively uses alcohol and smokes tobacco. Although she was born in the United States and has lived in the same state for her entire life, she has received no vaccinations since finishing high school, had not seen a medical practice until last year when she called to make an appointment, and could provide no medical records from her past. Which of the following recommendations is NOT appropriate at this time?

A. Smoking cessation

B. 23-valent pneumococcal vaccination

C. Herpes zoster vaccination

D. HPV vaccination

E. Colonoscopy

ANSWERS: What Would Gunner Jess/Jim Do?

1. WWGJD? A 77-year-old female is brought to the Emergency Department by her grandson, with pain in her arm after a fall. She had been exiting her apartment so that he could take her on some errands after a Saturday afternoon nap when she lost her balance and fell onto the sidewalk. Her past medical history is significant for hypertension, asthma, spinal stenosis, and type 2 diabetes mellitus, and her medications include lisinopril, hydrochlorothiazide, amlodipine, acetaminophen, tramadol, metformin, glyburide, zolpidem, albuterol, and fluticasone-salmeterol. Her vital signs are T 97.6, HR 89, BP 130/78, RR 16, SpO$_2$ 98% on room air. Finger stick blood glucose is 106. Radiographs of the right upper extremity show a simple, non-displaced fracture of the humerus. Vascular and neurologic exams of the right arm, forearm, and hand reveal no abnormalities. Head CT is also negative. She is to be discharged home with close follow-up with orthopedics. In order to prevent future falls, which of the following medications should be discontinued most?

Answer: D, Zolpidem.

Explanation: This is an elderly woman with multiple medical problems and polypharmacy who fractures her humerus due to a fall. Falls are often due to medication side effects and polypharmacy, and the challenge here is to discern which medication is both a likely offender and the least necessary for her. As her BP appears appropriate (indicating that hypotension is a less likely cause of her fall), and we are given no medical indication for her use of zolpidem, this medication is the most appropriate to discontinue. Zolpidem, a GABA agonist often used for the short-term treatment of sleep-onset insomnia, is a common cause of somnolence and difficulty with balance in the elderly population. For this reason, it is included in Beers List, which cautions against the use of certain medications in adults 65 and older.

A. Metformin → Incorrect. Metformin is both less likely to be causing falls than zolpidem and also more necessary for blood sugar control.

B. Lisinopril → Incorrect. Due to her normal BP, lisinopril is unlikely to be causing significant hypotension, and is indicated for treating her hypertension.

C. Glyburide → Incorrect. We are given no indication that her fall was caused by hypoglycemia and this drug is indicated for the treatment of her diabetes mellitus.

E. Albuterol → Incorrect. This drug is not associated with falls.

2. WWGJD? A 64-year-old male comes to your office for a follow-up appointment. You were the attending on the General Internal Medicine service that cared for him in the hospital two months ago. He was initially admitted for hypercarbic respiratory failure in the setting of a COPD exacerbation, which resulted in intubation. Unfortunately, he subsequently caught a ventilator-associated pneumonia, and respiratory cultures grew *Pseudomonas aeruginosa.* After a prolonged hospital stay and multi-modal treatment, he was discharged to a skilled nursing facility, where he remained until this past week. In the office, he appears well. His vital signs are T 98.4 HR 84 BP 134/80 RR 20 SpO$_2$ 94% on his home 2 L of oxygen by nasal cannula. He complains of difficulty hearing since his hospitalization, and, indeed, he displays a significant auditory deficit bilaterally. He denies vertigo, otalgia, tinnitus, nausea, and sinus pain and congestion. Which of the following medications given to him in the hospital most likely caused his new hearing deficit?

Answer: B, Gentamicin.

Explanation: This 64-year-old man has, per the question, endured medication-induced ototoxicity. Gentamicin is an aminoglycoside antibiotic often used in a synergistic manner with other antibiotics (especially in the treatment of drug-resistant Gram-negative rods, like *P. aeruginosa*). Aminoglycoside antibiotics are notorious for their ototoxicity (and nephrotoxicity), so gentamicin is the likely culprit here. None of the other choices are associated with hearing loss.

A. Cefepime → Incorrect. This is a fourth-generation cephalosporin often used in the treatment of *Pseudomonas.* It is not notorious for ototoxicity.

C. Methylprednisolone → Incorrect. This is a corticosteroid often used in treatment of COPD exacerbations. It is not notorious for ototoxicity.

D. Acetaminophen → Incorrect. This is a CNS-specific cyclooxygenase inhibitor often used as an antipyretic or pain reliever. It is not notorious for ototoxicity.

E. Ipratropium bromide → Incorrect. This is an anticholinergic medication often used in treatment of COPD exacerbations. It is not notorious for ototoxicity.

3. WWGJD? A 63-year-old female comes to your office for a follow-up appointment in February. You were the attending on the General Internal Medicine service that cared for her in the hospital last week. She had been admitted for a COPD exacerbation. She also has a history of hypertension and type 2 diabetes mellitus and actively uses alcohol and smokes tobacco. Though she was born in the United States and has lived in the same state for her entire life, she has received no vaccinations since finishing high school, had not seen a medical practice until last year when she called to make an appointment, and could provide no medical records from her past. Which of the following recommendations is NOT appropriate at this time?

Answer: D, HPV vaccination.

Explanation: This is a 63-year-old woman with multiple medical problems and limited medical care until recently. The HPV vaccine is currently approved for women up to 26 years of age, and so this patient falls outside of the recommended population to receive it. In addition, she has multiple illnesses and risks that require more immediate attention.

A. Smoking cessation → Incorrect. All patients using tobacco should be counseled on smoking cessation, regardless of age. The fact that the patient has COPD is NOT a reason to forego such counseling.

B. 23-valent pneumococcal vaccination → Incorrect. The PPSV23 is currently recommended for adults age less than 65 with chronic lung disease, active smoking, diabetes mellitus, and alcohol use disorder, among other risk factors. This patient, who smokes, has COPD, has diabetes mellitus, and may have alcohol use disorder, should receive the vaccine.

C. Herpes zoster vaccination → Incorrect. The herpes zoster vaccine is currently recommended to adults greater than 50 years of age.

E. Colonoscopy → Incorrect. Screening colonoscopy is recommended for adults beginning at age 50 (or 45, depending upon race and the guideline being used).

Immunologic Disorders

Hao-Hua Wu, Daniel Gromer, Leo Wang, and Rebecca Gao

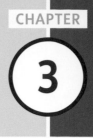

Introduction

Five to 10 questions on the shelf will be directly related to immunologic disorders, defined as abnormal processes that arise from a defective immune system. This chapter will be organized according to the United States Medical Licensing Examination (USMLE) Content Outline, which categorizes immunologic disorders into four sections: (1) Disorders Associated With Immunodeficiency, (2) HIV/AIDS, (3) Immunologically Mediated Disorders, and (4) Adverse Effects of Drugs on the Immune System.

Unlike Step 1, the medicine shelf will not test you directly on the normal immune system; you will not get questions on the difference between mast cells versus macrophages or the function of specific interleukins. However, a basic understanding of terminology associated with the immune system, such as MHC complexes or innate versus adaptive immunity, would be helpful.

This chapter is written with the assumption that the reader already has an adequate foundation of knowledge in normal processes of the immune system from either Step 1 studying or preclinical basic science courses. If you need further review, please refer to the video series linked in the Gunner Goggles app.

Make sure you know the buzz words associated with each disease. As a reminder, the buzz word section contains all the key clues within a question stem that you would need to ascertain a diagnosis or get the correct answer. Many of the immunologic disorders presented below, such as Wiskott-Aldrich syndrome (WAS) presenting with thrombocytopenia, bacterial infection, and eczema, are very rare, and clinicians rely on pathognomonic clinical clues in order to make the diagnosis.

As in other chapters, the diseases below are presented in the following format (Table 3.1): (1) Buzz Words, (2) Clinical Presentation, (3) Prophylaxis (PPx), (4) Mechanism of Disease (MoD), (5) Diagnostic Steps (Dx), and (6) Treatment and Management Steps (Tx/Mgmt).

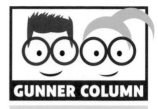

GUNNER COLUMN

QUICK TIPS

USMLE Content Outline Immune System Abnormal Processes, Page 5

99 AR

Immunology terminology, video series

TABLE 3.1 Type of Immunologic Deficiency Versus Types of Infections

Immunologic Deficiency	Types of Susceptible Infections
B-cell deficiency	Pyogenic bacteria, parasites, enteric bacteria and viruses (largely extracellular)
T-cell deficiency	Viruses, atypical mycobacteria, fungi, bacteria within the cell (largely intracellular)
Terminal complement deficiency	**Neisseria meningitides** and **Neisseria gonorrhoeae**

Disorders Associated With Immunodeficiency

Disorders associated with immunodeficiency are organized on the USMLE content by MoD. Organizing principle 1: This section is low yield for the medicine shelf because many of these disorders are congenital and disproportionately affect the pediatric population (which means these topics will be heavily tested on the Pediatrics shelf). However, the medicine shelf may present adult patients with the following immune deficiencies, and you will still need to know the buzz words. Organizing principle 2: Because most of these diseases are congenital or genetic, there are no prophylactic measures. Thus, most of the PPx sections will simply be "N/A." Instead, focus your attention on the Buzz Words, Dx, and Tx/Mgmt.

The humoral immune system is B-cell mediated and protects the body against extracellular microbes (e.g., pyogenic bacteria). Examples of disorders of humoral immune system include: common variable immunodeficiency (CVID), hyper-IgM syndrome, and Bruton agammaglobulinemia. The humoral immune system is also colloquially known as innate immunity.

The complement system is part of the innate immune system and defends the body against infection. Examples of disorders that arise due to defective complement proteins include terminal complement deficiency, and acquired and hereditary angioedema.

Phagocytes and natural killer (NK) cells are also part of the innate immune system and help defend the body against microbes such as bacteria. Examples of disorders that arise to defective phagocytic or NK cells include Chediak-Higashi disease.

Cell-mediated immunity is B- and T-cell mediated and protects the body against intracellular microbes (e.g., viruses, fungi). Examples include DiGeorge syndrome (DGS). Cell-mediated immunity is also known as adaptive immunity.

There are instances when diseases can present as a mix of B- and T-cell dysfunction; these diseases include severe combined immunodeficiency disease (SCID) and WAS.

Deficiency Primarily of Humoral Immunity
Common Variable Immunodeficiency

Buzz Words: Recurrent pulmonary infections/diarrhea + normal B cell number + reduced serum IgG/A/M.

Clinical Presentation: Typically presents in a 20–40 year old male or female with a chief complaint of infection, such as sinus or pulmonary infections. Patients who suffer from CVID have deficient number of B cells. Very similar to Bruton X-linked agammaglobulinemia; only difference is that the B cells in CVID are normal where as they are abnormal in Bruton. CVID may be associated with auto-immune disorders (i.e., SLE, RA) or gastric carcinoma. Official diagnosis of CVID is made by recurrent sinopulmonary infections + at least two of the following:

- Impaired immune response to immunizations
- Low levels of IgG (at least two standard deviations below the mean
- Low levels of IgA, IgM
- No other more likely immunodeficiency disorder

PPx: N/A

MoD: Unknown

Dx:

1. Complete blood count (CBC) with diff to look at white count
2. Measurement of antibody concentration in blood (IgG, IgA, IgM)
3. Flow cytometry
4. Serum protein electrophoresis

Tx/Mgmt:

1. Antibiotics for sinopulmonary infections
2. IVIG

Hyper-IgM Syndrome

Buzz Words: Recurrent sinopulmonary infections (e.g., acute otitis media, pneumonia, sinusitis, pneumocystis jiroveci) + elevated IgM (high in proportion to other Ig) + growth impairment

Clinical Presentation: HIGM is a rare, heterogeneous disease that is characterized by an increase in serum levels of IgM

99 AR

AR hyper-IgM: "At least 4 autosomal recessive forms involve a B-cell defect. In 2 of these forms (deficiency of activation-induced cytidine deaminase [AID] or uracil DNA glycosylase [UNG]), serum IgM levels are much higher than in the X-linked form; lymphoid hyperplasia (including lymphadenopathy, splenomegaly, and tonsillar hypertrophy) is present, and autoimmune disorders may be present. Leukopenia is absent."

and a concurrent deficiency in IgG, IgA, IgE. All types of HIGM involve a defect in the ability of B cells to undergo class-switch recombination, the process through which antibody heavy chains are replaced with other species. The most common cause involves X-linked mutations in CD40L, making the disease more prevalent in males. Clinical manifestations include: recurrent sinopulmonary infections and opportunistic infections (PCP, cryptosporidium).

PPx: Intravenous immunoglobulin (IVIG)

MoD: X-linked hyper-IgM: X-linked genetic defect in CD40 ligand on the surface of activated helper T cells → Absence of CD40 ligand = not helper T cell and B cell interaction → Absence of CD40 also → Inhibits plasma cell formation → inadequate immune response to pathogens

Dx:
1. CBC with diff to look at white count
2. Measurement of antibody concentration in blood (IgG, IgA, IgM)
3. Flow cytometry for presence of CD40 ligand
4. Genetic testing

Tx/Mgmt:
1. IVIG
2. Antibiotics like TMP/SMX
3. Hematopoietic stem cell transplantation

X-Linked Bruton (Agammaglobulinemia)
Buzz Words:
- Recurrent otitis media, pneumonia after 6 months of age + decreased B cells + no Ig abnormalities
- Pseudomonas infection + recurrent sinopulmonary infection + normal T cells + abnormal low B cells + low IgG, IgM, IgA + no germinal centers/no primary lymphoid follicles → Bruton
- Defective lymphocyte tyrosine kinase → Bruton
- Normal B cells + decreased immunoglobulins→ CVID

Clinical Presentation: Bruton agammaglobulinemia is characterized by recurrent bacterial infections due decreased B cells and low levels of immunoglobulins. Mycoplasma infection predisposed (not mycobacterium, which is Tb).

Be sure to differentiate Bruton agammaglobulinemia from CVID, which still has B cells (vs. X-linked Bruton has no mature B cells). Also, keep in mind that Bruton patients are susceptible to Mycoplasma infection and not mycobacterium (e.g., tuberculosis [TB]).

PPx: N/A

MoD (Fig. 3.1): X-linked recessive, Mutation to cytoplasmic tyrosine kinase known as Bruton tyrosine kinase (btk) → loss of signaling to turn pro-B/pre-B cells to mature B cells → only mu heavy chains produced; cannot move forward without btk → no B cells and all classes of immunoglobulin → no germinal centers and primary lymphoid follicles in lymph node

Dx: Serum electrophoresis shows low gamma globulin curve. Diagnosis is made if:

a. Onset of recurrent bacterial infections in first 5 years of life

b. Serum IgG, IgM and IgA values that are 2 SD below normal for age

c. Absent isohemagglutinins or poor response to vaccines

d. Less than 2% CD19 B cells in peripheral circulation

Tx/Mgmt: IVIG

IgA Immunodeficiency

Buzz Words: Rash on skin exposed area + sinopulmonary infections + ataxia low serum IgA + normal IgM/IgG → IgA deficiency in setting of ataxia/telangiectasia

- Recurrent respiratory infections or diarrhea + anaphylactic reaction to blood transfusion (itching, rash) leading to death → IgA deficiency (anti-IgA antibodies present in packed RBCs react with tiny amount of IgA in donor blood)

Clinical Presentation: IgA immunodeficiencies are associated with celiac disease, ataxia telangiectasia. Increased atopic allergy from frequent class switching to IgE. A minority of patients can develop anaphylactic reactions to blood or plasma products that contain IgA. This generally occurs only in patients with undetectable levels of serum IgA. (This clinical pearl, however, may be highlighted in board questions).

PPx: N/A

MoD: Decreased mucosal barrier of IgA → increased Giardia infections (GIs) and strep/H. flu infections (sinopulmonary).

Dx: Blood levels of IgA (<5–7 mg/dL).

Tx/Mgmt: IgA cannot be replaced. Manage infection and complications.

Deficiency/Dysfunction Primarily of Cell-Mediated Immunity

Cell-mediated immunity is immunity mediated by T cells. As stated in Table 3.1, defects in cell-mediated immunity

QUICK TIPS

Gamma globulin on electrophoresis demonstrates presence of immunoglobulin (so alpha1/beta1/beta2 globulins are part of hgb, while gamma globulin = immunoglobulin)

99 AR

IgA deficiency mnemonic

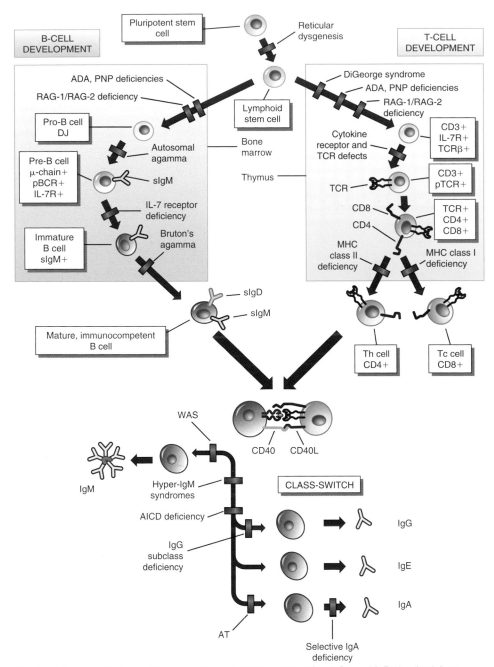

FIG. 3.1 X-linked Bruton (agammaglobulinemia). (From Huether S, McCance K. *Pathophysiology*, St Louis, 2010, Mosby.)

lead to largely intracellular pathogens and fungi. Use infectious etiology to differentiate defects in cell-mediated/adaptive and humoral/innate immunity.

22q11.2 Deletion Syndrome (DiGeorge)

Buzz Words:
- Immunodeficiency + hypocalcemia (hypoPTH) + cleft palate + congenital heart disease (truncus arteriosus)
- **Co**notruncal cardiac defects (truncus arteriosus, cyanosis)) + **A**bnormal facies (low set ears and micrognathia) + **T**hymic aplasia/hypoplasia + **C**left palate + **H**ypocalcemia → CATCH syndrome that is now known as DGS
- Interrupted aortic arch + recurrent fungal infection + small chin
- Viral + fungal infection + history of "tetany" + truncus arteriosus

Clinical Presentation: DiGeorge is now part of 22q11.2 deletion syndrome. However, since the National Board of Medical Examiners (NBME) sometimes recycles old questions, the term "DiGeorge syndrome" may come up. Clinical findings in patients with DGS stem from defects in the development of the pharyngeal pouch system.
- **C**ardiac Defects: most patients present with conotruncal/outflow tract defects including: interrupted aortic arch, truncus arteriosus, tetralogy of Fallot, septal defects, or vascular rings.
- **A**bnormal Facies: may include ear and ocular defects but these findings are not specific for DGS.
- **T**hymic Hypoplasia: the thymus can also be completely absent in DGS patients. The severity of the hypoplasia determines the degree of immunodeficiency. Patients can present with recurrent infections or symptoms of SCID.
- **C**left Palate
- **H**ypocalcemia: due to poor parathyroid development. Hypocalcemia in DGS patients can therefore be paired with low parathyroid hormone levels. Patients may present with seizures due to the hypocalcemia.

PPx: Avoid all live vaccines (e.g., rotavirus, MMR, varicella and intranasal influenza); killed or inactivated vaccines okay

MoD: Chromosome 22q11.2 deletion → Absence of third and fourth branchial pouch; third brachial pouch → thymus; fourth brachial pouch → parathyroid

99 AR
Truncus arteriosis video

99 AR
DiGeorge syndrome, abnormal facies video

Dx:
1. BMP to assess life-threatening hypocalcemia
2. CXR to confirm absence of thymus
3. Genetic testing
4. Candida intradermal test to r/o T-cell dysfunction

Tx/Mgmt:
1. Surgery to correct cardiac defects
2. Supportive treatment of additional defects

Severe Combined Immunodeficiency Disease

Buzz Words: Recurrent bacterial AND recurrent viral AND recurrent fungal infections + absent thymic shadow + absent lymph nodes/tonsils + absent T, B, and NK cells

Clinical Presentation: SCID is characterized by immunodeficiency due to a defective lymphoid cell (B and T cell) lineage. It can be thus caused by many different mechanisms; however, for the NBME shelf exams, adenosine deaminase (ADA) deficiency is the most commonly tested etiology. Patients typically present with recurrent infections from all different microbes (e.g., bacteria, viruses AND fungi) since both B and T cells are defective. Be sure to recognize that patients infected with many different bugs is indicative of SCID. Although this is more often seen in the pediatric population, you may get an adult SCID patient on the medicine shelf which the NBME will expect you to identify.

PPx: Neonatal screening with T-cell receptor excision test

MoD: Most commonly caused by ADA deficiency (Fig. 3.1); ADA catalyzes the reaction from pluripotent to lymphoid stem cell; without ADA no proliferation of B and T cells, although normal production of myeloid cells (i.e., neutrophils, macrophages)

Dx:
1. CBC with diff
2. Immunoglobulin levels
3. Flow cytometry to determine T-cell, B-cell, and NK cell counts
4. Measurement of ADA levels
5. Genetic testing for future siblings

Tx/Mgmt:
1. Antibiotics, antifungals, antivirals (depending on infection)
2. IVIG
3. ADA replacement if needed
4. Hematopoietic stem cell transplant

Wiskott-Aldrich Syndrome

Buzz Words: Young boy + eczema + thrombocytopenia + recurrent infections with encapsulated organisms + bruising/bleeding + low IgM + high IgA + IgE levels

Clinical Presentation: X-linked congenital disorder caused by mutation in the *WAS* gene, which plays an important role in linking T cell receptor signaling pathways to cytoskeletal rearrangement. Although patients initially have normal serum lymphocyte levels, both T- and B-cell counts decrease over time, therefore increasing infection susceptibility with age. Eczema is common within the first year of life. (This is often used as a clue to board questions.) WAS is also associated with B-cell lymphoma and leukemia.

PPx: N/A

MoD: Mutation of Wiskott-Aldrich syndrome protein (WASP) gene on short arm of X-chromosome (recessive) → T cells unable to reorganize actin cytoskeleton caused by WAS gene mutation → B-cell and T-cell disorder from X-linked recessive disorder.

Dx:

1. CBC (thrombocytopenia)
2. Measurement of antibody concentration in blood (low IgM but elevated IgA/IgE)
3. WAS in maternal male cousins, uncles or nephews
4. Poor antibody response to polysaccharides/polysaccharide vaccines: encapsulated bacteria: *Neisseria meningitidis, Streptococcus pneumoniae,* and *Haemophilus influenza*
5. T-Cell Studies: lymphocyte counts are generally normal early in life, but levels fall over time. T cells may also exhibit poor proliferative responses to mitogen

Tx/Mgmt: IVIG

Complement Deficiency

The complement system defends the body through a variety of mechanisms, such as opsonization. Deficiencies can be broken down into deficiencies of the classical pathway, alternative pathway and terminal complement pathway; it is important, however, to know that you do NOT need to have an in-depth knowledge of which complement proteins belong to which category. For the Medicine shelf, you only need to know three things related to complement deficiency: (1) patients with terminal complement deficiency present with disseminated *Neisseria* infections

99 AR

Wiskott Aldrich symptoms

MNEMONIC

Mr. Wiskott-Aldrich wears a TIE but no Matching shirt; T = thrombocytopenia, I = infection (bacterial), E = eczema, M = low IgM (even though other Ig are high)

(e.g., *Neisseria meningitidis* causing meningitis; *Neisseria gonorrhoeae* causing systemic infection), (2) Buzz Words and work-up of C1 esterase inhibitor deficiency, and (3) Buzz Words and work-up of hereditary angioedema. These topics may also appear on your Pediatric and Family Medicine shelf exams.

Terminal Complement Deficiency

Buzz Words: Recurrent meningococcal meningitis secondary to *N. meningitidis* OR recurrent *N. gonorrhoeae* infections

Clinical Presentation: This is the only type of complement deficiency you must be aware of for the Medicine shelf. Defects in the classical and alternative pathway lead to recurrent pyogenic infections in the patient; however, they would be too difficult to differentiate from other primary immunodeficiencies. Thus the NBME will only ask you to recognize the *Neisseria* and terminal complement deficiency connection; often the answer choice will just be "complement deficiency" not even specify "terminal."

PPx, MoD, Dx, and Tx/Mgmt: Do not need to know for Medicine shelf.

C1 Esterase Inhibitor Deficiency (Acquired Angioedema)

Buzz Words: Adult patient + first episode of edema following infection or dental procedure or trauma + rapid onset of facial edema + genital edema + tracheal edema + extremities edema + colicky ab pain from ab edema + no urticarial signs + associated with autoimmune or lymphoproliferative disease

Clinical Presentation: Acquired angioedema is when the C1 esterase inhibitor (C1-INH), which is responsible for regulating the levels of C2b and bradykinin to prevent swelling, is diminished by a noncongenital mechanism. Patients experience edema in many different areas of the body after an insult that activates the complement system. Most commonly, acquired angioedema is associated with autoimmune disorders that can produce an antibody directed at the C1 esterase inhibitor, although no one autoimmune disorder has distinguished itself in the literature.

PPx:
1. Avoid infections or events that trigger complement
2. Danazol
3. androgens
4. C1-INH infusions preoperatively

99 AR

List of disorders found to be associated with acquired angioedema

MoD: Acquired C1 esterase inhibitor deficiency secondary to destruction → elevated levels of C2b and bradykinin, which both have elevated levels of the edema-production factors. Similar to ACEi mechanism of causing edema from elevated levels of bradykinin

Dx: Serum complement levels

Tx/Mgmt: C1-INH infusions/concentrate

Hereditary Angioedema

Buzz Words: Young adult patient + **Recurrent** episodes of **edema following** infection or **dental procedure** or trauma + rapid onset of facial edema + acral (pertaining to peripheral parts such as LE and UE) extremities + genital edema + tracheal edema + abdominal edema (colicky pain) + **no urticarial**

Clinical Presentation: Hereditary angioedema is when there is a congenital defect in the C1 esterase inhibitor (C1-INH), which is responsible for regulating the levels of C2b and bradykinin to prevent swelling. The patients present the same as they would in acquired angioedema except folks with hereditary angioedema are more likely to present with recurrent episodes of swelling stemming from childhood.

PPx:
1. Avoid infections or events that trigger complement
2. Danazol
3. androgens
4. C1-INH infusions preoperatively

MoD: Acquired C1 esterase inhibitor deficiency caused by destruction → elevated levels of C2b and bradykinin, which both have elevated levels of the edema-production factors. Similar to ACEi mechanism of causing edema from elevated levels of bradykinin

Dx: Serum complement levels

Tx/Mgmt: C1-INH infusions/concentrate

Deficiency of Phagocytic Cells and Natural Killer Cells

Chediak-Higashi Syndrome

Buzz Words: Azurophilic granules in neutrophils + recurrent pyogenic infections + streaks of blonde hair + neutropenia + toddler

Clinical Presentation: Chediak-Higashi disease is caused by autosomal recessive defect in the neutrophil phagosome-lysosome fusion, which leads to recurrent bacterial

99 AR

Review article on hereditary angioedema

99 AR

Azurophilic granules in neutrophils

infections and other unique signs, such as oculocutaneous albinism.

MoD: Mutation causing defective microtubule → decreased degranulation + decreased chemotaxis + decreased granulopoiesis → giant lysosomes in neutrophils/lymphocytes from inability to clear lysosome content

- MoA of pyogenic infection in Chediak-Higashi: no phagolysosomes
- MoA of neutropenia: no microtubules for PMN division
- MoA of giant granules in granulocytes/platelets: since there is no microtubule transport of granules from Golgi to where they need to go, the granules just all pile up next to Golgi.
- MoA of defective hemostasis: granules in platelets are not properly functioning
- MoA of albinism: melanocytes make melanin in one cell at base and then passes melanin from cell to cell through microtubules.
- MoA of peripheral neuropathy: transport via microtubules to distal ends of neurons is defective.

Dx: CBC and blood smear show neutropenia and giant lysosomes in neutrophils.

Tx/Mgmt:
1. TMP/SMX for infection PPx
2. Vitamin C to prevent infection if taken daily

Chronic Granulomatous Disease

Buzz Words: Severe/recurrent infection with catalase positive bacteria/*Aspergillus* + NADPH oxidase deficiency

Clinical Presentation: The main problem in patients with CGD is an inability to kill phagocytized material via oxidative burst. In CGD, there is a defect in NAPDH oxidase, which leads to an inability to form O_2 radical and HOCl (bleach). The consequence of this defect is that patients with CGD cannot defend itself from catalase positive microbes, such as candida, aspergillus, listeria, staph, serratia, nocardia, pseudomonas cepacia, *Burkholderia cepacia*.

PPx: N/A

MoD: NAPDH oxidase defect caused by inability to form O_2 radical and eventually bleach (HOCl) → **impaired oxidative metabolism within phagocytes** → uncontrolled catalase-positive infections

Dx:
1. **Nitro blue tetrazolium test** (positive)
2. Flow cytometry

3. Cytochrome C reduction
4. Gram stain → numerous bacteria filled segmented neutrophils

Tx/Mgmt:
1. TMP-SMX 3 times a week to prevent infection
2. Gamma-interferon 3 times a week to prevent infection
3. Bone marrow transplantation (experimental but curative)

Leukocyte Adhesion Deficiency

Buzz Words: Delayed umbilical cord falling off + increased circulating PMNs + no PMNs in pus

Clinical Presentation: Leukocyte adhesion deficiency is divided into several types, each with its own mechanism. Although understanding the basic science was important for Step 1, the only thing you need to know for LAD on the Medicine and Pediatric shelf is how to recognize it in a question stem. The Buzz Word here is a patient with a history of delayed umbilical cord falling off (adult patient for Medicine shelf; pediatric patient for Pediatric shelf) and no PMNs found in pus. PPx, Dx, and Tx/Mgmt are not tested.

MoD:
- Type 1 is caused by mutation in gene encoding beta-chain of β2 integrins → defective leukocyte adhesion/migration
- Type 2 is caused by defective E- and P-selectin ligands mutation → defective adhesion/migration
- Increased PMNs found in the blood because of reserve of neutrophils typically stuck to endothelial cells in the lungs are released

Human Immunodeficiency Virus/Acquired Immune Deficiency Syndrome

HIV/AIDS is the most high-yield subsection of the immunologic disorders for the medicine shelf. This is because this is a disease that primarily affects adults, is well publicized, and is very well studied. Thus it is important to understand the clinical presentation, PPx, MoD, Dx, and Tx/Mgmt of HIV/AIDS.

Human Immunodeficiency Virus Infection and Acquired Immunodeficiency Syndrome

Buzz Words:
- Sexually active male or female + intravenous (IV)-drug user + enlarged inguinal lymph nodes (or generalized

QUICK TIPS

Positive nitroblue tetrazolium test = chronic granulomatous disease

99 AR

Leukocyte adhesion deficiency types graphic

lymphadenopathy + fever/recent sickness + sore throat + unspecified rashes → HIV (acute phase)

- *Toxoplasma* infection + *Cryptosporidium* infection, *Mycobacterium avium* infection, fungal infections *(Candida, Cryptococcus, Pneumocysitis jirovecii pneumonia, Histoplasma, Coccidioides)* + cytomegalovirus (CMV) + Kaposi sarcoma + lymphomas + encephalopathy + wasting syndrome → AIDS (CD4<200, considered late phase of infection)

Clinical Presentation: HIV is a double-stranded RNA virus that infects immune cells (e.g., CD4) by embedding themselves into DNA through reverse transcription. On the medicine shelf, patients can either present in the acute phase of illness (e.g., sore throat, generalized lymphadenopathy, fever) or late stage of illness aka with AIDS. AIDS is diagnosed if patient has a CD4 cell percentage ≤14%, CD4 count <200 per μL, and presence of AIDS defining condition.

For the medicine shelf, you will only encounter adults with HIV; congenital HIV buzz words will only be needed for Pediatrics. Be prepared to recognize the classic signs of acute illness as well as a few frequently tested AIDS-defining conditions, such as Kaposi sarcoma. You may also be tested on prevention techniques, Dx as well as treatment/management steps, although, unlike Step 1, you do not have to know the exact details of MoD and/or drug target of action (although we do encourage you to learn this for your patients and to impress your attendings!)

PPx: To understand prophylactic measures, know the common modes of HIV transmission: (1) sexual intercourse through genital, rectal, or oral fluids, (2) use of contaminated instruments or needles (e.g., IV drug users sharing needles), (3) maternal to fetus through breastfeeding or childbirth, and (4) blood transfusion. Thus to prevent HIV transmission:

1. Condom use
2. Avoidance of dirty needles
3. Treatment of pregnant patient to reduce HIV viral load and chance of vertical transmission
4. Screening of blood donors for HIV
5. HIV antibody testing for sexually active patients,
   vi. Stay updated with vaccinations (flu, HBV, pneumococcal, HPV, zoster)

MoD: HIV is a lentivirus capable of long-term latent infection and spread through semen and blood → HIV Env (envelope glycoprotein) binds to CD4 and chemokine coreceptors (CXCR4, CCR5) → HIV RNA w/ reverse transcriptase release into cell → HIV integration into genome and replication within cell → Lysis of infected cell to release of HIV and propagate infection

HIV infection leads to immunodeficiency by (1) loss of CD4 cells from direct cytotoxic effect, (2) infection of macrophages, dendritic cells and follicular dendritic cells, (3) decreased immune response caused by depletion of CD4 T cells.

Dx:

Initial diagnosis

1. HIV antibody testing
2. Nucleic acid amplification assays for HIV RNA level
3. ELISA±Western blot to confirm diagnosis

To monitor HIV

1. CD4 count (e.g., CBC with diff)
2. Plasma HIV RNA level
3. PPD or quantiFERON gold to r/o concomitant TB

Tx/Mgmt:

1. Combination treatment with antiretroviral therapy, for example, highly active antiretroviral therapy (HAART)
2. If AIDS (CD4 < 200/microL), TMP/SMX or dapsone to PPx against pneumocystis jiroveci
3. If AIDS (CD4 < 50), azithromycin/clarithromycin to PPx against *Mycobacterium avium-intracellulare* (MAC)
4. If HIV + suspicion of TB, start patient on isoniazid and pyridoxine (vitamin B6 to counter isoniazid side effects)
5. If concerned for fungal infections: fluconazole

Immunologically Mediated Disorders

In contrast to the "Disorders associated with immunodeficiency," in which the immune system is too weak to mount an adequate immune response, the "Immunologically mediated disorders" can be thought of as an overactive immune response. The actors in the immune system are responding too well to insults. Very high yield for the Medicine shelf. These topics will appear on multiple shelf exams. Hypersensitivity reactions will appear on prominently on the Pediatrics shelf and "Graft versus host disease" will be featured prominently on the Surgery shelf as well (Table 3.2).

Adverse Effects of Drugs on the Immune System

This section covers the medication side effects commonly tested on the Medicine shelf (Table 3.3). You will

99 AR

NIH treatment guidelines for HIV/AIDS

QUICK TIPS

Immune reconstitution inflammatory syndrome (IRIS) occurs when there is an immune reaction to subclinically detectable infection, even though CD4 count and HIV viral load improve. Self-limited and improves with steroids. Make sure to think of IRIS in a patient who appears to be getting sicker even though lab values paint a healthier picture.

QUICK TIPS

Definition of serum sickness syndrome: immune complex mediated hypersensitivity to nonhuman proteins

TABLE 3.2 Types of Hypersensitivity Reactions: Mechanisms and Examples

Hypersensitivity	Mediated by	Mechanism of Action	Example
Type 1	IgE	Allergen binds and cross links two IgE molecules attached to mast cells	Atopy/urticaria/anaphylaxis
Type 2	Antibodies	Antibody attack antigen	ABO incompatibility + Rh hemolytic disease
Type 3	Immune complex mediated	IgG or IgM antibodies form immune complexes → nonspecifically activates inflammatory process	Serum sickness syndrome (antibody-containing-blood mediated) Arthus reaction Serum sickness–like reaction (drug mediated)
Type 4	Cell mediated (T cell)	Prior exposure to allergen before developing reaction; reexposure activated cell-mediated response	allergic contact dermatitis from poison ivy, oak, or sumac

TABLE 3.3 Side Effects of Immunologic Drugs Tested on the Medicine Shelf

Immunologic Drug	Adverse Effect
Cyclosporine	Hirsutism, gum hypertrophy
Tacrolimus	Hypertension, hyperkalemia, nephrotoxicity, diabetes/glucose intolerance, tremor
Azathioprine	Diarrhea, leukopenia, toxicity of liver
Mycophenolate	Suppression of bone marrow
Methotrexate	Pulmonary fibrosis, hepatotoxicity, myelosuppression (reversed with leucovorin), mouth ulcers
Prednisone	Psychosis, Cushing-like symptoms (e.g., central obesity, hyperglycemia, etc.)

QUICK TIPS

Serum sickness syndrome versus serum sickness–like reaction; former is triggered when patient is given antibody-containing blood from another living source; serum sickness–like reaction is triggered by drugs

not have to memorize every side effect from that big table in First Aid from Step 1. Instead, focus only on the reactions, such as Jarisch-Herxheimer reaction, that may be seen in patients. Also focus on commonly given drugs that affect the immune system, such as prednisone, azathioprine, etc. because they will likely be tested on the medicine shelf. The good thing about drugs is that you will only need to know the Buzz Words (e.g., how to recognize a patient from the question stem) of drug reactions as well as a basic understanding of the drug mechanism of action. Very rarely will you be tested on Dx and treatment/management. The PPx for all of these reactions is to discontinue the drug.

Jarisch-Herxheimer Reaction

Buzz Words:
- Spontaneous abortion in pregnant mother with syphilis treated with penicillin
- Infection treated with antibiotic + myalgias, rigors, high fever post antibiotic administration + self-limiting

Clinical Presentation: Jarisch-Herxheimer reaction is a reaction to endotoxin-like products released by the death of harmful microorganisms within the body during antibiotic treatment (resembles bacterial sepsis). Can often be seen with penicillin treatment of congenital syphilis, but can occur with **any** antibiotic treatment for an organism.

PPx: Avoid antibiotic treatment when appropriate.

MoD: Unknown, but reaction likely secondary endotoxin-like products from microorganisms released into the blood stream

Dx: N/A

Tx/Mgmt: N/A

QUICK TIPS

fever + urticarial rash + polyarthralgia + lymphadenopathy (LAD) + viral infection + use of penicillin + amoxicillin + cefaclor → serum sickness–like reaction. Although serum sickness–like reaction is drug induced, it does not represent a true drug allergy because it is an immune complex mediated (type 3) reaction. Treat by withdrawing offending agent.

QUICK TIPS

Patient returned from trip to woods + itching/burning/oozing lesions of skin → allergic contact dermatitis from poison ivy → Type IV (cell-mediated) hypersensitivity

MNEMONIC

Azathioprine toxicity → the Liver Dies Leuking to get rid of Azathioprine

GUNNER PRACTICE

1. A 33-year-old man comes to the physician 2 days after an itchy rash developed on his hands, forearms, arms, and face. He reports returning from a recent camping trip and states how happy he was that he protected himself with ample sunscreen, a wide-brimmed hat, and copious amounts of bug spray. He recalls being adventurous and wading through "many bushes and leaves." His vital signs are within normal limits. On exam, there is a linear pattern of red papules and vesicles on his arms and face. Otherwise, no abnormalities are found. What is the mechanism for the rash seen on this patient?
   A. Hypersensitivity, type 1
   B. Hypersensitivity, type 2
   C. Hypersensitivity, type 3
   D. Hypersensitivity, type 4
   E. Jarisch-Herxheimer reaction

2. A 41-year-old male presents to the emergency department with a 5-day-old wound that has purulent drainage on his left thigh at the site of a previous surgical incision. He complains that his wounds "never seem to go away" and that this has sort of thing has been ongoing since he was little. He had a surgery to fix a left femoral neck fracture and reports that the operation had gone "just fine." Cultures of the purulent drainage show *Staphylococcus aureus* resistant to methicillin. His blood counts are within normal range but the nitroblue

tetrazolium test is positive. The appropriate treatments are then started. What is this patient's initial diagnosis?
A. Chronic granulomatous disease
B. Chediak-Higashi syndrome
C. Wiskott-Aldrich syndrome
D. DiGeorge Syndrome
E. Bruton agammaglobulinemia

3. A 29-year-old female with a history of HIV for 5 years comes to the physician for a follow-up appointment. She endorses being compliant with the medication and having no trouble controlling her symptoms. She is currently taking the HAART regimen and a proton pump inhibitor for GERD. CD4 counts that were last checked were near normal. She does however, endorse being around people who cough all the time recently, from her significant other to her parents who live nearby. What is the next most appropriate step?
A. Reassurance
B. Prescribe anxiolytic
C. PPD skin test
D. Spirometry
E. Chest x-ray

Notes

ANSWERS: What Would Gunner Jess/Jim Do?

1. WWGJD? A 33-year-old man comes to the physician 2 days after an itchy rash developed on his hands, forearms, arms, and face. He reports returning from a recent camping trip and states how happy he was that he protected himself with ample sunscreen, a wide-brimmed hat, and copious amounts of bug spray. He recalls being adventurous and wading through "many bushes and leaves." His vital signs are within normal limits. On exam, there is a linear pattern of red papules and vesicles on his arms and face. Otherwise, no abnormalities are found. What is the mechanism for the rash seen on this patient?

Answer: D. Hypersensitivity, type 4

Explanation: Given the patient's history, it is likely that he got poison ivy or poison oak from forays into nature. What gives it away are the clinical clues about being in direct contact with foliage and the fact that only the uncovered parts of the body were affected. The difficult part is remembering what type of hypersensitivity reaction poison ivy or poison provokes, which is actually a type 4 (cell-mediated) reaction. Be sure to remember these types of questions as they may also be on your Pediatrics shelf as well.

A. Hypersensitivity, type 1 → Incorrect. This is an IgE-mediated reaction that is often manifested by allergic responses.

B. Hypersensitivity, type 2 → Incorrect. This is an antibody-mediated reaction that is often times seen with blood type (ABO) incompatibility.

C. Hypersensitivity, type 3 → Incorrect. This is an immune complex mediated reaction (IgG and IgM, in particular) to blood containing preformed antibodies or with particular drugs.

E. Jarisch-Herxheimer reaction → Incorrect. There was no indication that a patient has taken an antibiotic for his troubles.

2. WWGJD? A 41-year-old male presents to the emergency department with a 5-day-old wound that has purulent drainage on his left thigh at the site of a previous surgical incision. He complains that his wounds "never seem to go away" and that this has sort of thing has been ongoing since he was little. He had a surgery to fix a left femoral neck fracture and reports that the operation had gone "just fine." Cultures of the purulent drainage show

Staphylococcus aureus resistant to methicillin. His blood counts are within normal range but the nitroblue tetrazolium test is positive. The appropriate treatments are then started. What is this patient's initial diagnosis?

Answer: A. Chronic granulomatous disease

Explanation: Right away, key words like nitroblue tetrazolium, should tell you what diagnosis this is. Do not worry about generating a broad differential here and comparing each answer choice. Once you see nitroblue tetrazolium, scan the rest of the clues to corroborate your suspicion of CGD, and then when you've made up your mind, answer appropriately. With these types of questions, it can be easy to get lost by looking at the answer choices before establishing a clear train of thought.

B. Chediak-Higashi syndrome → Incorrect. Nitroblue tetrazolium is not used to diagnose Chediak-Higashi. Also, patient did not have any of the classic symptoms of Chediak-Higashi, such as oculocutaneous albinism.

C. Wiskott-Aldrich syndrome → Incorrect. Although patient may have had recurrent bacteria infections, he did not have the eczema as would be expected in a Wiskott patient (e.g., TIE → thrombocytopenia, bacterial infection, and eczema).

D. DiGeorge Syndrome → Incorrect. Patient does not have the CATCH-22 congenital symptoms.

E. Bruton agammaglobulinemia → Incorrect. Patient appears to have a localized, yet compromised immune system. Bruton would likely present with more systemic symptoms.

3. WWGJD? A 29-year-old female with a history of HIV for 5 years comes to the physician for a follow-up appointment. She endorses being compliant with the medication and having no trouble controlling her symptoms. She is currently taking the HAART regimen and a proton pump inhibitor for GERD. CD4 counts that were last checked that she was near normal. She does however, endorse being around people who cough all the time recently, from her significant other to her parents who live nearby. What is the next most appropriate step?

Answer: C. PPD Skin test.

Explanation: It is recommended that all HIV patients at some point get tested for tuberculosis, because those two diseases are so intertwined. Thus the first step in PPx is to try to rule out TB early. PPD is the fastest and most cost-effective way to do so.

A. Reassurance → Incorrect. While reassurance may feel good for the patient, she still needs a PPD to rule out TB.

B. Prescribe anxiolytic → Incorrect. It is never appropriate to prescribe an anxiolytic without the proper indication. In this case, there was no indication the patient had pathologic worry (e.g., sleep disturbances, disturbance of daily activities, etc.)

D. Spirometry → Incorrect. No need for spirometry here, although may have use in patients with chronic disorders of the respiratory system, such as cystic fibrosis.

E. Chest x-ray → Incorrect. Although it may be tempting to rule out pneumonia, it is important to recognize that the patient herself is NOT coughing; she only complains about all the people around her that do. Thus, at this moment, she does not have respiratory pathology and would best be suited by administering the PPD.

Diseases of the Blood and Blood-Forming Organs

Leo Wang, Daniel Gromer, Sila Bal, Hao-Hua Wu, Rebecca Gao, and Nadia Bennett

Introduction

Chapter 4 covers the hematology/oncology that you will face on the medicine shelf. Despite the length of this chapter, you will only get 5–10 questions on this chapter on the medicine shelf, making it relatively lower yield than chapters on major organ systems. However, the organizing principles in this chapter apply to many other chapters, so it is recommended to know the content well for the shelf exam.

This chapter is divided into several sections that highlight the various pathologies that can occur in the blood, ranging from infections to clotting problems to cancer. As a rule, complete blood count (CBCs) and peripheral blood smears play major diagnostic roles in the workup of many of these diseases. As such, recognizing normal CBC values and peripheral blood smears can go a long way for the shelf exam. Bone marrow aspirates are used for many blood disorders, and it will be helpful to also have a sense of what normal marrow looks like. For specific diseases such as coagulopathies, understand principles behind PT, aPTT (discussed later).

Infections of the Blood

This chapter covers various types of infections of the blood. The concepts applied herein are relatively general and go a long way. Blood cultures in general should always be ordered for suspected infections.

Bacterial Infections of the Blood

Buzz Words: Bacteria (or other infectious agent) in bloodstream + high/low temp, high heart rate (HR), respiratory rate (RR) + high leukocyte count

Clinical Presentation: Sepsis is a spectrum that ranges from bacteremia all the way to septic shock. Bacteremia is defined as the presence of bacteria in the bloodstream. It can have no accompanying symptoms and is diagnosed based on the presence of bacteria from blood cultures. Bacteria in the bloodstream can lead

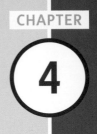

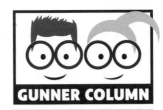

GUNNER COLUMN

to systemic inflammatory response syndrome (SIRS), which is the presence of two or more of the following:
1. Temp >38°C or <35°C
2. HR >90 bpm
3. RR >20 or PCO_2 <32
4. Leukocytes >12,000 or <4000 or >10% immature

Sepsis is defined as the presence of SIRS with a documented source of infection (such as pneumonia, meningitis). Severe sepsis is defined as the additional presence of end organ damage from hypoperfusion or hypotension. Septic shock (SBP <90) is defined as the presence of the aforementioned, with refractory hypotension that does not respond to fluids.

Prophylactic (PPx): Treat underlying infection.

Mechanism of Disease (MoD): Release of proinflammatory cytokines that trigger a cascade of events leading to hemodynamic compromise

Diagnostic Steps (Dx):
1. Culture of blood and/or infection site,
2. Detailed physical exam/imaging for source of infection

Treatment/Management (Tx/Mgmt):
1. Aggressive fluid resuscitation
2. Broad-spectrum antibiotics

Viral Hemorrhagic Fever (Ebola, Marburg Virus)

Buzz Words: Fever + bleeding from venipuncture sites + decreased function of liver and kidneys

Clinical Presentation: This will typically present with viral hemorrhagic fever syndrome (capillary leak, bleeding diathesis, circulatory compromise leading to shock). Most of the time, the bleeding is caused by disseminated intravascular coagulation (DIC). Ebola and Marburg virus are filoviruses.

PPx: Ebola and Marburg are spread nosocomially; airborne precautions should be taken; practice careful hygiene in areas with Ebola outbreak.

MoD: Thought to emerge from fruit bat or primate leading to human infection and dissemination from direct contact with body fluids, objects (needles, syringes), and semen

Dx:
1. Clinical history
2. ELISA testing, polymerase chain reaction (PCR), virus isolation
3. IHC testing

Tx/Mgmt: Supportive

FOR THE WARDS

The guidelines are currently changing, and many people now use qSOFA for sepsis, since they think SIRS criteria may be too sensitive a measure.

Chikungunya Virus

Buzz Words: Fever + joint paint within 7 days of mosquito bite + travel to Africa, Asia, Europe

Clinical Presentation: This is a virus transmitted to people by mosquitos, leading to a very classic joint pain presentation. There is a low yield for the medicine shelf, so the ability to recognize this disease is usually the extent to which you will be tested.

PPx: Prevent mosquito bites (insect repellant, long sleeves).

MoD: Virus spread by *Aedes albopictus* or *Aedes aegypti* and replication in human epithelial, endothelial, fibroblasts, and macrophages. Virus can be spread by mosquito from person to person.

Dx: Viral RNA/antibodies to virus

Tx/Mgmt: Supportive. Most patients recover, but it can lead to a chronic infection.

Dengue Fever

Buzz Words: Retro-orbita

l pain + muscle/joint pain + mosquito exposure within 7 days + hemorrhage + rash

Clinical Presentation: Dengue fever is also called "breakbone" fever that describes the muscle/joint pain that accompanies it. The infection with the Dengue virus, an arbovirus, leads to a hemorrhagic fever that can also cause leukopenia and thrombocytopenia.

PPx: Prevent mosquito bites (insect repellant, long sleeves); vaccine is available in some countries; avoid nonsteroidal antiinflammatory drugs (NSAIDs).

MoD: Virus spread by *Aedes albopictus* or *Aedes aegypti* and replication in human epithelial, endothelial, fibroblasts, and macrophages. Virus can be spread by mosquito from person to person.

Dx:

1. Physical exam
2. CBC
3. Blood cultures
4. PCR
5. ELISA (viral antigens/antibodies)

Tx/Mgmt:

1. Supportive
2. Blood transfusions
3. Acetaminophen, not NSAIDS (NSAIDs aggravate risk of bleeding)

QUICK TIPS

Chikungunya from the Makonde language means "bend up," describing contorted posturing of affected individuals due to joint pain.

 AR

WHO dengue fever fact sheet

Malaria microscopy

Malaria

Buzz Words: Cyclical/irregular fevers (e.g., fever every 48–72 hours) + anemia + jaundice + splenomegaly + endemic area (Africa)

Clinical Presentation: Malaria is a mosquito-borne disease caused by a parasite of the Plasmodium species. The most common cause of death is by *Plasmodium falciparum*, as vivax, ovale, and malariae cause mild disease. Malaria replicates in red blood cells (RBCs), leading to a hemolytic anemia. A classical finding in malaria is paroxysm, where cold/shivers alternate with fever/sweating that repeats every 2 days. Initial infection with malaria is usually severe; individuals can get immunity and get milder infections as they age.

PPx:
1. Mosquito control,
2. doxycycline, mefloquine, atovaquone/proguanil—plasmodium-resistant species
3. chloroquine/hydroxychloroquine—plasmodium sensitive species
4. dapsone/primaquine/quinine

MoD: Infected *Anopheles* female mosquito transmits malaria sporozoites to humans through the bloodstream, which travel to liver for a 2-week incubation period. Symptoms begin after 2–4 weeks. If infected with *Plasmodium vivax* and *Plasmodium ovale*, patients may get symptoms months after exposure due to activation of hypnozoites in the liver.

Dx:
1. Recent travel history
2. CBC
3. Giemsa stained blood smear
4. Antigen rapid detection tests

Tx/Mgmt:
1. Chloroquine
2. In resistant areas, use artemisinin combination therapy (ACT) or atovaquone-proguanil
3. Quinine and mefloquine

Babesiosis

Buzz Words: Fever + hemolytic anemia (jaundice, pallor) + hepatosplenomegaly + no rash or lymphadenopathy + tick exposure in May–September

Clinical Presentation: This infection is endemic to the Northeastern United States and Europe. Babesia infects RBCs and lyses them, leading to a hemolytic anemia (Fig. 4.1). Fever can sometimes be cyclical, and will lead

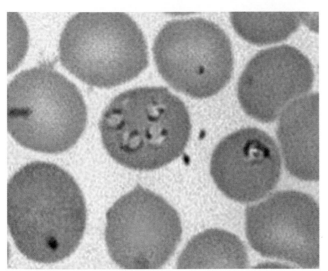

FIG. 4.1 Babesia in red blood cells. (From Centers for Disease Control and Prevention Public Health Image Library. Provided by Steven Glenn.)

to specifically no rash of lymphadenopathy (unlike Borrelia). Other nonspecific findings include headaches and myalgias.

PPx: N/A

MoD: This infection is transmitted by the *Ixodes* tick, which is the same as Borrelia (Lyme disease). Therefore suspect Babesia in patients with Lyme disease as well. Merozoites (reproductive form of Babesia) from Babesia invade and lyse RBCs, leading to a severe, prolonged hemolytic anemia.

Dx:
1. CBC (anemia, thrombocytopenia)
2. Blood cultures (Giemsa or Wright blood smear)
3. Liver function tests (LFTs)

Tx/Mgmt: Atovaquone + azithromycin

Infections of Lymphoid Tissue

Lymphadenitis

Buzz Words: Red, tender skin over lymph node + swollen or tender lymph nodes + tender red streaks

Clinical Presentation: This is an infection of the lymph nodes. In most situations, this term is used interchangeably with lymphadenopathy, although they are functionally different. Lymphadenopathy is a disease process that increases the size or consistency of the lymph nodes, whereas lymphadenitis refers to an inflammatory disease process from underlying infection. Unlike lymphadenopathy, lymphadenitis spreads quickly and can become lymphangitis. It can also lead to complications like abscess formation, cellulitis, and sepsis.

PPx: Proper hygiene

MoD: Infection from various agents that causes infection/inflammation of one or more lymph nodes

Dx:
1. Physical exam
2. Lymph node biopsy
3. Blood cultures

Tx/Mgmt:
1. Treat underlying infection
2. Analgesics
3. NSAIDs

Lymphangitis images

Lymphangitis

Buzz Words: Reddening of skin + warmth/swelling + inflammation of lymph gland + raised border over affected area + fever + history of trauma

Clinical Presentation: Inflammation of the lymphatic system, including bone marrow, spleen and thymus. Typically caused by an infected wound and invasion of lymph *system, most commonly caused by Strep pyogenes, Staph aureus, and Sporothrix schenckii.*

PPx: Treat precipitating infection

MoD: Infection of wound site leading to lymphoid spread to lymphatic organs like bone marrow, spleen, thymus.

Dx:
1. Physical exam
2. Biopsy of affected area
3. Culture of affected area
4. Blood culture

Tx/Mgmt:
1. Antibiotics
2. Analgesics
3. NSAIDs

Bubonic Plague (Yersinia pestis)

Buzz Words: Exposure to fleas + endemic area + sudden onset fever + painful lymph node + headache + bleeding

Clinical Presentation: This is a disease caused by flea exposure in areas like Africa. Hosts of this bacteria include rodents or cats.

PPx: Killed vaccine available

MoD: *Y. pestis* enters the bloodstream via the flea and enters the lymphatic system, leading to swollen lymph nodes. They are able to evade macrophages and precipitate an intense inflammatory response that leads to fever, headache.

Dx:
1. Blood culture
2. PCR/ELISA

Tx/Mgmt: Streptomycin/gentamicin

Cat Scratch Disease (Bartonella henselae)

Buzz Words: Tender, swollen lymph nodes occurring near site of bite or scratch from cat + generalized malaise

Clinical Presentation: This is an infection by a gram-negative bacillus that you get from scratches from a flea-infested cat. Commonly found in children. In very rare cases, cat scratch disease can cause meningitis, encephalitis, endocarditis, and other very mortal complications. Immunocompromised patients may get bacillary angiomatosis or bacillary peliosis.

PPx: Take flea control measures after handling cat/feces.

MoD: Systemic symptoms caused by widespread dissemination of *B. henselae* following inoculation (most commonly cat scratch). Can also lead to lymphadenitis.

Dx:
1. Blood cultures
2. PCR
3. Warthin-Starry stain (microbial cultures)

Tx/Mgmt:
1. Azithromycin, doxycycline, or ciprofloxacin

Immunologic and Inflammatory Disorders

This section covers various immunologic pathologies that can occur in the blood. These concepts are eclectic but high yield. In particular, autoimmune hemolytic anemia, thrombocytopenic thrombotic purpura (TTP), and hemolytic uremic syndrome (HUS) are frequently tested on the medicine shelf.

Cryoglobulinemia (Essential Mixed Cryoglobulinemia)

Buzz Words: Purpura + joint pains + itching + weakness

Clinical Presentation: This is a disease where the blood accumulates immunoglobulins that become insoluble at lower body temperatures and precipitate out. This typically causes blockage of blood vessels, leading to vaso-occlusion, infarctions, and gangrene. In many cases, this is considered a vasculitis. It is separated into three types based on the type of immunoglobulins present:

- Type I: monoclonal IgM, related to multiple myeloma
- Type II: polyclonal IgG, monoclonal IgM or IgA; the combination of these antibody components form complexes
- Type III: polyclonal IgM and IgG
- Type II and III are referred to as "mixed cryoglobulinemia," and when there is no precipitating cause, it is called "Essential Mixed Cryoglobinemia."

PPx: Present exposure to cold temperatures

MoD: Causes of cryoglobulinemia: Glomerulonephritis, multiple myeloma, leukemia, lupus, rheumatoid arthritis, hepatitis B, human immunodeficiency virus (HIV)

Dx:
1. CBC—cryoglobulins precipitate out at cold temperatures
2. Blood complement levels
3. LFTs

Tx/Mgmt:
1. Treat underlying cause
2. Immunosuppressants (steroids, cyclophosphamide, azathioprine)
3. Rituximab
4. Plasmapheresis

Autoimmune Hemolytic Anemia

Buzz Words: Anemia symptoms (fatigue, pallor, jaundice) + jaundice from hemolysis

Clinical Presentation: This is a disease caused by production of autoantibodies (IgG or IgM) toward RBCs. It is separated into **warm** which is more common than **cold**. Warm occurs with **IgG** and only at 37°C—it leads to **extravascular** hemolysis and **splenic** sequestration of RBCs. Cold occurs with **IgM** and only at 0°C—it leads to **intravascular** hemolysis and **liver** sequestration of RBCs.

PPx: Avoid cold exposure in Cold AIHA.

MoD: In both cases, they elevate IgG or IgM, respectively, binding to RBC membranes, which leads to hemolysis and sequestration of RBCs.

- **Warm AIHA:** Primary—idiopathic, secondary—lymphomas, leukemias (especially chronic lymphocytic leukemia [CLL]), malignancies, collagen vascular diseases, methyldopa
- **Cold AIHA:** Idiopathic, infectious mononucleosis, *Mycoplasma pneumoniae*, leukemias (CLL)

Dx:

1. Coombs test (Fig. 4.2)
   - Coating with IgG → Warm AIHA
   - Coating with complement → Cold AIHA
2. Positive cold agglutinin titer
3. Spherocytes in warm AIHA

Tx/Mgmt: No treatment necessary in most cases

- Warm AIHA
  1. Glucocorticoids
  2. Splenectomy
  3. Immunosuppressants
  4. Tx anemia—RBC transfusions, folic acid supplementation
- Cold AIHA
  1. Avoid cold exposure
  2. Tx anemia—RBC transfusions
  3. Immunosuppressants

QUICK TIPS

Glucocorticoids are never indicated in cold AIHA.

Direct Coombs test/Direct antiglobulin test

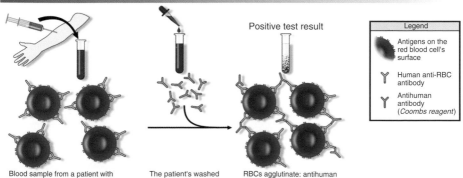

Positive test result

Legend

Antigens on the red blood cell's surface

Human anti-RBC antibody

Antihuman antibody (*Coombs reagent*)

Blood sample from a patient with immune mediated haemolytic anaemia: antibodies are shown attached to antigens on the RBC surface.

The patient's washed RBCs are incubated with antihuman antibodies (Coombs reagent).

RBCs agglutinate: antihuman antibodies form links between RBCs by binding to the human antibodies on the RBCs.

Indirect Coombs test/Indirect antiglobulin test

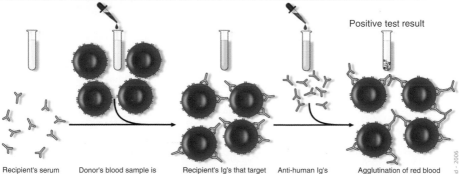

Positive test result

Recipient's serum is obtained, containing antibodies (Ig's).

Donor's blood sample is added to the tube with serum.

Recipient's Ig's that target the donor's red blood cells form antibody-antigen complexes.

Anti-human Ig's (*Coombs antibodies*) are added to the solution.

Agglutination of red blood cells occurs because human Ig's are attached to red blood cells.

© Ariǝ Rad - 2006

FIG. 4.2 Coombs test. (From Wikimedia Commons. https://commons.wikimedia.org/wiki/File:Coombs _test_schematic.png. Created by A. Rad—Own work. Used under the Creative Commons Attribution Share Alike 3.0 Unported License and the Gnu Free Documentation License.)

99 AR

PNH diagram

Paroxysmal Nocturnal Hemoglobinuria

Buzz Words: Back, abdominal or leg pain + evidence of pancytopenia (platelet, white blood cell [WBC] or RBC dysfunction) + bright red blood in urine in the morning

Clinical Presentation: Paroxysmal nocturnal hemoglobinuria (PNH) is a disease of young adults (aged 35–40) and leads to a chronic intravascular hemolysis, leading to anemia, pancytopenia, and sometimes may cause thrombosis in the venous system. In rare cases, PNH can progress to myelofibrosis, myelodysplasia, aplastic anemia, and even leukemia (3%–5%).

PPx: N/A

MoD: Anchoring proteins normally link complement inhibitors to RBC, WBC, and platelet membranes to prevent complement-mediated destruction. In PNH, HSC develops a mutation and lose these anchoring proteins, and, as a result, lysis of RBC, WBC, and platelets ensues. This is an acquired disorder that affects acute lymphoblastic leukemia (ALL) blood cells.

Dx:
1. CBC, low Hb, elevated LDH, elevated bilirubin, decreased haptoglobin (for intravascular hemolysis)
2. Blood cells in sugar water → complement-mediated lysis
   - If positive, Ham's test → acidified serum triggers complement-mediated lysis of blood cells
3. Gold standard: Flow cytometry for surface proteins CD55 and CD59

Tx/Mgmt:
1. Steroids therapy (prednisone)
2. Bone marrow transplantation

MNEMONIC

FATRN (Fever, Anemia, Thrombocytopenia, Renal Dysfunction, Neurologic Dysfunction)

Thrombotic Thrombocytopenia Purpura

Buzz Words: Fever + anemia + thrombocytopenia + renal dysfunction + neurologic dysfunction + schistocytes

Clinical Presentation: TTP is a rare disease that causes small blood clots to form in the circulation. Microthrombi can shear RBCs, which can lead to hemolytic anemias and schistocytes.

PPx: N/A

MoD: TTP is caused by a deficiency ADAMTS13, a metalloprotease that cleaves von Willebrand factor (vWF). In its absence, vWF builds up, leading to spontaneous activation and aggregation of platelets causing thrombosis, and thrombocytopenia from consumption of platelets during this thrombotic process. Most cases are idiopathic, but can be linked to ADAMTS13.

Dx:
1. CBC (low platelets)
2. PT/aPTT (normal)
3. Bleeding time (elevated)
4. ADAMTS13 activity testing

Tx/Mgmt:
1. Plasmapheresis
2. Rituximab
3. Caplacizumab (vWF blocking antibody)
4. LDH levels to measure disease progression (hemolysis)

Hemolytic Uremic Syndrome

Buzz Words: Hemolytic anemia (jaundice, fatigue, pallor) + thrombocytopenia + renal dysfunction + schistocytes + child

Clinical Presentation: This is a medical emergency consisting of a triad of hemolytic anemia, thrombocytopenia, and renal dysfunction, and is usually associated with previous infection, especially from EHEC 0157:H7, Campylobacter, or Shigella (Shiga toxin). Toxins damage kidneys and can activate platelets, leading to microthrombi that can shear RBCs, leading to schistocytes and a hemolytic anemia.

PPx: Hygiene to prevent food-borne illness.

MoD: Toxins damage kidney/activate platelets → kidney damage, platelet activation, and microthrombi formation

Dx:
1. Physical exam
2. CBC/BMP
3. UA/UCx
4. Blood culture
5. Rule out TTP via ADAMTS13 levels

Tx/Mgmt: Supportive. Do NOT administer antibiotics, as these can elevate Shiga toxin.

Neoplasms

Neoplasms are some of the most commonly tested concepts on the medicine shelf. Neoplasms in the blood are organized into leukemias versus lymphomas. Leukemias are cancers of the blood, whereas lymphomas are cancers of the lymph. Although these distinctions exist, the lines are actually more blurry than they may seem. Lymphomas are cancers that affect the lymph nodes, whereas leukemias are cancers that affect the blood and bone marrow. However, it is important to recognize that leukemias can infiltrate the lymph, just as lymphomas can infiltrate the bone marrow.

Lymphomas are typically broken down into Hodgkin versus non-Hodgkin lymphoma. Hodgkin lymphoma carries a significantly better prognosis. Leukemias are also broken down as chronic or acute. Remember that chronic leukemias involve mature cells, whereas acute leukemias tend to involve immature cells. Leukemias are also myelogenous or lymphoid in origin, indicating their origin cell line in hematopoiesis. Use these organizing principles to remember the differences between the different cancers, and focus on the buzz words to differentiate specific facets between the different cancers. Key buzz words include things like smudge cells, Auer rods, elevated basophils, Reed-Sternberg cells, etc.

Acute Lymphoblastic Leukemia

Buzz Words: Child + Recurrent infections + easy bleeding/bruising + hepatosplenomegaly + elevated WBC

Clinical Presentation: ALL is the most common malignancy for children under the age of 15. It presents with general features of leukemia, which include symptoms from lymphoblast infiltration of bone marrow. Low RBCs gives anemic symptoms include pallor. Low platelets lead to bleeding. Lack of functional WBCs lead to recurrent infections. Hepatosplenomegaly is a common presenting finding as well. ALL is the leukemia that is MOST responsive to therapy and carries the best prognosis.

PPx: N/A

MoD: Acquired mutation in lymphocyte progenitor leading to clonal proliferation that infiltrates bone marrow, decreasing RBCs, platelets, and neutrophils

Dx:

1. CBC
   - Normal to elevated WBCs
   - Low RBC
   - Low platelets
   - Low neutrophils
2. Bone marrow biopsy
   - Replacement of marrow by neoplastic lymphoblasts

Tx/Mgmt:

1. Treat recurrent infections
2. Chemotherapy (most children go into complete remission)

Acute Myelogenous Leukemia

Buzz Words: Adult + recurrent infections + easy bleeding/bruising + hepatosplenomegaly + elevated WBC

99 AR
ALL blood smear

Clinical Presentation: This is a neoplasm of myeloid progenitor cells and mostly occurs in adults.

PPx: Prevent exposure to radiation, alkylating agents. Acute myelogenous leukemia (AML) risk is elevated in patients with Down syndrome. Acute promyelocytic leukemia (APML) is a subtype consisting of t(15;17) that causes pancytopenia.

MoD: Acquired mutation from radiation, alkylating agents, or other causes leads to abnormal, clonal proliferation of myeloid progenitors (blasts). In APML, t(15;17) causes a PML-RAR-Alpha fusion protein that binds to the retinoic acid receptor and prevents myeloid differentiation.

Cleveland Clinic AML overview

Dx:

1. CBC
   - Normal to elevated WBCs
   - Low RBC
   - Low platelets
   - Low neutrophils (especially prominent in APML)
2. BMP
   - Hyperkalemia
   - Hyperuricemia
3. Bone marrow biopsy
   - Replacement of marrow by neoplastic myeloblasts
   - Presence of Auer rods in APML, granular materials, taking the shape of needles (Fig. 4.3)
4. Peripheral blood smear

Tx/Mgmt:

1. Treat recurrent infections,
2. Chemotherapy (all-trans retinoic acid for APML)
3. Bone marrow transplantation

Chronic Lymphocytic Leukemia/Small Lymphocytic Leukemia

Buzz Words:
- Incidental finding, most people asymptomatic at diagnosis + generalized painless lymphadenopathy + splenomegaly + recurrent infections + >50 years
- Advanced disease findings: fatigue, weight loss, pallor, easy bruising

Clinical Presentation: This is the MOST common leukemia occurring after the age of 50 and the most common leukemia in the Western world. However, it is the least aggressive leukemia. CLL is synonymous with SLL (small lymphocytic leukemia), a B-cell cancer.

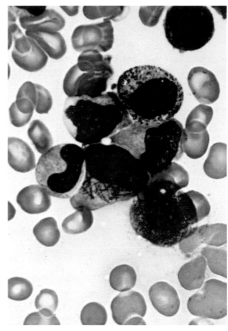

FIG. 4.3 Auer rods. (From Wikimedia Commons. https://common-s.wikimedia.org/wiki/File:Faggot_cell_in_AML-M3.jpg by the Armed Forces Institute of Pathology (AFIP) [Public domain].)

PPx: N/A

MoD: Lymphocytes acquire a mutation that leads to a monoclonal proliferation that are morphologically mature but functionally deficient.

Dx:

1. CBC
   - Elevated WBC >50,000
   - Low platelets, neutrophils, RBCs
2. Peripheral blood smear—gold standard
   - Elevated WBCs, mature, small
   - Smudge cells—"fragile" cells broken when placed on a slide (Fig. 4.4)
3. Bone marrow biopsy
   - Infiltrating lymphocytes in bone marrow

Tx/Mgmt:

1. Observation
2. Chemotherapy

Chronic Myelogenous Leukemia

Buzz Words: Fatigue + weight loss/anorexia/early satiety + elevated basophils, but most commonly is asymptomatic + greater than 60 years

CLL smudge cells

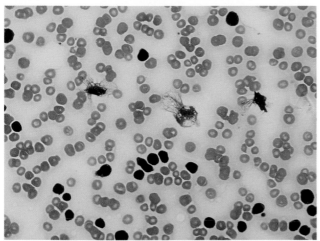

FIG. 4.4 Smudge cell. (From Wikimedia Commons. https://comm ons.wikimedia.org/w/index.php?curid=20525320 By Dr Graham Beards—Own work, CC BY-SA 3.0. Used under the Creative Commons Attribution-Share Alike 3.0 Unported license. https://creativec ommons.org/licenses/by-sa/3.0/deed.en.)

Clinical Presentation: Chronic myelogenous leukemia (CML) is abnormal growth of granulocytes and elevates platelet count, RBC count; in the initial stage, neutrophils initially accumulate other granulocytes as well. CML occurs in three phases:
- Chronic phase: Few blasts, no symptoms, lasts months to years
- Accelerated phase: Peripheral blood presents lots of immature blasts, lots of platelets, increased symptoms with drops in healthy blood cells
- Blast crisis: Blasts increase, resistant to chemotherapy, and growth begins to resemble acute leukemia

PPx: N/A

MoD: All CML cells have a translocation between chromosome 9 and 22, called the "Philadelphia chromosome," creating a fusion gene called BCR-ABL, which provides a constant growth signal to CML cells.

Dx:
1. CBC
2. Cytogenetic studies
3. FISH
4. PCR
5. Blood smear
   - Lymphocytosis, specifically granulocytosis
   - Elevated basophils is often associated with CML

6. Bone marrow biopsy
   - Hypercellular marrow; myeloid hyperplasia in marrow, but you don't see all blasts—you actually see all different levels of maturation.
   - Megakaryocytes are small "micromegakaryocytes" "hypolobated."
7. Monitoring CML (in order of increasing sensitivity): WBC, cytogenetic studies, FISH, PCR
   - Complete hematologic response (CHR)— normalized CBC and peripheral blood, limited prognostic significance
   - Cytogenetic response—0% Ph+ cells, major response 1%–35% Ph+ cells, partial response: >35% Ph+ cells
   - Major molecular response—greater than 3 log reduction in BCR-ABL transcripts, MMR at 1 year predicts 100% progression free survival at 5 years

Tx/Mgmt:

1. Imatinib/Gleevec
   a. Bind in ATP binding sites, cessation of downstream signaling and killing of these cells
2. Second generation tyrosine kinase inhibitors
3. Bone marrow transplant

Hodgkin Lymphoma

Buzz Words: Painless lymphadenopathy + spread to adjacent nodes + B symptoms (fever, night sweats, weight loss) + hepatomegaly + splenomegaly

Clinical Presentation: Burkitt's occurs in individuals between the age of 15–30 and in individuals over the age of 50. There are four subtypes (in order of prevalence):
- Nodular sclerosis: Reed-Sternberg cells in collagen envelope pools (tumor nodules)
- Mixed cellularity: Reed-Sternberg cells among many pleomorphic cells
- Lymphocyte predominant: Primarily B cells, few Reed-Sternberg cells
- Lymphocyte depleted: No reactive cells, worst prognosis

Hodgkin's lymphoma is further staged based on lymph node spread:
- Stage I—single lymph node
- Stage II—two or more lymph nodes on same side of diaphragm
- Stage III—lymph nodes on both sides of diaphragm
- Stage IV—presence in extralymphatic organs

For each stage, A or B is selected:

- A—asymptomatic
- B—symptomatic (B symptoms: fever, night sweats, weight loss)

PPx: N/A

MoD: Unclear, acquired mutation → proliferation of B cells

Dx:

1. Lymph node biopsy for Reed-Sternberg cell (B cell phenotype; Fig. 4.5)
   - Inflammatory cell infiltrate must be present— these are lymphocytic reaction to Reed-Sternberg cells
2. Chest x-ray (CXR), computed tomography (CT) scan—lymph node involvement
3. Bone marrow biopsy—bone marrow infiltration
4. CBC—leukocytosis and eosinophilia

Tx/Mgmt:

1. Radiation therapy for stage I, II, and IIIA
2. Chemotherapy for stage IIIB and IV
   a. ABVD: Doxorubicin, bleomycin, vinblastine, dacarbazine
   b. Stanford V: Doxorubicin, bleomycin, vinblastine, vincristine, mechlorethamine, etoposide, prednisone

Non-Hodgkin Lymphoma

Buzz Words: Painless lymphadenopathy + B symptoms (fever, chills, night sweats)

Clinical Presentation: NHL is a cancer of lymphoid cells that causes proliferation of T cells, B cells, or natural killer (NK) cells, often with extranodal involvement. It usually presents as a rapidly growing, painless mass that

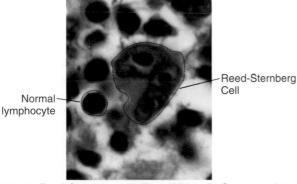

FIG. 4.5 Reed-Sternberg cell. (From Wikimedia Commons. https://commons.wikimedia.org/w/index.php?curid=5580965 By Unknown—National Cancer Institute, AV Number: CDR576466, Public Domain.)

is associated with autoimmune disorders. This mass can sometimes compress on surrounding vasculature, causing problems like superior vena cava (SVC) syndrome, facial plethora, or respiratory distress. It is overall much more common than Hodgkin lymphomas.

PPx: N/A

MoD: Acquired mutation in lymph cells that causes proliferation of T cells, B cells, or NK cells that invade surrounding lymph tissue

Dx:

1. Lymph node biopsy

Tx/Mgmt:

1. Chemotherapy
2. Radiation therapy (except in pediatric populations)

Burkitt Lymphoma

Buzz Words: EBV exposure + rapidly growing mass in jaw + "starry sky appearance"

Clinical Presentation: Burkitt lymphoma is a disorder of B cells, causing their proliferation within germinal centers of lymph nodes. Burkitt lymphoma affects children and young adults, leading to a very typical enlarging jaw mass. It is associated with immunodeficiencies, which can precipitate EBV infection that is thought to lead to Burkitt lymphoma.

PPx: N/A

MoD: EBV infection stimulates translocation of chromosomes 8 and 14 in B cells and lead to a constitutively active c-Myc oncogene. Other less common translocations all include chromosome 8 for c-Myc.

Dx: Tumor biopsy showing starry sky appearance (Fig. 4.6)

Tx/Mgmt: Chemotherapy with rituximab

T-cell Lymphoma

Buzz Words: Rash + generalized lymphadenopathy + lytic bone lesions

Clinical Presentation: This is a cancer of CD4 T cells occurring in elderly individuals from the Caribbean or Japan. It presents with lytic bone lesions, a rash, and generalized lymphadenopathy. It is associated with HTLV-1.

PPx: N/A

MoD: Acquired mutation → proliferation of mature CD4+ T cells

Dx:

1. Lymph node biopsy
2. Flow cytometry (CD4 T cell proliferation)

Tx/Mgmt: Chemotherapy

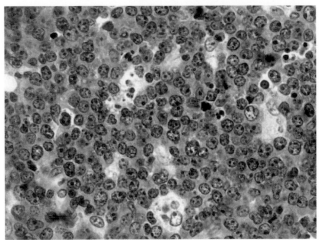

FIG. 4.6 Starry sky appearance in Burkitt's. (From Wikimedia Commons. http://visualsonline.cancer.gov/details.cfm?imageid=4156, Public Domain, https://commons.wikimedia.org/w/index.php?cur id=859300)

Multiple Myeloma

Buzz Words: Hypercalcemia (stones, bones, abdominal groans, psychiatric overtones) + renal failure + anemia + back pain + recurrent infections

Clinical Presentation: Multiple myeloma is a cancer of plasma cells, leading to production of a monoclonal antibody of a single isotype (IgG or IgA). It is twice as common in African Americans as in Caucasians, and eventually malignant plasma cells overtake the bone marrow, resulting in pancytopenia in advanced disease. Lytic lesions from proliferation of these plasma cells occur in many bones, leading to bone pain in the lower back, chest, and jaw (Fig. 4.7). Renal failure is caused by deposits of Bence Jones protein (Ig light chain) in the renal tubules. Recurrent infections are common due to dysfunction of both antibodies and leukocytes.

PPx: N/A

MoD: Etiology unclear; acquired mutation leading to proliferation of plasma cells

Dx:
- Serum/urine protein electrophoresis (SPEP/UPEP)
  - Monoclonal spike of a single antibody isotype (IgG > IgA); this spike is called M protein
- X-rays to detect boney lytic lesions
- Bone marrow biopsy greater than 10% plasma cells

MNEMONIC

Multiple Myeloma—CRAB (**C**alcium, **R**enal, **A**nemia, **B**one)

gg AR

Multiple myeloma electrophoresis bands

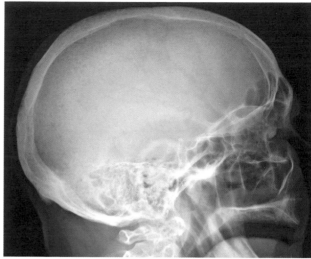

FIG. 4.7 Lytic lesion. (From Wikimedia Commons. https://common s.wikimedia.org/w/index.php?curid=49320711 Created By James Heilman, MD—Own work, CC BY-SA 4.0. Used under the Creative Commons Attribution-Share Alike 4.0 International license.)

- Peripheral blood smear (rouleaux formation of RBC stacks on top of each other; Fig. 4.8)
- Urinalysis—elevated Bence Jones protein

Tx/Mgmt:
1. Autologous HSC transplantation
   - Chemotherapy cannot be started if you are considering HSC, as it would then preclude you
2. Alkylating agents (chemo)
3. Radiation therapy—last resort

Monoclonal Gammopathy of Unknown Significance

Buzz Words: M Spike + asymptomatic

Clinical Presentation: This is an incidental finding of an M spike from SPEP/UPEP without any clinical features. May occur in patients with family history of monoclonal gammopathy of unknown significance (MGUS) or MM.

PPx: N/A

MoD: Premalignant proliferation of plasma cells that has NOT YET progressed to multiple myeloma

Dx:
1. SPEP/UPEP
2. Bone marrow biopsy
3. X-rays (rule out lytic lesions)

Tx/Mgmt: Observation (risk of development into multiple myeloma)

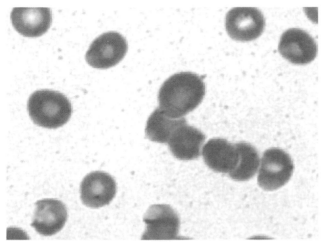

FIG. 4.8 Rouleaux. (From Wikimedia Commons. https://commons.wikimedia.org/w/index.php?curid=23406655 Created by Gabriel Caponetti—Own work, CC BY-SA 3.0. Used under the Creative Commons Attribution-Share Alike 3.0 Unported license.)

Myelofibrosis

Buzz Words: Splenomegaly + hepatomegaly + increased risk of infections + weakness, fatigue, anemia + easy bruising/bleeding

Clinical Presentation: Neoplastic proliferation of mature myeloid lineage cells (megakaryocytes predominantly), leading to excessive PDGF production, which causes extensive fibrosis of bone marrow. This is a chronic leukemia and often leads to defects in WBCs, RBCs, and platelets. This disease occurs in those aged 50–60.

PPx: N/A

MoD: JAK2 kinase mutation → myeloid lineage proliferation → extensive fibrosis of bone marrow → deficiency in WBCs, RBCs, and platelets. Precipitating chemicals and radiation include benzene and toluene; 25% of patients have calreticulin (CALR) mutation.

Dx:
1. CBC
2. X-ray and MRI
3. Bone marrow biopsy—gold standard
4. Peripheral blood smear
   - Leukoerythroblastic peripheral blood smear— nucleated RBCs, teardrops cells, left shifted granulocytes, including blasts
5. Genetic testing

Tx/Mgmt:
1. Most patients who are asymptomatic only require monitoring
2. Ruxolitinib—targeting JAK2 mutation
3. Blood transfusions,
4. Androgen therapy—stimulate RBC production
5. Thalidomide
6. Splenectomy

Myelodysplastic Syndrome

Buzz Words: Incidental finding, asymptomatic + previous history of chemotherapy or radiation therapy

Clinical Presentation: This is an often asymptomatic disease characterized by the absence of RBCs, WBCs, and platelets. It is typically found in older individuals and is caused by a problem with the bone marrow in producing blood cells.

PPx: N/A

MoD: Mutation in HSCs, leading to ineffective production of RBC, platelets, and WBCs. Secondary to radiation therapy, chemotherapy, or genetic problems like Fanconi anemia and Bloom syndrome.

Dx:
1. CBC
2. Peripheral blood smear (dysplasia in >20% blasts)
3. Bone marrow biopsy (dysplasia in >20% blasts)

Tx/Mgmt:
1. Immunosuppression
2. Chemotherapy
3. Bone marrow transplantation

Waldenstrom Macroglobulinemia (Lymphoplasmacytic Lymphoma)

Buzz Words: M spike + peripheral neuropathy + hepatosplenomegaly + recurrent bleeding + fatigue, weight loss + lymphadenopathy + torturous retinal veins

Clinical Presentation: This is a cancer of B cells producing too much IgM. Too much IgM in the blood leads to hyperviscosity (torturous retinal veins on retinal exam). It can also lead to anemia from infiltration of bone marrow, or can lead to platelet deficits due to platelet clumping. IgM can also lead to cryoglobulinemia. There are no lytic lesions, unlike multiple myeloma.

PPx: N/A

MoD: Somatic mutation in MYDD88 in B cells leading to uncontrolled, clonal proliferation. Also associated with autoimmune disease and environmental factors.

Dx:
1. CBC
2. SPEP/UPEP (M spike)
3. Bone marrow biopsy (plasma cell infiltration)
4. Flow cytometry

Tx/Mgmt:
1. Observation, most patients asymptomatic
2. Plasmapheresis (decreases hyperviscosity)
3. Rituximab, chemotherapy

Anemia

Anemia should be approached systematically as microcytic (MCV < 80), macrocytic (MCV > 100), and normocytic anemias, corresponding to small, large, and normal sized RBCs, respectively (Fig. 4.9). There are different causes for each, and the MCV should be one of the first things looked at when making a diagnosis. Causes of microcytic anemia include iron deficiency, thalassemias, sideroblastic anemia/lead poisoning. Causes of macrocytic anemia include B12 and folate deficiency, alcoholism/liver failure, kidney disease, and certain drugs. Normocytic anemia is further classified into hemolytic versus nonhemolytic anemias, and on the basis of whether these hemolytic processes occur extravascularly or intravascularly. They can also be caused by intrinsic or extrinsic processes, respectively. These diseases are outlined as follows. A hemolytic anemia can easily be recognized by a few key features: elevated bilirubin, decreased haptoglobin, increased LDH. Clinical features will include jaundice and pallor.

Khan Academy anemias overview

Microcytic Anemia

Buzz Words: Microcytic anemia + elevated ferritin + decreased Fe/TIBC + malignancy + autoimmune conditions

Clinical Presentation: Microcytic anemia with elevated ferritin (storage form of iron) but decreased serum iron levels. TIBC decreased. Can be seen in the setting of malignancy and autoimmune conditions. Patients will present with fatigue, weakness, pallor in setting of autoimmune disorders, endocarditis, malignancy.

PPx: N/A

MoD: Chronic disease state → Elevated acute phase reactants (hepcidin) → Hepcidin pushes iron into storage form in order to prevent bacterial access to iron → Decreased free iron causes decreased hemoglobin production → Microcytic anemia

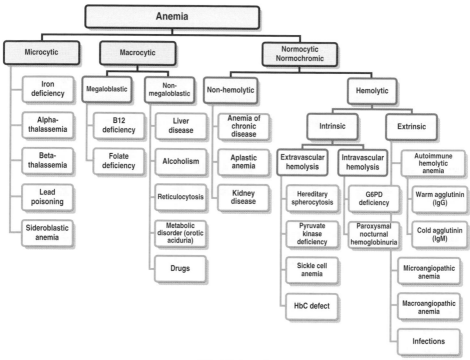

FIG. 4.9 Anemia.

Dx:
1. CBC
2. Peripheral blood smear
   - Microcytic anemia
3. Iron studies
   - Elevated ferritin, decreased serum iron, decreased TIBC
4. Acute phase reactants
   - Elevated hepcidin

Tx/Mgmt:
1. Treat underlying cause; otherwise, there is no treatment for asymptomatic anemia
2. EPO if symptomatic
3. Transfusion if severely decreased hemoglobin

G6PD Deficiency

Buzz Words: Hemolysis and jaundice after fava bean or sulfa antibiotics in African Americans

Clinical Presentation: G6PD deficiency is the most common red cell enzymopathy. It is inherited in an X-linked recessive pattern, and females only get it from lyonization (X-chromosome inactivation). There are two common variants:

- G6PD A → present in 10% of AA males, decreased activity only in aged RBCs, less severe disease
- G6PD B → present in 5% of Mediterranean and Asians, decreased activity in all RBCs

G6PD is precipitated by an acute event that induces oxidant stress; such events include acute illness, exposure to certain drugs or chemicals (naphthalene, sulfa antibiotics), or fava bean ingestion.

PPx: Avoid triggers of G6PD deficiency, as listed previously.

MoD: Glutathione is responsible for reducing oxidant free radicals in RBCs; generation of glutathione requires G6PD. In G6PD deficiency, there is decreased glutathione rendering hemoglobin susceptible to oxidant free radicals. This denatures Hb and form intracellular Heinz bodies; macrophages in the spleen remove Heinz bodies and form "bite cells," causing hemolysis.

Dx:

1. CBC
2. G6PD biochemical assay, tested several months after acute event; don't measure during acute event, because those with A disease may have "normal" levels due to selective destruction of older cells

Tx/Mgmt: RBC transfusions for acute episodes

99 AR

GRPD management

Pyruvate Kinase Deficiency

Buzz Words: Anemia + cholelithiasis + splenomegaly + jaundice precipitated by stress/illness + Northern European/Japanese

Clinical Presentation: PK deficiency occurs in both autosomal dominant and recessive inheritance patterns, although recessive is more common. This leads to hemolysis, which will cause anemia. Breakdown of RBCs can lead to cholelithiasis, splenomegaly, and jaundice.

PPx: Prevent precipitating factors.

MoD: PK deficiency is caused by a mutation in the PKLR gene, which is important in glycolysis. This causes less ATP in RBCs, and as a result leads to cell death and extravascular hemolysis under conditions in which high levels of ATP are needed.

Dx:

1. CBC (elevated reticulocytes)
2. Bilirubin levels

Tx/Mgmt:

1. Monitoring for most patients.
2. In severe cases, blood transfusions/splenectomy

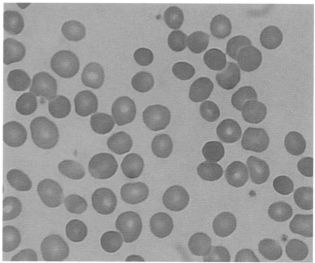

FIG. 4.10 Spherocytes on blood smear. (From Wikimedia Commons. https://commons.wikimedia.org/wiki/File:Hereditary_Spherocytosis_smear_2010-03-17.JPG Created by Paulo Henrique Orlandi Mourao. Used under the Creative Commons Attribution-Share Alike 3.0 Unported license [http://creativecommons.org/licenses/by-sa/3.0 or GFDL http://www.gnu.org/copyleft/fdl.html].)

Hereditary Spherocytosis

Buzz Words: Jaundice + pallor + fatigue + familial pattern + spherocytes on blood smear (Fig. 4.10)

Clinical Presentation: This is a commonly tested disease and cause of anemia and extravascular hemolysis. The unique shape of RBCs in hereditary spherocytosis is very characteristic, and it is this unique shape that causes them to be targeted by the spleen.

PPx: N/A

MoD: Autosomal dominant disease caused by defect in **spectrin** or other RBC structural proteins. As a result, RBCs lose surface area but NOT volume, leading to spherical shape. Spherical RBCs are destroyed in the spleen, leading to extravascular hemolysis.

Dx:
1. Osmotic fragility test
   • Tests ability for RBCs to swell in hypotonic solutions; spherocytes have less membrane integrity and rupture more easily
2. CBC (elevated MCHC, reticulocyte count)
3. Peripheral blood smear (spherocytes)
4. Coombs test to rule out (r/o) AIHA (warm AIHA also leads to spherocytes)

Tx/Mgmt: Splenectomy

Hereditary Elliptocytosis (Ovalocytosis)

Buzz Words: Hemolytic anemia (pallor, jaundice) + elliptocytes on blood smear + splenomegaly + gallstones

Clinical Presentation: This is the baby brother of hereditary spherocytosis. It is a relatively benign inherited disease that gets passed down in various patterns of inheritance. In this disease, RBCs take on a spheroid shape and get cleared by the spleen, leading to a hemolytic anemia.

PPx: Folate supplementation

MoD: Various mutations (most common is Spectrin) in the RBC cytoskeleton destabilize them. Of note, ALL RBCs assume an ellipsoid shape when they pass through capillaries. However, they can rearrange themselves to a normal configuration once outside. In hereditary elliptocytosis, these RBCs never rearrange themselves and retain that shape permanently and are later removed by the spleen.

Dx:
1. CBC
2. Blood smear (>25% of RBCs are ellipsoid)
3. Osmotic fragility testing
4. Bilirubin levels

Tx/Mgmt:
1. Monitoring, most patients are asymptomatic
2. Tx cholelithiasis with cholecystectomy if pain is problematic
3. Splenectomy in severe cases
4. Folate supplementation

Methemoglobinemia

Buzz Words: Cyanosis (blue/gray skin, lips) + normal pulse oximetry reading + lightheadedness + chocolate colored blood

Clinical Presentation: Methemoglobinemia is a problem in which iron in hemoglobin is oxidized, impairing oxygen delivery to tissues. It can also be an inherited condition, in which methemoglobin is unable to be reduced due to a missing enzyme.

PPx: Prevent use of dapsone and topical anesthetics (lidocaine), especially in children.

MoD: Iron is overoxidized, compromising its function in heme and in carrying oxygen. As a result, patients become cyanotic. Congenital disorder arises from deficiency in NADH-cytochrome b5 reductase, which cannot convert oxidized iron back to the reduced state.

QUICK TIPS

Amyl nitrate is a treatment for cyanide poisoning that induces methemoglobinemia.

Dx:
1. Physical exam
2. Co-oximeter detection of methemoglobin
3. Arterial blood gas

Tx/Mgmt:
1. Supplemental oxygen (hyperbaric in severe cases)
2. Methylene blue
3. Transfusion

Sickle Cell Disease

Sickle cell is arguably the single most commonly tested hematologic disease that appears on every standardized exam available, including the medicine shelf. This is a disease worth knowing cold.

Buzz Words: Painful fingers and toes in the young African American child + fatigue, pallor + shortness of breath (acute chest) + familial pattern + splenic atrophy

Clinical Presentation: Sickle cell is an autosomal recessive trait that causes the formation of Hemoglobin S. Hemoglobin S is prone to "sickling" under low oxygen states, which leads to a plethora of complications that arise from hemolysis and sickling in inappropriate places. Vaso-occlusion can occur when sickled RBCs obstruct capillary beds and lead to ischemia, infarction, and necrosis of organs.

One of the most commonly infarcted organs is the **spleen**, which will lead to **splenic atrophy**. Many sickle cell patients are therefore functional asplenics. Lack of spleen function renders these patients susceptible to encapsulated organisms, most commonly *Strep pneumo* and *H. Flu*. In some cases, splenic sequestration can occur, where sickled cells get sequestered in the spleen, leading to huge falls in hemoglobin and eventual circulatory failure.

Acute chest syndrome is a common finding in patients with SCD, where sickled RBCs occlude the capillaries in the lungs, leading to respiratory compromise and hypoxemia. Dactylitis is an early finding in patients with sickle cell, which is characterized by painful fingers and toes due to sickled RBC occlusion of their vasculature. Sickle cell patients can also have aplastic crises, where an infection by Parvovirus B19 (or other agents) leads to rapid degradation of RBCs, leading to abrupt declines in RBC count that can be life threatening. Other complications of sickle cell include priapism, cholelithiasis (bilirubin breakdown → gallstones), stroke, renal papillary necrosis, ulcers, osteomyelitis pulmonary hypertension

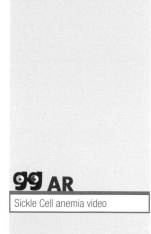
99 AR
Sickle Cell anemia video

→ right heart failure, and opioid tolerance and addiction. Frequently ask yourself why each of these complications happen as a means to better learn them. The precipitant behind everything anyone can get from sickle cell is vaso-occlusion and hemolysis.

PPx:

1. Daily penicillin prophylaxis as child for *S. pneumo*
2. Vaccination for *S. pneumo*, *H. Flu*, *Meningococcus*
3. Anti-malarial chemoprophylaxis in areas endemic
4. Counseling for parents with sickle trait/disease

MoD: Glutamic acid (hydrophilic) to valine (hydrophobic) substitution of the beta-globin gene leads to sickling (hydrophobic amino acids like to aggregate) inherited in autosomal recessive fashion. Oxygen tension normally leads to high elasticity, allowing RBCs to pass through capillary beds. In sickled states, oxygen tension is unable to enhance RBC elasticity due to the aggregated, sickled beta-globin. This leads to hemolysis and vaso-occlusive crises.

Dx:

1. CBC; low Hb, high reticulocyte count
2. Sodium metabisulfite induced RBC sickling
3. Hb electrophoresis
4. UA, UCx, CXR, blood cultures for infection workup

Tx/Mgmt:

1. Folic acid
2. Patient-controlled analgesia for vaso-occlusion
3. Oxygen supplementation, transfusion for acute chest crisis
4. **Hydroxyurea** → elevated HbF production (fetal hemoglobin has higher affinity for O_2);
5. Blood transfusions; (6) bone marrow transplant (curative)

Sideroblastic Anemia

Buzz Words: Anemia + hepatosplenomegaly + sideroblasts on blood smear + isoniazid or lead exposure

Clinical Presentation: This is caused by abnormalities in RBC iron metabolism, where iron cannot get incorporated into hemoglobin despite normal iron levels. This results in sideroblasts, which are abnormal, nucleated RBCs that have iron that has accumulated in mitochondria surrounding the nucleus (Fig. 4.11). Resultant iron (cannot be incorporated into Hb) buildup can lead to iron deposition in heart, liver, and kidney, leading to failure.

QUICK TIPS

A random complication of sickle cell that gets frequently tested is osteomyelitis. The most common cause is *Salmonella*.

QUICK TIPS

The reason sickle cell still exists is because it is protective against malaria spread. This happens because malaria infects RBCs, but patients with sickle cell trait actually have increased RBC turnover, leading to increased malarial death.

QUICK TIPS

But just because sickle cell is protective against malaria does not mean malaria is not a problem for patients. In fact, patients with sickle cell are vulnerable to malaria, and malaria is the most common cause of sickle crises in countries where malaria is endemic.

99 AR

Sideroblastic anemia video

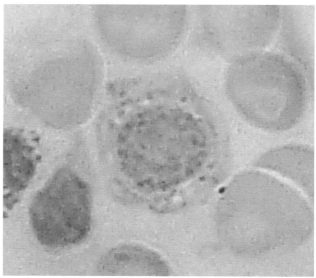

FIG. 4.11 Sideroblasts. (From Wikimedia Commons. Created by Paulo Henrique Orlandi Mourao. Used under the Creative Commons Attribution-Share Alike 3.0 Unported license [http://creativecommons.org/licenses/by-sa/3.0] or GFDL [http://www.gnu.org/copyleft/fdl.html].)

PPx: Prevent lead exposure.

MoD: Inherited or acquired causes of iron metabolism leading to iron buildup in RBC mitochondria and other organs. This leads to functional anemia (decreased RBCs because unable to incorporate iron into Hb) with anemic symptoms. Iron in other body areas leads to potential end organ failure.
- Inherited causes of sideroblastic anemia:
  - X-linked or autosomal recessive
- Acquired causes of sideroblastic anemia:
  - Drugs (chloramphenicol, isoniazid, alcohol)
  - Lead exposure
  - Collagen vascular disease
  - Myelodysplasia

Dx:
1. CBC (low Hb/Hct)
2. High iron, high ferritin, normal or low TIBC, high transferrin
3. Peripheral smear (abnormal RBC size and basophilic stippling)
4. Bone marrow biopsy (ringed sideroblasts in marrow with Prussian blue stain)

Tx/Mgmt:
1. Remove precipitants,
2. Pyridoxine (for isoniazid-induced sideroblastic anemia)
3. Desferrioxamine (to chelate iron)

Thalassemias

Buzz Words:

- Target cells + Mediterranean descent → beta thalassemia
- HbA2 + HbBarts/HbH + Southeast Asian → alpha thalassemia

Clinical Presentation: Thalassemias are a microcytic anemia of varying severity. In severe cases, patients may exhibit signs of extramedullary hematopoiesis with a crew-cut appearance of skull on x-ray, chipmunk facies due to facial bone involvement, and hepatosplenomegaly. Thalassemias generally presents a few months after birth, as HbF is protective.

PPx: Prenatal genetic testing

MoD: The major hemoglobin found in adults is hemoglobin A, composed of 2 alpha and 2 beta chains. Thalassemia is an inherited mutation in the alpha or beta globin chain of hemoglobin, resulting in decreased hemoglobin synthesis. Both forms lead to increased hemolysis and extramedullary hematopoiesis with resultant enlarged bones.

- Alpha thalassemia is more commonly seen in Southeast Asian populations, with four variations:
  - 1–2, gene deletions result in normal or mild anemia.
  - Three, gene deletions result in Barts (HgH) disease: severe anemia with a chain that binds strongly to oxygen similar to fetal Hb
  - Four, gene deletions are unsustainable with life, resulting in hydrops fetalis
- Beta thalassemia is more commonly seen in Mediterranean populations.
  - Heterozygotes will have beta thalassemia minor and present with mild microcytic anemia.
  - Homozygotes will have Cooley anemia with hepatosplenomegaly, bone marrow hyperplasia with thalassemia face. These patients may require lifelong transfusions resulting in secondary hemochromatosis (iron overload).

Dx:

1. CBC
2. Hemoglobin electrophoresis with **HbA2** or **HbF** and little/no **HbA**
3. Peripheral smear shows microcytic, hypochromic RBCs with target cells (Fig. 4.12)

Tx/Mgmt:

1. Observation if asymptomatic
2. Iron supplementation for hemolysis
3. Blood transfusions

Thalassemia overview

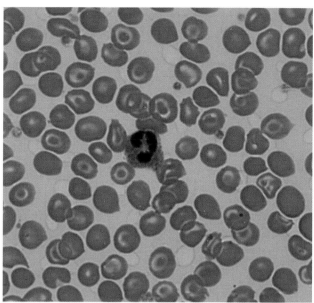

FIG. 4.12 Target cells. (From Wikimedia Commons. https://com mons.wikimedia.org/wiki/File:Target_cells_and_spherocytes.jpg. Created by Dr Graham Beards. Used under the Creative Commons Attribution-Share Alike 3.0 Unported license [http://creativecommon s.org/licenses/by-sa/3.0].)

Anemia from Blood Loss

Buzz Words: Normocytic anemia + source for bleeding (heavy menstrual bleeding)

Clinical Presentation: Normocytic anemia, **most common cause of anemia overall.** May see spoon shaped nails or diminished attention. Occurs in setting of recent trauma or surgery. Bleeding into the retroperitoneal space or the thigh is often missed. If iron deficiency from chronic blood loss, will appear as microcytic anemia.

PPx: N/A

MoD: Blood loss → increased reticulocyte formation + decrease in iron levels necessary to produce new RBCs → iron deficiency leads to worsening anemia. Blood loss may be secondary to cow's milk, peptic ulcer disease (PUD), inflammatory bowel disease (IBD), or Meckel's.

Dx:
1. CBC
2. Iron studies (low ferritin if iron deficiency from chronic blood loss)
3. Identify bleeding source via imaging

Tx/Mgmt:
1. Management of the source
2. Iron supplementation for several months if there was evidence of iron deficiency on iron studies
3. Transfusion if Hb <7 with symptoms (dyspnea, dizziness, severe fatigue)

Cytopenias

Aplastic Anemia

Buzz Words: Pancytopenia + low reticulocyte count

Clinical Presentation: Varies based on severity. Common manifestations include fatigue, bleeding, and infection. Can be precipitated by recent parvovirus B19 infection, which likes to infect the bone marrow. Fanconi anemia is an autosomal recessive congenital aplastic anemia with renal dysfunction, absent thumb and radius, short stature, and hyperpigmentation.

PPx: N/A

MoD: Injury to hematopoietic stem cells caused by infection, autoimmune damage, inherited disorders, or drugs → pancytopenia

Dx:
1. CBC (low reticulocyte count)
2. Bone marrow biopsy (empty)

Tx/Mgmt:
1. Remove causative agents
2. Marrow stimulating factors, including GM-CSF, G-CSF, and EPO may be used.
3. Transfusion if severe

Leukopenia

Buzz Words: Decreased WBC count + recurrent infection

Clinical Presentation: Leukopenia is an isolated decrease in WBC count.

PPx: N/A

MoD: Leukopenia occurs secondary to a number of conditions, including radiation therapy, myelofibrosis, aplastic anemia, autoimmune conditions (lupus), infections, or HIV. Drugs can also cause leukopenia, and some examples include immunosuppressants or chemotherapeutic agents. Agranulocytosis is the isolated decrease in neutrophils, and will be tested, as this is a common manifestation of the antipsychotic clozapine.

Dx: CBC

Tx/Mgmt: Treat underlying cause

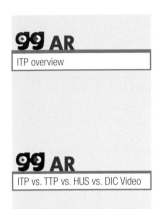

99 AR
ITP overview

99 AR
ITP vs. TTP vs. HUS vs. DIC Video

QUICK TIPS
ITP gets confused with TTP a lot. The biggest difference is the lack of anemia, renal, or neurologic findings in ITP.

99 AR
Polycythemia vera presentation and differential

Immune Thrombocytopenic Purpura

Buzz Words: Petechiae/purpura + thrombocytopenia + s/p viral infection/immunization + increased megakaryocytes on biopsy + easy bruising/bleeding

Clinical Presentation: This is a disease characterized by low platelet counts that leads to petechiae/purpura. ITP typically is an autoimmune process that occurs secondary to infection or immunization. One characteristic finding is large numbers of megakaryocytes (platelet precursor) on bone marrow biopsy.

PPx: N/A

MoD: Various conditions like infection/immunization cause antibodies to form against platelets toward GPIIb-IIIa (fibrinogen receptor) or GPIb-Ix (von Willebrand factor receptor); these antibodies cause platelets to be cleared by splenic macrophages and Kupffer cells in the liver.

Dx:
1. CBC (low platelet count)
2. Rule out secondary causes of low platelets (leukemia, cirrhosis, lupus, HIV, vWF deficiency, etc.)
3. PT/aPTT (normal)
4. Bleeding time (elevated)

Tx/Mgmt:
1. Steroids
2. Rho(D) immune globulin
3. Immunosuppressants (azathioprine, mycophenolate), IV IG
4. Thrombopoietin receptor agonists (stimulate platelet production) such as romiplostim or eltrombopag
5. Splenectomy

Polycythemias

Polycythemia Vera

Buzz Words: High hemoglobin + clotting + kidney stones + sweating + itching after shower + hepatosplenomegaly + GI bleeding + hypertension

Clinical Presentation: This is the malignant proliferation of hematopoietic stem cells, leading to endogenous erythroid colony (EEC) formation. This is only disorder in which erythroid colonies grow in absence of erythropoietin, leading to increased RBC mass. Polycythemia vera or primary polycythemia is a disease caused by a mutation in hematopoiesis, leading to increased RBCs.

Secondary **polycythemia** is a mechanism by which RBC mass is increased, due to some underlying signal. It can be a compensatory mechanism in the case of hypoxemia, chronic obstructive pulmonary disease (COPD), congestive heart failure (CHF), sleep apnea, and pulmonary hypertension, where increased RBC count can overcome deficiencies in oxygenation of tissue. It can also be caused by erythropoietin producing liver, kidney, and adrenal cancers.

PPx: N/A

MoD: Recurrent activated mutation in JAK2 V617F, important in signaling through cytokine receptors, phosphorylates STAT proteins to increase proliferation; once it does this, you don't need erythropoietin to signal through JAK2

Dx:
1. Workup or rule out secondary causes as described previously
2. CBC (hematocrit > 50)
3. Serum EPO levels
4. Elevated B12
5. Bone marrow biopsy

Tx/Mgmt:
1. Therapeutic and repeated phlebotomy
2. Aspirin
3. Chemotherapy (hydroxyurea)
4. Interferon
5. JAK2 inhibitors

Essential Thrombocythemia (Essential Thrombocytosis)

Buzz Words: Clots or bleeding, but most patients are asymptomatic

Clinical Presentation: This is a rare problem when your body produces too many platelets, leading to too much clotting. This disease is rare and occurs in five people per million. The median age at diagnosis is 60 years, but 20% of patients are less than 40 years old. Unlikely to be tested on the medicine shelf, as this is an incidental finding that appears randomly for most patients.

PPx: N/A

MoD: JAK2 V617F occurs in 50%–60%, Mpl515 (thrombopoietin receptor activation mutation) mutations occur in 5%; patients must be BCR-ABL negative (because sometimes CML can cause high platelets also)

Dx:
1. CBC (elevated platelet count)
2. Bone marrow biopsy (clustered megakaryocytes)

Tx/Mgmt:
1. Observation
2. Aspirin
3. Hydroxyurea
4. Interferon

Coagulation Disorders

Coagulation disorders are some of the highest yield concepts on the medicine shelf, and you will likely get at least two to three questions testing some kind of coagulopathy. This is only because coagulation disorders are everywhere and every kind of doctor, in and outside of internal medicine, will deal with these at some time in their lives. Mastering coagulation disorders requires a firm understanding of the coagulation cascade but is not absolutely necessary if you are short on time. At the least, a minimum understanding should include which coagulation factors prolong PT, which prolong PTT, and which prolong both.

Next, recognize an important distinction between platelet function and clotting cascade—together, these terms come together to form **coagulation**. Platelets are important in forming an **initial platelet plug**. Platelets are activated by biomolecules released from sites of injury like ADP, thromboxane A2, von Willebrand factor, and collagen. Platelets are then bound to each other by fibrinogen through the GPIIbIIIa receptor. Remembering these steps will help you in both identifying pathologies and drug targets. Unfortunately, platelet plugs are very weak and require the support of the fibrin mesh that forms from the coagulation cascade. Thus, after platelet plug formation, the coagulation cascade is activated and forms a cross-linked fibrin clot that is much stronger to support the entire wound healing process. Bleeding time is a measure of how long it takes to form this platelet plug, and is strictly a measure of platelet activity or amount. PT/aPTT are tests of the clotting factors themselves, and do not tell you anything about platelets.

Recognizing these fundamental differences between platelet activation and clotting are vital to understanding how deficiencies in either are tested. Platelet activation is required only in areas where a weak plug would be sufficient to stop bleeding. Thus low pressure venous sites tend to exhibit deficiencies in platelets to a greater degree. This will manifest with mucosal bleeding from more outward sites prominent with easily damaged venous vasculature such as the GI tract, nasal or gingival mucosa, or the uterus. Conversely, arterial sites tend to exhibit

gg AR

Easy way to memorize the coagulation cascade (PPT)

deficiencies in clotting factors to a greater degree. This is because platelets are already insufficient for maintaining a blood clot in the high-pressure arterial system. As such, injury depends on the clotting cascade (Fig. 4.13). As a result, deficiencies in members of the clotting cascade such as in hemophilia lead to more serious deep bleeds, such as in the joints or brain.

As an organizing principle, most coagulopathies are diagnosed from CBC, PT, aPTT, and bleeding times. Treatments should be commensurate with the underlying pathologies, which should be anticoagulants in hypercoagulable states, and procoagulants in hypocoagulable states. This should be intuitive.

Hypocoagulable States

The following diseases cause hypocoagulable states, which means the coagulation system is NOT functioning and leads to bleeding. These diseases will be characterized by low levels or dysfunction of components within the coagulation cascade. This can range from the factors themselves to platelets to fibrinogen to von Willebrand factor. The workup for these diseases will always begin with a CBC, PT/aPTT, and bleeding times based on an initial clinical suspicion, and further testing is available for specific genetic abnormalities.

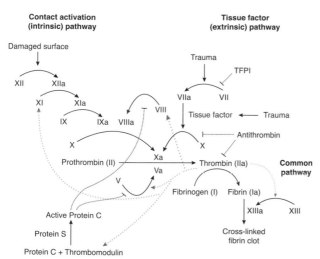

FIG. 4.13 Coagulation cascade. (From Wikimedia Commons. http s://commons.wikimedia.org/wiki/File:Coagulation_full.svg. Created by Joe D. Used under GFDL [http://www.gnu.org/copyleft/fdl.html], CC-BY-SA-3.0 [http://creativecommons.org/licenses/by-sa/3.0/] or CC BY-SA 2.5-2.0-1.0 [http://creativecommons.org/licenses/by-sa/2.5-2.0-1.0].)

Remember that deficiencies in platelets will lead to decreased bleeding times, whereas deficiencies in clotting factors will decrease PT/aPTT. Deficiencies in platelets (vWF, Bernard-Soulier, Glanzmann Thrombasthenia) tend to lead to bleeding from mucosal surfaces, where platelet activation plays a more important role. Deficiencies in coagulation factors (hemophilia A, B) tend to lead to bleeding in deeper, more serious sites, such as the joints and brain. See the previous paragraph for a more detailed explanation for why this phenomenon occurs. Treatment for the majority of these diseases is usually to replace missing procoagulation components.

Disseminated Intravascular Coagulation

DIC video

Buzz Words: Ecchymosses, petechiae, purpura + bleeding from mucosal surfaces (GI tract, gingival, oral mucosa) + surgical procedure bleeding + current infection, malignancy or obstetric complication + elevated PT/aPTT + increased bleeding time/low platelets + increased fibrin split products/D-dimers

Clinical Presentation: DIC is a condition in which microthrombi are formed in your body, consuming all your platelets and coagulation factors, leading to bleeding. This is usually occurring secondary to infection. DIC is characterized as a hypocoagulable process caused by a transient hypercoagulable induced by some precipitating factor.

PPx: N/A

MoD: Pathologic, transient activation of the coagulation cascade leading to microthrombi that disseminate throughout the circulation, consuming platelets, fibrin, and coagulation factors. The absence of these factors leads to hypocoagulability and eventual hemorrhage. This is a paradoxical disease in which bleeding and thrombosis are **occurring at the same time.** This pathologic activation that starts this sequelae can be caused by infection (most common), obstetric complications, major tissue injury, malignancy, shock, or rattlesnake venom.

Dx:

1. CBC, PT/aPTT
   a. Platelet count is decreased
   b. PT/aPTT are elevated
   c. Bleeding is elevated
2. Fibrin split products (elevated)
3. D-dimers (elevated)
4. Fibrinogen levels (decreased)
5. Peripheral blood smear (schistocytes from shearing of RBCs by microthrombi)

QUICK TIPS

The diagnostic findings from DIC should be intuitive. If too many microthrombi are forming, there should be evidence of elevated D-dimers and fibrin split products. As a result of these microthrombi, coagulation factors, fibrinogen, and platelets are consumed, leading to elevated PTT, aPTT, decreased fibrinogen, decreased platelet count, and resultant elevated bleeding time.

Tx/Mgmt:
1. Manage precipitating condition
2. Supportive measurements for severe hemorrhage
   a. FFP
   b. Platelet transfusions
   c. Cryoprecipitate
   d. Heparin

Hemophilia A

Buzz Words: Knee joint bleeding at early age + intracranial bleeding + hematuria + familial pattern

Clinical Presentation: X-linked recessive disorder from missing factor VIII. The most common sign is joint bleeding, also known as hemarthrosis, which can lead to joint destruction. However, bleeding can occur in other areas, and the most common cause of death in these patients is intracranial bleeding.

PPx: Prevent trauma.

MoD: Deficiency in factor VIII (FVIII) leads to defect in intrinsic pathway → hypocoagulability

Dx:
1. CBC
2. PT/aPTT (prolonged PTT)
3. Low VIII levels; normal vWF

Tx/Mgmt:
1. Analgesia and immobilization for acute hemarthrosis
2. FVIII replacement
3. DDAVP ? leads to endothelial secretion of vWF, which is a carrier for FVIII and protects it

Hemophilia B

Buzz Words: Knee joint bleeding at early age + intracranial bleeding + hematuria + familial pattern

Clinical Presentation: X-linked recessive disorder; rarer than hemophilia A but presents identically; caused by deficiency in factor IX.

PPx: Prevent trauma.

MoD: Deficiency in factor IX leads to defect in intrinsic pathway → hypocoagulability

Dx:
1. CBC
2. PT/aPTT (prolonged PTT)
3. Low VIII levels

Tx/Mgmt:
1. Analgesia and immobilization for acute hemarthrosis
2. FVIII replacement

99 AR
Hemophilia video

MNEMONIC
Hemophilia **AEIGHT** for Factor Eight

QUICK TIPS
DDAVP does NOT work for hemophilia B

Hypofibrinogenemia/Afibrinogenemia (Factor I deficiency)

Buzz Words: Umbilical cord bleeding at birth + surgical bleeding (GI, oral mucosa) + splenic rupture + intracranial hemorrhage

Clinical Presentation: Defect in factor I (fibrinogen) that is required to become activated during the coagulation cascade. This leads to a hypocoagulable state.

PPx: Prevent trauma, avoid antiplatelets, aspirin/NSAIDs

MoD: Fibrinogen is important for both forming fibrin during the cascade and for cross-linking platelets during initial platelet plug formation. Thus this is a defect in both coagulation cascade and platelet activation. Defects in fibrinogen can also be acquired during diseases like cirrhosis.

Dx:
1. CBC
2. Fibrinogen levels
3. PT/aPTT (both elevated)
4. Bleeding times (elevated)
5. Thrombin time (elevated)

Tx/Mgmt:
1. Cryoprecipitate,
2. Factor I concentrate
3. Antifibrinolytics (tranexamic acid, aminocaproic acid)

Von Willebrand Disease

Buzz Words: Recurrent nosebleeds + cutaneous bleeding + gingival bleeding + bleeding after dental procedures + menorrhagia + GI bleeding + elevated bleeding time

Clinical Presentation: vWF disease is a common, autosomal dominant disease leading to deficiency in vWF. vWF plays two roles; it binds to platelets to allow them to adhere to vessel walls, and is a carrier for factor VIII that prevents it from degradation. Thus vWF plays two procoagulant roles that, when missing, leads to a hypocoagulable state. There are three kinds, in order from most to least common:
- Type 1—decreased levels
- Type 2—dysfunctional, but normal levels
- Type 3—missing vWF (severe)

PPx: Avoid aspirin/NSAIDS → overbleeding

MoD: vWF is secreted from megakaryocytes and endothelial cells that protects FVIII in the blood from degradation and is also part of aggregating platelets by allowing them to adhere to endothelial cells after

von Willebrand disease video

injury. In vWF disease, vWF is missing or defective, leading to an inability for platelets to aggregate and for FVIII to partake in the coagulation cascade. This leads to problems primarily with mucosal bleeding, where the most common sign is recurrent nosebleeds (epistaxis).

Dx:
1. CBC
2. PT/aPTT
3. Bleeding time (elevated)
4. Decreased vWF and factor VIII activity
5. Ristocetin platelet aggregation (platelets will not aggregate)

Tx/Mgmt:
1. DDAVP—causes endothelial cells to secrete vWF
2. Factor VIII concentrates

Bernard-Soulier Syndrome (Hemorrhagiparous Thrombocytic Dystrophy)

Buzz Words: Bleeding after dental procedures + easy bruising + nosebleeds + menorrhagia

Clinical Presentation: This is a rare deficiency in platelets that causes large platelets, and another name for this is *giant platelet disorder.* Like vWF disease and Glanzmann thrombasthenia, this disease leads to mucosal bleeding that is characteristic of platelet problems.

PPx: Avoid aspirin/NSAIDs or antiplatelet drugs.

MoD: This is caused by a defect in GPIb-Ix on platelets caused by mutations in GP1BA, GP1BB, or GP9 that prevents the GPIb-IX receptor from forming. This is the receptor for vWF that allows vWF to activate platelets and for platelets to adhere to vWF on the endothelium.

Dx:
1. CBC (low platelet count)
2. PT/aPTT
3. Bleeding time (elevated)
4. Blood smear (abnormally large platelets)
5. Ristocetin platelet aggregation

Tx/Mgmt:
1. Platelet transfusion
2. Tranexamic acid for mucosal bleeding

Glanzmann Thrombasthenia

Buzz Words: Excessive bleeding after dental procedure OR mucosal membrane bleeding (frequent nosebleeds, GI bleeding, menorrhagia) + petechiae + prolonged

bleeding time + normal platelet count + normal PT/
aPTT + autosomal inheritance pattern → Glanzmann's
thrombasthenia

Clinical Presentation: Autosomal recessive disease, causing
a defect in fibrinogen receptor on platelets (GPIIb-IIIa),
leading to platelet hypoactivity

PPx: Do not take antiplatelet drugs or NSAIDs.

MoD: GPIIb-IIIa is required to bind to fibrinogen and
cross-links platelets into a platelet plug, stabilizing
initial thrombus formation. The absence of functional
GPIIb-IIIa leads to a deficit in the ability to form the initial platelet plug, and therefore leads to failure to form
a thrombus upon injury, which is most prominent in
mucosal vasculature.

Dx:

1. Examine for petechiae/ecchymoses
2. CBC
3. PT/aPTT
4. Bleeding time
5. Flow cytometry
6. Antibody levels to GPIIb-IIIa
7. Ristocetin platelet aggregation (platelets will not
   aggregate)

Tx/Mgmt:

1. Avoid antiplatelet agents
2. If actively bleeding → platelet transfusions
   (leukocyte depleted)
3. Vaccinate against Hep B (due to multiple
   transfusions)
4. Oral contraceptives to control menorrhagia
5. Recombinant factor VII (children refractory to
   platelet transfusions)

Hypercoagulable States

The following diseases cause hypercoagulable states,
which means the coagulation system is functioning and
working in overdrive. These diseases will be characterized
by high levels of components that can induce the coagulation cascade OR low levels/dysfunction in components
that inhibit the coagulation cascade. The workup for these
diseases will always begin with a CBC, PT/aPTT, and
bleeding times based on an initial clinical suspicion, and
further testing is available for specific genetic abnormalities. In most of these diseases, prophylaxis, treatment, and
management will consist of anticoagulation with heparin
and warfarin.

Heparin-Induced Thrombocytopenia/Thrombosis

Buzz Words: Low platelets following heparin administration + enlargement of clots or formation of new clots (deep vein thrombosis [DVTs])

Clinical Presentation: This is a disease where heparin-platelet complexes are recognized by autoantibodies, leading to platelet activation and clot formation. Resultantly, it is another disease where platelet levels are LOW while there is an overall hypercoagulable state.

PPx: Avoidance of heparin

MoD: Heparin finds to platelet factor 4 (PF4) on platelets. This complex is recognized by autoantibodies in circulation, which form immune complexes that can do two things:
1. activates platelets, leading to microthrombi, and
2. platelet removal by macrophages in the spleen, leading to thrombocytopenia

Dx:
1. CBC (low platelets)
2. ELISA for heparin/PF4 complexes
3. Doppler sonography to detect DVTs

Tx/Mgmt:
1. Discontinue heparin
2. Switch to other anticoagulants (danaparoid, fondaparinux, bivalirudin, argatroban)
   - Avoid warfarin because of increased risk of warfarin-induced skin necrosis

Warfarin-Induced Skin Necrosis

Buzz Words: Skin necrosis 3+ days after warfarin administration + hypercoagulability + obese, middle-aged woman

Clinical Presentation: This is a disease in which a usually obese, middle-aged woman on anticoagulants (warfarin) presents with pain and redness in some area of their skin, leading to petechiae and then purpura. The most common sites are breasts, thighs, and buttocks, all of which are surrounded with a lot of subcutaneous fat.

PPx: Prevent large loading doses of warfarin and bridge with heparin.

MoD: Warfarin inhibits vitamin K dependent factor synthesis, which includes Factor II, Factor VII, Factor IX, Factor X, and Protein C and S. Protein C and S have the shortest half-lives (3–6 hours, 30 hours, respectively) and are depleted the fastest of all the factors. Therefore, during early warfarin administration, patients actually exhibit a pro-coagulant state due to the fact that they have lost

gg AR
Homocystinemia overview

anticoagulant factors and have not yet lost their procoagulants. This will manifest in hypercoagulability in the skin, leading to ischemia and necrosis.

Dx:
1. CBC
2. PT/aPTT/INR

Tx/Mgmt:
1. Discontinue warfarin and reverse with vitamin K
2. Administer heparin to prevent further clotting
3. FFP, activated protein C

Homocysteinemia

Buzz Words: High homocysteine + recurrent thrombosis

Clinical Presentation: This is a disease caused by abnormally high levels of homocysteine in the blood and urine. This can lead to thrombosis and a hypercoagulable state, but can also lead to neuropsychiatric illness and fractures.

PPx: Prevent deficiency in B6, B9, and B12; alcohol consumption can precipitate homocysteinemia.

MoD: Can be caused by deficits in B6, B9, and B12 or deficiency in 5-MTHF reductase → these all elevate homocysteine levels; homocysteinemia is also related to a rare disease called homocystinuria, an autosomal recessive deficiency in cystathionine beta synthase. Elevated homocysteine levels damage endothelial lining of blood vessels, leading to thrombosis and coagulation.

Dx:
1. CBC
2. B6, B9, B12 levels
3. Complete medical evaluation

Tx/Mgmt:
1. Supplement B6, B9, B12
2. Taurine supplementation

Hypoplasminogenemia

Buzz Words: Recurrent DVT/PE + low plasminogen + family history

Clinical Presentation: This is an extremely rare disease characterized by plasminogen deficiency and impaired fibrinolysis, leading to hypercoagulability and fibrin rich membranes forming at sites of wound healing. It can also be acquired secondary to conditions that consume plasminogen, including DIC, malignancy, or trauma.

PPx: Warfarin anticoagulation

MoD: Plasminogen gets activated into plasmin, which cleaves fibrin from clots into fibrin degradation products. When plasminogen is missing, clots cannot get broken down, leading to a hypercoagulable state.

Dx:

1. CBC
2. PT/aPTT
3. Plasminogen levels (decreased)

Tx/Mgmt:

1. Treat underlying cause or acute DVT/PE, if applicable
2. Warfarin for recurrent DVT/PE

Antithrombin III Deficiency

Buzz Words: Recurrent DVT/PE + repetitive intrauterine death + requiring higher doses of heparin or heparin resistance

Clinical Presentation: Autosomal dominant deficiency in ATIII, which is an inhibitor of thrombin. A deficiency leads to thrombin hyperactivity and hypercoagulability. A common finding is heparin resistance or requiring high doses of heparin, since heparin requires active ATIII to work.

PPx: Screen family members.

MoD: Mutation 1q23-q25 causes low or dysfunctional ATIII

Dx:

1. CBC + ATIII levels
2. Rule out liver/kidney disease

Tx/Mgmt: IV ATIII replacement

Protein C/S Deficiency

Buzz Words: Recurrent DVT or PE at young age + family history

Clinical Presentation: Protein C and S are two major cofactors that downregulate the clotting cascade. Protein C cleaves activated FV and FVIII. Protein S is a co-factor for protein C. Their absence promotes a recurrent hypercoagulable state that presents with venous thromboembolisms.

PPx: Heparin/warfarin to prevent recurrent DVTs

MoD:

- Protein C deficiency
  - Congenital (autosomal dominant)
  - Acquired (warfarin, DIC, liver disease)
- Protein S deficiency
  - Congenital
  - Acquired (OCPs, pregnancy, nephrotic syndrome)

99 AR

Antithrombin III deficiency overview

QUICK TIPS

Protein S deficiency is an underlying cause of DIC (see above).

Dx:
1. CBC
2. PT/aPTT
3. Protein C/S activity/antigen assays

Tx/Mgmt:
1. Tx DVT/PE with heparin
2. Protein C and S replacement
3. Liver transplant in severe cases

Factor V Leiden

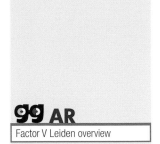

Factor V Leiden overview

Buzz Words: Recurrent episodes of DVT (leg pain after long periods of immobility) or PE (shortness of breath) + occurring before age of 40 + thrombosis in unusual sites + family history

Clinical Presentation: Factor V Leiden is a hypercoagulable state that causes recurrent thromboembolic events, thrombosis in weird sites, and usually occurs in younger individuals who have a family history of such events.

PPx: Warfarin in individuals with 2+ thromboembolic events

MoD: This is a disease caused by a mutation in the factor V gene that renders factor V unable to be inactivated by protein C—therefore, factor V is always activated and leads to a hypercoagulable state that presents with DVT, PE, or thromboses in sites like the mesentery.

Dx:
1. Coagulation testing with APC resistance assay (patient cannot be on anticoagulants)
2. Genetic testing for Factor V Leiden

Tx/Mgmt:
1. Tx for DVT/PE (Heparin)
2. 2+ thromboembolic events → lifetime Warfarin anticoagulation

Antiphospholipid Syndrome (Lupus Anticoagulant, Anticardiolipin)

Antiphospholipid mnemonic

Buzz Words: Repeat arterial and venous thromboses + stroke/TIA + lupus + intrauterine death or intrauterine growth restriction + placental infarctions

Clinical Presentation: Antiphospholipid antibodies lead to recurrent venous/arterial thromboses, presenting with complications like recurrent DVT/PE, stroke, and other conditions. A common presenting finding is a pregnancy complication, such as intrauterine death. APLS is categorized into primary versus secondary. Primary APLS is idiopathic in nature. Secondary APLS is caused by conditions like lupus.

PPx: N/A

MoD: Phospholipids are part of all cell membranes. Antiphospholipid antibodies are antibodies made against these components of all cell membranes. Sometimes, these phospholipids take on specific names, like cardiolipin. Anticardiolipin antibodies are antibodies toward a specific phospholipid in the mitochondrial (and hence they are also antimitochondrial) and are elevated in diseases, including SLE and syphilis. These bind to ApoH, activating it, leading to inhibition of protein C. Protein C is then unable to exert its anticoagulant effect on the clotting cascade. Lupus anticoagulant is an antiphospholipid that binds to prothrombin, activating it to form thrombin leading to a pro-coagulant state. They also target beta2-microglobulin, which also leads to thrombosis. The lupus anticoagulant is a PRO-coagulant in vivo, despite its name. It receives its name for its function in vitro, where it increases PTT.

> **QUICK TIPS**
>
> Another confusing part of the lupus anticoagulant is that most people with it actually don't have lupus.

Dx:
1. CBC
2. PT/aPTT
3. Mixing test
   a. Lupus anticoagulant will inhibit clotting in normal plasma
4. Serologic testing (ELISA)

Tx/Mgmt:
1. Observation
2. Lifelong anticoagulation

Prothrombin G20210A Mutation

Buzz Words: Caucasian/European + recurrent DVT + PE + elevated plasma prothrombin

Clinical Presentation: Common

PPx: Test family members, women should not take oral contraceptive pills (OCPs)

MoD: Caused by single nucleotide polymorphism of guanine to adenine in the noncoding region of the prothrombin gene. This mutation stabilizes the mRNA of prothrombin, leading to improved synthesis and hypercoagulability.

Dx: PCR for G to A polymorphism

Tx/Mgmt:
1. Tx acute DVT/PE
2. Most patients do not require treatment
3. Lifetime anticoagulation with heparin/warfarin in serious cases

Reactions to Blood Components

Blood transfusions are listed as Tx/Mgmt for various complications listed in this chapter. Recognizing the various processes that can go wrong during a blood transfusion can go a long way (Table 4.1).

Traumatic, Mechanical, and Vascular Disorders

This section includes miscellaneous disorders involving mechanical and vascular disorders that affect the blood and lymph.

Cardiac Valve Hemolysis

Buzz Words: RBC fragmentation (schistocytes) + previous cardiac valve replacement + anemia (fatigue, pallor) + increased indirect bilirubin

Clinical Presentation: Cardiac valve hemolysis leads to a hemolytic anemia that will elevated bilirubin, LDH, and decrease haptoglobin. It will also present with traditional symptoms of anemia such as jaundice, fatigue, and pallor.

PPx: Valve replacement for malfunctioning valves

MoD: Intravascular RBC shearing due to malfunctioning heart valves or VADs, platelet microthrombi in TTP, or fibrin shearing across vessels as seen in DIC.

Dx:
1. CBC
2. Peripheral smear with fragmented RBCs

Tx/Mgmt:
1. Treat underlying defect
2. In the case of prosthetic valve damage, replace the valve
3. Folic acid or iron supplementation to optimize RBC production

Splenic Rupture/Laceration

Buzz Words: Pain radiating to the left shoulder (Kehr sign) + hypotension and signs of blood loss + LUQ pain + splenomegaly

Clinical Presentation: Splenic rupture/laceration can occur in the history of recent trauma or sports injury, and is more likely to occur in setting of history of malaria or recent mononucleosis infection. Malaria can also cause nontraumatic splenic rupture.

PPx: N/A

TABLE 4.1 Common Transfusion Reactions

Reaction	Signs and Symptoms	Mechanism	Treatment	Comments
Febrile Nonhemolytic Transfusion Reaction	Fever, chills, headache, malaise, flushing	Host antibodies against donor MHC antigens or due to cytokines from leukocytes in donor blood	May need to discontinue transfusion, but usually fever resolves in 15–30 minutes without specific treatment. Acetaminophen may be used.	Most common transfusion reaction. Can be prevented with leukocyte filters or irradiation.
Hemolytic Transfusion Reaction	Fever, chills, pain at the infusion site, dark urine, nausea, shock	ABO incompatibility with host antibodies against antigens on donor red blood cells	Immediately discontinue transfusion and administer fluids	Most severe reaction
Allergic Transfusion Reaction	Urticaria, pruritus	Allergic reaction to plasma proteins in transfused blood	Symptomatic treatment with antihistamines. Does not require discontinuing the transfusion	Can be prevented with antihistamine pretreatment
Anaphylactic Transfusion Reaction	Urticaria, angioedema, wheezing, laryngeal edema, abdominal pain, hypotension, shock	Host antibodies against IgA antibodies in the donor plasma	Immediately discontinue transfusion and administer epinephrine	Usually seen in patients with IgA deficiency. Can be prevented by administering washed or IgA deficient products
TRALI (Transfusion Related Acute Lung Injury)	Dyspnea, hypoxemia, bilateral chest infiltrates	Donor antibodies to MHC class I or class II or human neutrophil antigens. Activated neutrophils cause endothelial damage.	Immediately discontinue transfusion and provide airway support	Most common cause of transfusion associated death
TACO (Transfusion Associated Circulatory Overload)	Dyspnea, pulmonary edema, hypertension, peripheral edema	Rapid volume expansion	Supportive. Diuretics can be used.	Seen in elderly patients with heart failure or anemia. Can be prevented with slower transfusions and diuretics.

MoD: Direct impact to spleen leading to rupture/laceration and bleeding.

Dx:

1. CT if stable
2. Peritoneal lavage and surgery

Tx/Mgmt:

1. Surgical intervention
2. Hemodynamic stabilization
3. Transfusions

Splenic Infarct

Buzz Words: Fibrotic spleen in sickle cell patients + acute onset + LUQ abdominal pain

Clinical Presentation: Often accompanied by fever, nausea/vomiting, leukocytosis, and splenomegaly. Suspect in patient with history of Gaucher disease (marked splenomegaly), sickle cell disease, hypercoagulability, embolic disease.

PPx: N/A

MoD: Occlusion of one or more branches of the splenic artery results in infarction of splenic tissue

Splenic infarction radiology

Dx: CT abdomen with contrast

Tx/Mgmt:

1. Pain management
2. If rupture or abscess formation may require surgical intervention or transfusion

Splenic Abscess

Buzz Words: LUQ pain + persistent fever (despite antibiotics) + splenomegaly

Clinical Presentation: May also be accompanied by left pleural effusions or splenic infarcts due to septic emboli. Suspect in setting of endocarditis, recent infection, with antibiotic treatment.

PPx: N/A

MoD: Splenic infection secondary to septic emboli, most commonly from endocarditis

Dx: CT abdomen with contrast

Tx/Mgmt:

1. Antibiotics
2. Splenectomy

Effects/Complications of Splenectomy

Buzz Words: Sepsis secondary to encapsulated organisms + splenectomy/functional asplenia (sickle cell patients) + fever

PPx: Pneumococcal, meningococcal, and *Haemophilus influenzae* type b vaccines

MoD: The spleen plays an important role in humoral immunity and bacterial clearance. As such, asplenia results in increased risk of severe bacterial sepsis secondary to encapsulated organisms most notably *Streptococcus pneumoniae*, *H. influenzae*, and *Neisseria meningitides*. Physicians should have a high suspicion for encapsulated bacteria in these patients.

Dx: Blood culture if febrile

Tx/Mgmt: Broad coverage with ceftriaxone and hospital admission if febrile

Hypersplenism

Buzz Words: Splenomegaly (LUQ mass) + thrombocytopenia, anemia, neutropenia

Clinical Presentation: Hypersplenism is an overactive spleen. It can be caused by a number of things, but some of the most common are cirrhosis, lymphoma, and TB. In most cases, this will accompany splenomegaly, a large spleen. The consequence of hypersplenism is **pancytopenia.** Be wary of hypersplenism in patients with sickle cell, for whom hypersplenism can induce a sickle cell crisis.

PPx: N/A

MoD: The spleen clears the blood of circulating RBCs, platelets, and neutrophils. Hyperactivity of the spleen will lead to anemia, thrombocytopenia, and neutropenia, respectively with associated symptoms of fatigue/pallor, easy bleeding, and recurrent infections.

Dx:
1. Physical exam
2. CBC
3. Consider liver, bone marrow, or lymph node biopsy for precipitating conditions

Tx/Mgmt:
1. Supportive
2. Transfusions
3. Splenectomy

Adverse Effects of Drugs on the Hematologic and Lymphoreticular System

See Table 4.2.

TABLE 4.2 Adverse Effects of Drugs on the Hematologic and Lymphoreticular System

Name	MoA	Uses	Side Effects	Notes
Heparin (LMWH = enoxaparin, dalteparin)	Lowers activity of thrombin and FX	PE, DVT, ACS, MI	Bleeding, HIT	Follow PTT, use in pregnancy
Bivalirudin	Inhibits thrombin	PE, DVT, AFib, HIT	Bleeding, no reversal agent	
Warfarin	Inhibits carboxylation of vitamin K-dependent factors (II, VII, IX, X, C/S)	PPx VTE, AFib	Bleeding, P450 interactions, warfarin-induced skin necrosis	Follow PT/INR, do not use in pregnancy Reverse with vitamin K.
Apixaban, Rivaroxaban	Inhibit factor X	DVT, PE, Stroke PPx in AFib	Bleeding	Do not require monitoring
tPA, rPA, streptokinase	Convert plasminogen to plasmin, cleaving thrombin and fibrin	MI, stroke, severe PE	Bleeding	Elevates PT, aPTT, no change in plt count Contraindicated in patients who you suspect might bleed, Tx overdose with aminocaproic acid
Clopidogrel, prasugrel, ticagrelor, ticlopidine	Block ADP receptor on platelets, preventing platelet activation	ACS/MI	Neutropenia, TTP	
Cilostazol/dipyridamole	PDEIII inhibitor, inhibits platelets	Claudication, PPx stroke, TIA, angina	Nausea, headache, flushing, hypotension	
Abciximab, eptifibatide, tirofiban	Binds to GPIIb/IIIa on platelets, prevents fibrinogen crosslinking and activation	Angina, stenting	Bleeding, thrombocytopenia	II x III = CIX (GPIIbIIIa for abciximab); ept**fib**atide, tiro**fib**an for fibrinogen blocking
Hydroxyurea	Inhibits DNA synthesis	Melanoma, sickle cell (elevates HbF)	Myelosuppression	
Azathioprine, 6-mercaptopurine	Inhibits purine synthesis	Organ rejection, RA, IBD, SLE	Myelosuppression, GI, liver toxicities	
Cladribine	Inhibit purine synthesis	Hairy cell leukemia	Myelosuppression, nephrotoxicity	
Cytarabine	Inhibits pyrimidine synthesis	Leukemia/lymphoma	Pancytopenia	
5-Fluorouracil	Inhibits thymidine synthesis	Various solid cancers	Myelosuppression	Enhanced with leucovorin

TABLE 4.2 Adverse Effects of Drugs on the Hematologic and Lymphoreticular System—cont'd

Name	MoA	Uses	Side Effects	Notes
Methotrexate	Inhibits thymidine synthesis	Solid/liquid cancers, autoimmune disease	Myelosuppression, hepatotoxicity, pulmonary fibrosis	
Bleomycin	Causes DNA damage	Hodgkin lymphoma	Pulmonary fibrosis	
Dactinomycin	Causes DNA damage	Solid cancers in children	Myelosuppression	
Doxorubicin	Causes DNA damage	Solid/liquid cancers	Dilated cardiomyopathy "Rubin has a big heart"	Dexrazoxane to chelate iron, PPx cardiac toxicity
Busulfan	Causes DNA damage	CML	Myelosuppression, pulmonary fibrosis, hyperpigmentation	
Cyclophosphamide, ifosfamide	Causes DNA damage	Solid/liquid cancers	Myelosuppression, hemorrhagic cystitis	
Nitrosureas (-ustine)	Causes DNA damage	Brain tumors	CNS toxicity	
Cisplatin, carboplatin	Causes DNA damage	Solid cancers	Nephrotoxicity, ototoxicity, neuropathy	
Paclitaxel	Prevents mitosis (binds microtubules)	Solid cancers	Myelosuppression, neuropathy	
Vincristine, vinblastine	Prevents mitosis (bind tubulin)	Solid and liquid cancers	Vincristine: neuropathy (but not vinblastine)	
Etoposide, teniposide	Inhibits topoisomerase, prevents DNA unwinding	Solid and liquid cancers	Myelosuppression	
Irinotecan, topotecan	Inhibits topoisomerase, prevents DNA unwinding	Solid cancers	Myelosuppression	
Bevacizumab	VEGF antibody	Solid tumors	Bleeding	
Imatinib	Inhibits BCR-ABL	CML	Rash, liver toxicity	
Rituximab	Inhibits CD20 on B cells	Lymphomas, RA	PML (JC virus)	

CML, Chronic myelogenous leukemia; *CNS*, central nervous system; *DVT*, deep vein thrombosis; *GI*, gastrointestinal; *PML*, promyelocytic leukemia; *TTP*, thrombocytopenic thrombotic purpura.

GUNNER PRACTICE

1. A 23-year-old female is brought by her roommate to the emergency department after she became unable to speak fluent sentences for 10 minutes. She has resumed talking at her normal pace, and relates 4 days of progressive fatigue, nausea, and "feeling warm." She has a medical history of mild, persistent asthma, for which she takes albuterol and inhaled fluticasone. Her vital signs are T 100.9 HR 110 BP 123/82 RR 17 SpO_2 98% on room air. On examination, she appears tired and pale. She has several red-purple spots on her arms and legs that do not blanch with pressure. Blood cultures are sent and pending. Laboratory evaluation reveals Hgb 8.7, PLT 12,000, Cr 1.3, LDH 1530, Haptoglobin 6, normal PT and PTT, and a negative Coombs test. Urine hCG is negative, and her peripheral blood smear is shown below. What is the next best step in management? (Fig. 4.U01)
   A. Transfuse packed red blood cells
   B. Initiate empiric vancomycin and cefepime
   C. Initiate rituximab
   D. Initiate plasma exchange
   E. Give aspirin

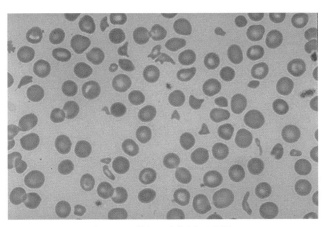

Courtesy Edward C. Klatt, MD.

2. A 67-year-old woman is brought to the emergency department by her friend, who found her lying in bed, soaked in urine, and difficult to arouse. She has a history of well-controlled hypertension and mild COPD, for which she takes albuterol, tiotropium, fluticasone-salmeterol, and hydrochlorothiazide. A diagnosis of urinary tract infection is made, and after 2 days of broad-spectrum antibiotics, she has returned to her baseline

mental status. At this point, she relates that she has had 3 months of fatigue, and has recently noticed her urine is foamy and her legs and back seem swollen. Initial labs show Hgb 10.2, MCV 86, Cr 1.9, Ca 11.3, and ESR 48. Her peripheral blood smear is shown as follows. What is the most likely diagnosis? (Fig. 4.U02)

A. Polycythemia vera
B. Multiple myeloma
C. Hereditary spherocytosis
D. Clear cell renal cell carcinoma
E. Myelofibrosis

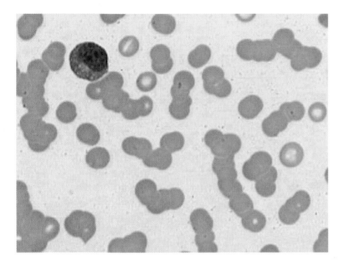

3. A 34-year-old male is brought to the emergency room by his husband for a fever. Three months ago, he was hit by a car that jumped onto the curb. He required exploratory laparotomy, splenectomy, and open reduction and internal fixation of his right tibia and fibula. His husband states that he was recovering well and had returned to work until today, when he "felt warm" and began shaking uncontrollably every few minutes. His vital signs are T 103.6 HR 134 BP 78/32 RR 26 SpO$_2$ 96% on room air. On exam, the patient is ill-appearing and stuporous with warm extremities. The surgical sites are clean, dry, and intact, and full exam yields no other abnormal findings. Blood cultures are acquired, a central venous catheter and multiple peripheral venous catheters are placed, and he is started on vancomycin, ceftriaxone, intravenous fluids, and norepinephrine. Initial labs show WBC 28,000, Cr 2.3, ALT 1578, and Lactate 4.3. Chest x-ray is unrevealing, as is CT of the abdomen and pelvis. Despite rapid transfer to the ICU, aggressive

blood pressure support, and intubation, he dies in the middle of the night. The following morning, what are his blood cultures most likely to show?

A. *Candida albicans*
B. *Bacteroides fragilis*
C. *Rhizopus* spp.
D. *Mycobacterium tuberculosis*
E. *Streptococcus pneumoniae*

Notes

ANSWERS: What Would Gunner Jess/Jim Do?

1. WWGJD? A 23-year-old female is brought by her roommate to the emergency department after she became unable to speak fluent sentences for 10 minutes. She has resumed talking at her normal pace, and relates 4 days of progressive fatigue, nausea, and "feeling warm." She has a medical history of mild, persistent asthma, for which she takes albuterol and inhaled fluticasone. Her vital signs are T 100.9 HR 110 BP 123/82 RR 17 SpO_2 98% on room air. On examination, she appears tired and pale. She has several red-purple spots on her arms and legs that do not blanch with pressure. Blood cultures are sent and pending. Laboratory evaluation reveals Hgb 8.7, PLT 12,000, Cr 1.3, LDH 1530, Haptoglobin 6, normal PT and PTT, and a negative Coombs test. Urine hCG is negative, and her peripheral blood smear is shown below. What is the next best step in management? (see Fig. 4.U01)

Answer: D, Initiate plasma exchange.

Explanation: This patient most likely has TTP, a micro-angiopathic hemolytic anemia (MAHA) characterized by ADAMTS13 depletion. The classic pentad of symptoms involves fever, anemia, thrombocytopenia, renal injury, and neurologic dysfunction, but the whole pentad is a rare finding. The peripheral smear shows schistocytes, which are indicative of MAHA. The low temperature, stable blood pressure, and normal PT and PTT make DIC due to sepsis unlikely, the negative pregnancy test rules out HELLP, and the normal range blood pressure rules out malignant hypertension. Thus the most likely possibilities are hemolytic-uremic syndrome (HUS) and TTP. The patient's age and minimal kidney injury argue for TTP and against HUS, which is classically seen in children during an EHEC 0157:H7 infection. As TTP is generally progressive and fatal without treatment, suspected cases should undergo plasma exchange immediately.

A. Transfuse packed red blood cells → Incorrect. The most important aspect of initial management in suspected TTP is plasma exchange.

B. Initiate empiric vancomycin and cefepime → Incorrect. The patient does not likely have DIC due to sepsis, and there is no evidence supporting antibiotic treatment for HUS. In fact, giving antibiotics to children with EHEC O157:H7 may increase the risk of HUS.

C. Initiate rituximab → Incorrect. While this is sometimes given as adjunctive treatment for TTP, it should not replace plasma exchange as initial management.

E. Give aspirin → Although TTP does result in part from platelet aggregation, plasma exchange is the first-line treatment for TTP patients.

2. WWGJD? A 67-year-old woman is brought to the emergency department by her friend, who found her lying in bed, soaked in urine, and difficult to arouse. She has a history of well-controlled hypertension and mild COPD, for which she takes albuterol, tiotropium, fluticasone-salmeterol, and hydrochlorothiazide. A diagnosis of urinary tract infection is made, and after 2 days of broad-spectrum antibiotics, she has returned to her baseline mental status. At this point, she relates that she has had 3 months of fatigue, and has recently noticed her urine is foamy and her legs and back seem swollen. Initial labs show Hgb 10.2, MCV 86, Cr 1.9, Ca 11.3, and ESR 48. Her peripheral blood smear is shown below. What is the most likely diagnosis? (see Fig. 4.U02)

Answer: B, Multiple myeloma.

Explanation: This is a 67-year-old woman who presents with a UTI and is found to have fatigue and complaints concerning for nephrotic syndrome. She has a normocytic anemia, renal insufficiency, hypercalcemia, and an elevated ESR, as well as rouleaux formation on her peripheral blood smear. This is a classic presentation of multiple myeloma (MM). The renal insufficiency with possible nephrotic syndrome is more likely due to AL amyloidosis or monoclonal immunoglobulin deposition disease (MIDD), as opposed to myeloma cast nephropathy, which can result in Bence-Jones proteinuria but does not usually cause significant albuminuria. The rouleaux (and ESR elevation) is due to hypersecretion of immunoglobulin by the myeloma cells, leading to hyperviscosity. Of note, multiple myeloma often results in compromised immunity. This patient is presenting with two common and life-threatening complications of MM, infection, and renal injury.

A. Polycythemia vera → Incorrect. The patient is anemic, not polycythemic, and many of her complaints and lab findings are not explained by this answer choice.

C. Hereditary spherocytosis → Incorrect. While this would lead to anemia, it is not consistent with the patient's other findings. In addition, this would likely be discovered long before the age of 67, and does not appear as such on peripheral smears.

D. Clear cell renal cell carcinoma → Incorrect. While this can lead to renal injury and hypercalcemia, it is more often correlated with polycythemia than anemia (due to erythropoietin secretion), and would not result in this peripheral smear.

E. Myelofibrosis → Incorrect. This would not be consistent with all of the patient's complaints and findings. Additionally, we are given no information about other cytopenias, and a classic peripheral smear finding of myelofibrosis is the dacryocyte, or tear drop cell.

3. WWGJD? A 34-year-old male is brought to the emergency room by his husband for a fever. Three months ago, he was hit by a car that jumped onto the curb and required exploratory laparotomy, splenectomy, and open reduction and internal fixation of his right tibia and fibula. His husband states that he was recovering well and had returned to work until today, when he "felt warm" and began shaking uncontrollably every few minutes. His vital signs are T 103.6 HR 134 BP 78/32 RR 26 SpO$_2$ 96% on room air. On exam, the patient is ill-appearing and stuporous with warm extremities. The surgical sites are clean, dry, and intact, and full exam yields no other abnormal findings. Blood cultures are acquired, a central venous catheter and multiple peripheral venous catheters are placed, and he is started on vancomycin and ceftriaxone, intravenous fluids, and norepinephrine. Initial labs show WBC 28,000, Cr 2.3, ALT 1578, and Lactate 4.3. Chest x-ray is unrevealing, as is CT of the abdomen and pelvis. Despite rapid transfer to the ICU, aggressive blood pressure support, and intubation, he dies in the middle of the night. The following morning, what are his blood cultures most likely to show?

Answer: E, *Streptococcus pneumoniae.*

Explanation: This patient dies of overwhelming sepsis 3 months after splenectomy. He has no obvious focus of infection on exam, and we are not given any information to indicate that he is otherwise immunocompromised or specifically susceptible to any of the other offered choices. Splenectomy can result in an increased risk of infection with encapsulated bacteria, especially *S. pneumoniae.*

A. *Candida albicans* → Incorrect. While this fungus would indeed fail to respond to vancomycin and ceftriaxone, we are given no indication that he is particularly susceptible to this organism.

B. *Bacteroides fragilis* → Incorrect. *B. fragilis* is an anaerobic bacterium, found especially in the colon, that can cause both localized infection and sepsis, but this is usually due to some derangement in the gut or gut wall. Since CT of the abdomen and pelvis does not indicate an obvious intraabdominal source of infection, this is less likely to be the offending organism.

C. *Rhizopus* spp. → Incorrect. Mucormycosis classically results during the immunocompromised state (including high blood glucose with diabetes mellitus). We have no indication of such a state, and no focus of infection that would make mucormycosis more likely (rhinocerebral, pulmonary, cutaneous, etc.).

D. *Mycobacterium tuberculosis* → Incorrect. The various clinical courses of tuberculosis tend to be indolent. The disseminated form, miliary tuberculosis, would likely be visible on chest x-ray and/or CT abdomen and pelvis. We are not given any risk factors for TB or dissemination of TB.

Diseases of the Nervous System and Special Senses

Cody Nathan, Leo Wang, Hao-Hua Wu, Rebecca Gao, and Chuang-Kuo Wu

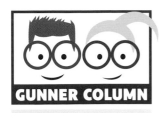

GUNNER COLUMN

General Principles for Diseases of the Nervous System and Special Senses

A solid understanding of diseases of the nervous system is high yield, not only for the shelf exam but also for Step 2 CK. The length of this chapter is due to the large breadth of content within the realm of nervous system diseases. We will help you focus on the most high-yield information on the Medicine shelf exam. Paying close attention to the buzz words, the treatment options (especially for the life-threatening diseases) will be most helpful for the test.

The main diseases of the nervous system can be remembered using the acronym "DVITAMINS". This stands for Degenerative, Vascular, Infectious/Inflammatory, Trauma, Autoimmune, Metabolic, Inherited, Neoplastic, Seizure. Knowing the age of the patient is a quick and easy way to help build your differential diagnosis based on these pathologic states. Degenerative diseases are those that cause a progressive loss of neurons and result in declined function. They tend to occur in adults and include conditions such as Alzheimer's disease, Parkinson's disease, Huntington disease, and vascular diseases (strokes). Being able to identify risk factors for stroke helps treat and prevent strokes from occurring.

Infectious/inflammatory disease can affect children and young adults. This process includes high-yield diseases such as meningitis, herpes simplex virus, and Guillain-Barré syndrome (GBS). Trauma mainly occurs in young adults, but may also affect the elderly population because they are prone to falls. The most high-yield topics related to trauma include subdural and epidural hematomas as well as spinal cord injuries. Autoimmune diseases are most common in young adults and include diseases such as multiple sclerosis (MS) and myasthenia gravis (MG). Metabolic and inherited diseases are often diagnosed in infants and young children. Some inherited diseases that tend to show up on the shelf exam are Friedreich ataxia, Duchenne muscular dystrophy, and neurofibromatosis. However, remember that not all inherited diseases show symptoms at birth, and some metabolic diseases (i.e., uremia, hepatic encephalopathy) are not caused by genetic problems.

Neoplasms can occur at any age and should always routinely be considered in the differential diagnosis, given its devastating effects and insidious onset. The most common neurologic neoplasms tested on the exam include glioblastoma multiforme (GBM), medulloblastoma, metastatic cancers of brain, and pituitary adenomas. Finally, seizures can occur in children with genetic propensity towards epilepsy and in adults who have suffered an insult to the brain, such as stroke, trauma, infection, or cancer. Seizures are often a symptom of an underlying pathology within the brain.

Knowing the nine broad categories of neurologic diseases will help you to organize your differential diagnosis as you take the exam. While understanding neuroanatomy in detail is not important, knowing the major regions and their functions will help. At least have an understanding about the difference between the central and peripheral nervous system, the functions of each lobe of the brain, and the organization of pathways within the spinal cord. Having this general understanding will help answer questions that include the interpretation of imaging, such as magnetic resonance imaging (MRI) and computed tomography (CT) scans. We have included examples of neuroimaging that tends to be high yield for the shelf exam. Spend extra time studying the areas that you may feel weakest in and supplement your reading with practice questions to solidify your knowledge.

Infectious, Immunologic, and Inflammatory Disorders

The most important topics to focus on are the different clinical signs and various causes of meningitis (Table 5.1). Be familiar with how to differentiate bacterial, viral, and fungal meningitis. The main factors that will help with this include the age of the patient, the cerebrospinal fluid (CSF) findings, and the comorbidities (such as HIV). Knowing the most common causes of meningitis within each of these categories will also help guide management. Otherwise, other inflammatory conditions within the nervous system are very buzzword heavy such as "triphasic spike and wave" on electroencephalogram (EEG) in CJD.

Acute Bacterial Meningitis

Age will help guide your differential diagnosis in terms of the cause of bacterial meningitis. For instance, knowing that Listeria is common in infants and the elderly means

TABLE 5.1 Causes (in Descending Order of Frequency) of Meningitis

Neonates (<6 months)	Children (6 months–6 years)	Adults (6–60 years)	Elders (>60 years.)
GBS	*Streptococcus pneumoniae*	*S. pneumonia*	*S. pneumoniae*
GNR (*Escherichia coli*)	*Neisseria meningitidis*	*N. meningitides*	GNR
Listeria monocytogenes	*Haemophilus influenza*	—	Listeria monocytogenes

GBS, Guillain-Barré syndrome.

that if a patient within these age groups presents with signs of meningitis you should make sure to add ampicillin to the empiric treatment regimen to cover Listeria. The most common cause of meningitis is *Streptococcus pneumoniae*, so always keep this high on the differential when considering the cause of meningitis. MRSA is a relatively rare cause of meningitis and is seen in situations where a foreign body has been found in the brain, such as after surgery. A lumbar puncture (LP) is usually a good idea to help differentiate the cause of meningitis, unless there is evidence for elevated intracranial pressure (ICP).

Buzz Words:

- Photophobia + altered mental status + nausea/ vomiting + seizures + Kernig (in supine position, passive extension of the knee from flexed elicits pain) and Brudzinski sign (flexion of neck causes spontaneous flexion at the hips)
- Petechiae, maculopapular rash, young adult → *Neisseria meningitides*

Clinical Presentation: The classic triad: headache, fever, and nuchal rigidity. Patients, such as college students in dorms or soldiers in military barracks, are at greater risk for meningitis due to living in close proximity with others. In an unimmunized child, put a stronger consideration to *Haemophilus influenzae*. Think of Listeria in elderly or pregnant patients that eat cheese or other unpasteurized dairy products.

PPx:

- Vaccines against *Neisseria meningitidis* and *H. influenzae* type B (HiB) for children and immunity-compromised adults (i.e., after splenectomy)
- Exposed contacts in *N. meningitidis* receive PPx with ceftriaxone, rifampin, or ciprofloxacin.

99 AR
Kernig Sign

99 AR
Brudzinski sign

MNEMONIC
- **K**ernig = **K**nee
- **B**rudzinski = **B**ottom (hips)

MoD:

- Bacteria from feces or skin → nasal cavity → meninges → infection and inflammation
- Most common in children and adults
- Bacteria from bloodstream → meninges → infection and inflammation

Dx:

1. Obtain CT before LP due to risk of brain herniation if any of the following are present: papilledema, history of intracranial mass, immunocompromise, or focal neurological deficits. In these patients, an LP creates negative pressure in the CSF, potentially causing brain herniation
2. LP (prior to starting antibiotics) -> increased opening pressure, increased PMNs, increased protein, decreased glucose
3. CSF and blood cultures

Tx/Mgmt:

1. Dexamethasone treatment is recommended to be given before the antibiotic treatment first to decrease inflammation → prevents neurologic sequelae (i.e., hearing loss, seizures, focal neurologic deficits, intellectual impairment)
   a. Steroid treatment should be given before or at the same time with antibiotics
2. Antibiotic regimen by age group
   a. Infants: ampicillin + 3rd generation cephalosporin *or* ampicillin + aminoglycoside
   b. Children and adults: 3rd generation cephalosporin, vancomycin
   c. Elderly and immunocompromised: 3rd generation cephalosporin, vancomycin, ampicillin
3. Supportive: analgesics, antipyretics, antiemetics

Acute Viral Meningitis (Aseptic Meningitis)

Buzz Words: Exanthema + coxsackievirus + herpangina + pleurodynia → echovirus aseptic meningitis

Clinical Presentation: A young child in the summer was recently diagnosed with hand-foot-mouth disease. He now complains of a headache and stiff neck, and has a fever.

Acute viral meningitis is mainly caused by enteroviruses, arboviruses, and herpesviruses. Arboviruses and some herpesviruses may present with encephalitis, which is an infection of the brain parenchyma (meningoencephalitis). The difference between meningitis and meningoencephalitis is that encephalitis almost always

CSF analysis in different types of meningitis

causes altered consciousness. The viral infection usually gets into the brain through the blood; therefore, it initially causes transient meningitis and then develops into encephalitis. Enteroviruses are the most common cause of viral meningitis, and most cases occur during the summer. Overall, viral meningitis is less common than bacterial meningitis.

PPx: Hand hygiene, mosquito repellent, polio vaccine

MoD:

- Viral infection outside of brain → hematogenous spread → meninges
- Feces → nasal cavity → meninges → infection and inflammation (e.g., polio)
- Retrograde spread along peripheral nerves → meninges (e.g., herpes)

Microbiology:

Most common cause of viral meningitis:

1. **Enteroviruses:** Coxsackievirus (most common), poliovirus, echovirus
2. **Herpesviruses:** Herpes simplex (HSV)1, HSV-2, varicella zoster virus, Epstein-Barr virus (EBV), cytomegalovirus (CMV)
3. **Arboviruses:** LaCrosse, West Nile, St. Louis, eastern equine encephalitis virus, western equine encephalitis virus
4. HIV

Dx:

1. LP
   - Normal/high opening pressure
   - Increased lymphocytes
   - Increased/normal protein
   - *Normal glucose* (most important for DD from bacterial infection)
   - If Xanthochromia (red blood cells [RBCs] in CSF) is present, it usually caused by HSV meningoencephalitis (destructed brain lesions in the temporal lobe)
2. CSF/blood culture with CSF polymerase chain reaction (PCR)

Tx/Mgmt:

1. Acyclovir
2. Ganciclovir/Foscarnet for suspected CMV
3. Supportive: analgesics, antipyretics, antiemetics

Fungal Meningitis

Buzz Words:

- Signs of pulmonary infection (e.g., productive cough) + spelunking + Ohio Valley + bats → histoplasmosis

- Southwestern US, Mexico, Central America + erythema nodosum → coccidiomycosis
- AIDS → *Cryptococcus*

Clinical Presentation: Chronic, increasingly severe headache, stiff neck, and, rarely, fever in a traveler to an endemic area. When a patient suffers from fungal meningitis, symptoms and signs usually develop for weeks or months (subacute or chronic). You should immediately be thinking that the patient is often an immunocompromised host. In particular, *Cryptococcus* is most prevalent in elderly patients with diabetes mellitus or in HIV patients with a CD4 count less than 100/μL. For those patients who are not immunocompromised, use the patient's location to guide you. For instance, histoplasmosis is prominent in the Ohio valley, whereas coccidiomycosis will predominate in California (southern)/Arizona/New Mexico (Southwestern states).

PPx: Cryptococcal antigen screening (blood test) in AIDS with CD4 <100 cells/μL

MoD: Inhalation of spores → pulmonary infection → hematogenous spread → meninges
- *Cryptococcus* sp. = spores in pigeon droppings, soil
- *Histoplasma capsulatum* = bat or bird droppings
- *Coccidia* sp. = spores in dust

Dx:
- LP
  - CSF-Latex agglutination for Cryptococcal antigen in LP
  - Eosinophilia in coccidiomycosis)
  - India Ink for Cryptococcus (Fig. 5.1)

Tx/Mgmt:
- Cryptococcus
  1. Amphotericin B
  2. Flucytosine & fluconazole
- Histoplasmosis, coccidiomycosis:
  1. Amphotericin B

Spirochetal Meningitis (Neurosyphilis)

Buzz Words: Argyll-Robertson pupil + ataxia + neuropathies + dementia + gummas, Romberg sign + neurogenic bladder + hydrocephalus + Charcot joint + aortic root aneurysm

Clinical Presentation: An adult with a history of sexually transmitted infections (STIs) complains of headache, confusion, and a stiff neck. It is rare for a patient with syphilis to develop meningitis, especially now with the widespread availability of penicillin. Nevertheless, it may still be tested. Use the other symptoms of the patient to guide your diagnosis. Look at clinical signs, such as

QUICK TIPS

Request an India Ink stain on the CSF smear slide to visualize Cryptococcus diagnosis - every time on the shelf

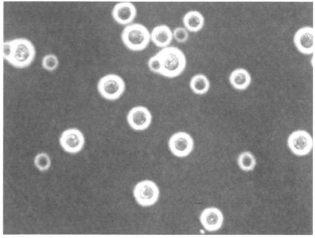

FIG. 5.1 India ink stain of cryptococcus. (From Microbewiki.kenyon.edu. https://microbewiki.kenyon.edu/images/thumb/1/14/Cneoindiaink.jpg/300px-Cneoindiaink.jpg.)

gummas (nodular, granulomatous skin lesion)—a sign of tertiary syphilis and pupils that accommodate but do not react (Argyll Robertson—AR pupils; "prostitute's pupils").

PPx: None

MoD: Untreated syphilis → meningitis after 1–2 years with hydrocephalus → potential stroke → paresis (10 years) with declining function → tabes dorsalis (20 years)

Dx:
1. LP
2. RPR/VDRL (nonspecific)
3. FTA-AB (more specific)
4. MRI/EEG

Tx/Mgmt: Penicillin G

Protozoal/Helminth Meningitis

Buzz Words: Food consumption + Asia, Hawaii + snails/slugs + LP with eosinophilia → acute eosinophilic meningitis

Clinical Presentation: Another rare form of meningitis (often with encephalitis—i.e., ameba eating the brain) that is low yield. The key finding here is the high eosinophilic count in the CSF. The majority of cases are caused by the nematode *Angiostrongylus cantonensis.* Patients are infected by ingesting larvae, which can penetrate the gastrointestinal (GI) tract and make its way to the meninges through hematogenous spread

PPx: None

MoD: Ingestion of larvae from *Angiostrongylus cantonensis, Baylisascaris procyonis, Gnathostoma spinigerum, Strongyloides stercoralis* → GI tract penetration → hematogenous spread → meninges

Dx: LP with culture

Tx/Mgmt: Supportive (do NOT give anthelminthic therapy)

Acute Encephalitis

Buzz Words: HSV-1 + temporal lobe lesion + headache + fever + seizures

Clinical Presentation: Encephalitis is defined as inflammation of the brain causing abnormal brain function. When it is associated with viral infection it is due to direct infection of neural cells, which ultimately causes inflammation and cellular destruction. The most common cause of viral encephalitis is herpesvirus. It is important to recognize that a patient with herpesvirus encephalitis is prone to seizures originating from the temporal lobe. Encephalitis differs from meningitis in that meningitis does not cause cerebral malfunction. In other words, a patient with meningitis may have headache, but they typically do not have altered mental status, focal neurologic deficits, or personality changes as seen in encephalitis. If a patient has features of both meningitis and encephalitis, it is called meningoencephalitis.

PPx: None

MoD: HSV-1 and arboviruses are the most common causes.

Dx:
1. LP
   a. Lymphocytosis and elevated RBCs
   b. CSF for HSV PCR
2. CT or MRI demonstrating lesions in the temporal lobe or orbitofrontal cortex

Tx/Mgmt: Intravenous (IV) acyclovir

Herpes encephalitis radiographs

Subacute Sclerosing Panencephalitis

Buzz Words: Myoclonus + ataxia + quadriplegia + spasticity

Clinical Presentation: Subacute sclerosing panencephalitis (SSPE) is an example of chronic (subacute) encephalitis because of untreated measles infection (extremely rare now). This is a devastating disease that is preventable with the measles, mumps, and rubella (MMR) vaccination. Keep this on your differential when you see "unvaccinated" in the question stem. A classic patient is an unvaccinated 17-year-old who was infected with measles when he was 7. He is now presenting with mood and personality changes, headaches, and seizures.

PPx: Vaccinate against measles.

MoD: Replication of untreated measles virus in neurons and glial cells → progressive neurodegenerative disease 7–10 years after measles infection.

Dx:

1. LP
2. Measles antibodies
3. MRI (increased T2 signal)
4. EEG (non-specific slowing, high voltage sharp slow waves 3–8 seconds)

Tx/Mgmt: No cure for this disease

- Detected early (extremely difficult): immunomodulators (interferon) and antivirals (isoprinosine and ribavirin) are suggested
- Detected late: supportive therapy (i.e., antiseizure therapy)

Prion Disease

Buzz Words: Startle myoclonus + rapidly altered mental status + memory impairment + triphasic spikes on EEG ("burst" EEG) + (positive CSF) 14-3-3 protein + elevated Tau protein in CSF

Clinical Presentation: Although this is a rare neurologic condition, it is extremely high yield for the exam due to its devastating course. Pay close attention to the buzzwords in this section; recognizing these will help you come to the diagnosis and save time when answering questions. A typical patient may be a 54-year-old pathologist who presents with altered mental status and random jerks and seizures.

PPx: Avoid infected human or animal tissue.

MoD: Mechanisms include prion protein caused by sporadic (unknown etiology), familial (mutated protein), or iatrogenic (tissue infection from someone else) mechanisms → misfolding of proteins in neurons causing misfolding of other proteins → death after the diagnosis can be from 6 months to 2 years.

99 AR

Video of CJD

Dx:

1. LP
   a. 14-3-3 protein
   b. Tau protein
2. MRI (DWI/T2-FLAIR signal changes in caudate and putamen and cortical ribbon sign)
3. EEG (periodic sharp wave complex)

Tx/Mgmt: Supportive care is the only treatment for prion disease

Opportunistic Central Nervous System Disorders Associated With Human Immunodeficiency Virus/ Acquired Immunodeficiency Syndrome

Buzz Words: Dementia + HIV + progressive neurologic deficit → progressive multifocal leukoencephalopathy (PML)

Clinical Presentation: John Cunningham (JC) virus is commonly found in the general population; but only immunocompromised patients, such as those with HIV/AIDS or patients who had received chemotherapies, are at risk of reactivation of the virus and then developing the brain infection. It is the *reactivation* of JC virus that can ultimately cause PML. The disease has an insidious progression and may cause multiple focal findings of the MRI depending on where the demyelination occurs within the central nervous system (CNS). There is no specific cure for this infection. In HIV/AIDS, optimization of highly active antiretroviral therapy (HAART) to control HIV is crucial to maintain immunity and avoid this infection. A typical patient may be a 36-year-old female with poorly controlled HIV infection and MS who complains of altered mental status, blurry vision, altered gait, and weakness of her left arm and leg.

PPx: None

MoD:
- Reactivation of JC virus in immunocompromised hosts → infection of oligodendrocytes → demyelination of CNS white matter
- Natalizumab (the treatment for MS) → increased risk of PML in immunocompromised patients (MS patients)

Dx:
1. LP (CSF PCR for JC virus)
2. MRI (white matter demyelination)
3. Brain biopsy is gold standard but not necessary for diagnosis

Tx/Mgmt:
1. Optimization of HIV therapy
2. Stop immunosuppressive therapy
3. Supportive

Immunologic and Inflammatory Disorders

Myasthenia gravis (MG) and MS are the highest yield topics within immunologic and inflammatory disorders. Both of these diseases can present in a variety of ways. In order to distinguish the clinical features, it helps to have a solid understanding of the disease mechanism. Treatment is important when it comes to these two topics because there are differences in acute and chronic treatment. Additionally, pay close attention to the dangerous aspects of the diseases, especially MG, because it can cause respiratory distress and ultimately death.

Myasthenia Gravis

Buzz Words: Ptosis with sustained upgaze or double vision + difficulty chewing + slurred speech + thymoma + worse with repeated activity (at end of day) or improves with rest

Clinical Presentation: A common topic tested on exams is differentiating between MG and Lambert Eaton syndrome, which are both neuromuscular junction disorders. MG is an autoimmune condition characterized by autoantibodies against the post-synaptic acetylcholine (cholinergic) nicotinic receptor whereas Lambert Eaton is caused by antibodies against pre-synaptic cholinergic receptors. In MG, the patient gets weaker with repetitive movements, whereas in Lambert Eaton the weakness often improves after repetitive movements are done to a degree. Finally, Lambert Eaton is often a paraneoplastic syndrome associated with small cell lung cancer, whereas MG is an autoimmune disorder often associated with thymomas. Bimodal distribution 20–30s then peaks again in 60–80s, females > males.

PPx: None

MoD: Autoimmune condition whereby antibodies attack the *post-synaptic* acetylcholine receptor of the NMJ → blocks the action of acetylcholine & downregulates the receptors → lower chance of nerve impulse at the NMJ → weakness with repeated use of muscle (Fig. 5.2)

Dx:

1. Physical exam
   - Weakness of facial muscles after sustained activity (ptosis with sustained upgaze)
   - Improved strength after period of rest
2. Serum anti-acetylcholine receptor antibodies
3. Increased strength with acetylcholinesterase inhibitors (neostigmine and ephodrium)
4. Electromyography (EMG)
   - Slow repetitive nerve stimulation (decremental response)
   - Single fiber electromyography showing increased jitter (most sensitive clinical test)
5. CT chest for thymoma

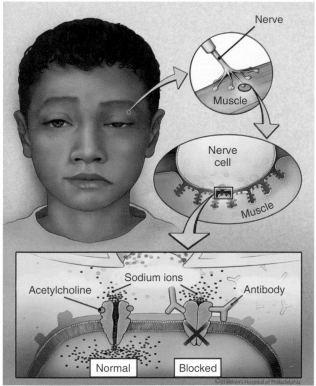

FIG. 5.2 Image of antibodies attacking post-synaptic Ach receptor. (From www.chop.edu. http://www.chop.edu/sites/default/files/myas thenia-gravis-neuromuscular-junction-illustration-773x949.png.)

Tx/Mgmt:
1. Symptomatic treatment with acetylcholinesterase inhibitors (neostigmine, pyridostigmine)
2. Chronic immune modulating agents (corticosteroids, azathioprine)
3. Rapid treatment for crisis (plasma exchange, IVIG, intubation/ventilation)
4. Thymectomy (may provide remission of symptoms in patients without thymoma but it must be performed in patients with a thymoma)

Lambert Eaton Syndrome

Buzz Words: Proximal > distal muscle weakness that improves with activity + autonomic dysfunction + ataxia

Clinical Presentation: Middle-aged adults presenting with progressive muscle weakness. May have underlying small cell lung cancer (most common) or Hodgkin lymphoma. Some patients have an autoimmune instead of a neoplastic cause.

QUICK TIPS

Myasthenia Gravis = Postsynaptic Ach, weakness worsens with movement versus Lambert Eaton = Presynaptic Calcium channels, weakness improves with movement

PPx: None

MoD: Antibodies against presynaptic voltage gated calcium channels → decreased Ca influx → release of Ach from presynaptic terminal

Dx:

1. Clinical presentation
2. Antibodies to voltage gated calcium channels
3. EMG

Tx/Mgmt:

1. Treat underlying malignancy
2. Acetylcholinesterase inhibitors (i.e., pyridostigmine)
3. IVIG
4. Prednisone
5. Supportive (respiratory failure may occur late in the course)

Multiple Sclerosis

Buzz Words: Optic neuritis + internuclear ophthalmoplegia + symptoms worsened by hot bath + Lhermitte sign

Clinical Presentation: A classic patient: a 15- to 45-year-old, female > male, presents with loss of vision in her left eye for 3 weeks after a viral illness, but the vision loss resolved. Six months later, she had weakness in her left leg for several weeks, which also resolved.

MS can present in a variety of ways but understanding the underlying disease process and the clinical course (e.g., relapsing—remitting pattern) help to make sense of the clinical presentation. Recognizing the MRI of a patient with MS is high yield for the shelf exam. Additionally, pay close attention to treatment modalities in terms of which will shorten the duration of an attack (steroids) versus those that decrease the number of future attacks (immune modulating therapy). Keep this high on the differential, especially if the patient is a young adult presenting with multiple neurologic findings separated by space (different locations of lesions in the CNS) and time (different onset times of separated attacks).

PPx: None

MoD: Combination of genetics + environment → T cell mediated autoimmune destruction of oligodendrocytes, demyelination within CNS, axonal degeneration → lesions within the brain and spinal cord

Dx:

1. History and physical exam: neurologic deficits separated by space and time (lesions in separate white matter regions that happened at different times)

QUICK TIPS

MS is more common in women and in people who live farther away from the equator

QUICK TIPS

Lhermitte's sign = electrical sensation down back and limbs when neck is flexed

2. MRI: T2 hyperintense periventricular white matter lesions (lesions also present in corpus callosum, cerebellar peduncles; Fig. 5.3)
3. LP: CSF with oligoclonal bands – different from the serum pattern. Increased CSF IgG synthesis not always found) + elevated CSF protein (during acute attack).

Tx/Mgmt:

1. Acute: steroids (shorten duration of symptoms) and plasmapheresis
2. Chronic immune modulating therapy: injectable medicines – interferon (IFN)-1alpha, IFN-1beta (decrease the rate of relapses), glatiramer (peptides mimic the basic myelin protein; modulating the immune reactivity), natalizumab (antibody against alpha 4-integrins), oral medicines (i.e., fingolimod), and others
3. Symptomatic therapy: baclofen for spasticity, anticholinergics for urinary urgency, antidepressants for depression

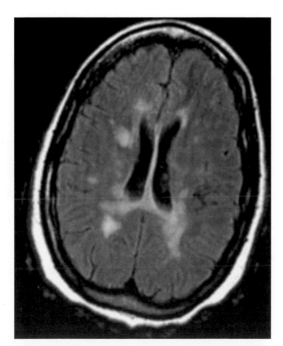

FIG. 5.3 Dawson's fingers = demyelinated plaques that spread outward from the corpus callosum (seen on magnetic resonance imaging). (From Howard J, Trevick S, Younger D: Epidemiology of multiple sclerosis. *Neurol Clin* 34(4):919–939, 2016.)

Internuclear Ophthalmoplegia

Buzz Words: Loss of eye adduction on contralateral lateral gaze + nystagmus of abducting eye → (Fig. 5.4).

Clinical Presentation: In a young adult think MS; in an elderly adult think ischemic infarction. Patients may have double vision with eye movements.

PPx: None

MoD: Damage to the medial longitudinal fasciculus (usually 2/2 MS, stroke)→ inability of CN VI to communicate with CN III → activation of CN VI causes ipsilateral lateral rectus stimulation but contralateral CN III does not stimulate medial rectus → nystagmus of abducting eye, inability of contralateral eye to abduct

Dx:

1. Extraocular muscle exam
2. MRI to rule out MS

Tx/Mgmt:

1. Treat underlying cause
2. Patching for symptomatic relief of diplopia

INO explanation

Optic Neuritis

Buzz Words: Difficulty distinguishing **colors** + decreased pupil reactivity + central scotoma ± papillitis

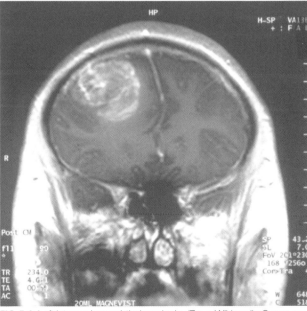

FIG. 5.4 Left internuclear ophthalmoplegia. (From Wikimedia Commons. Used under [GFDL (http://www.gnu.org/copyleft/fdl.html) or CC-BY-SA-3.0 (http://creativecommons.org/licenses/by-sa/3.0/)]. Used under the Creative Commons Attribution-Share Alike 3.0 Unported license.)

Clinical Presentation: A 32-year-old female with MS presents with **painful** loss of vision over hours to days.

PPx: None

MoD: Demyelination of white matter within the optic nerve

Dx:

1. Clinical presentation
2. MRI demonstrating demyelination
3. Visual evoked potentials showing delayed conduction of optic nerve
4. LP may show elevated protein

Tx/Mgmt:

1. IV methylprednisone
2. MS management (e.g., IFN-beta) if MRI demonstrates evidence of demyelination

Transverse Myelitis

Buzz Words: Urinary retention + sensory level deficit + MRI signal changes of the spinal cord (across segments of cervical vs. thoracic vs. lumbar spinal cord).

Clinical Presentation: Not as high yield of a topic compared to MS and myasthenia, but it is closely correlated with MS. If a patient presents with what looks like MS, but also has lesions within the spinal cord, then immediately think of transverse myelitis. A typical patient may be a 20-year-old female with rapid onset motor, sensory, and/or autonomic dysfunction.

PPx: None

MoD: Autoimmune driven demyelination of the white matter within the spinal cord—usually preceded by viral infection or commonly in the setting of MS

Dx:

1. History/physical (acute onset motor, sensory, autonomic dysfunction)
2. MRI (focal demyelination in spinal cord)
3. LP (CSF shows pleocytosis and sometimes increased protein)

Tx/Mgmt:

1. High dose steroids
2. Plasmaphoresis if refractory to steroids

Central Nervous System Neoplasms

Never underestimate neoplasms as they can present in a variety of ways in a wide age range. There is less emphasis on histology and more emphasis on clinical features and imaging findings when it comes to CNS neoplasms on the shelf exam. The skull contains a limited small space and is

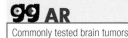

occupied by brain parenchyma, vessels/blood, and CSF. Thus, when a tumor is present in the brain it causes increased ICP, so think of tumors when a patient presents with severe headache with nausea, vomiting, and papilledema.

Additionally, tumors can destroy the cortices of the brain, which can lead to seizures.

Keep in mind that metastatic brain tumors are the most common type of brain tumors; so think of an extracranial primary source when a patient has a tumor within the brain. Also remember the common neoplasms that metastasize to the brain (melanoma, breast, renal cell carcinoma [RCC], lung, colon). Primary tumors, though less common than metastatic tumors, still come up on the shelf exam. The best way to decide which tumor is the culprit is to pay attention to the location (supratentorial, posterior fossa, etc.) and the patient.

Malignant

The most commonly tested malignant tumor is the GBM. The prognosis is very poor for these patients, which is why it is critical to recognize and diagnose this type of neoplasm. If you see an MRI with a giant tumor crossing the corpus callosum think GBM.

Glioblastoma Multiforme
Buzz Words: Butterfly (crosses corpus callosum) + personality changes (involving bilateral prefrontal lobes) + GFAP + astrocyte stain → GBM (Fig. 5.5)

Clinical Presentation: A middle-aged adult with a headache (specifically a headache that often occurs right after waking up in the morning), sudden focal seizures, subacute focal neurologic deficit (i.e., weakness, numbness). Patient may also have signs/symptoms if elevated ICP (i.e., headache worse when leaning forward, papilledema, nausea, vomiting, etc.)

PPx: None

MoD: Arises from astrocytes (grade IV astrocytoma) → spreads along the white matter

Dx:
1. Head MRI
2. Brain biopsy (pseudopalisading cells, necrosis, hemorrhage)

Tx: Surgery and chemoradiation

Pilocytic Astrocytoma
Buzz Words: Benign + posterior fossa (cerebellum) + GFAP positive

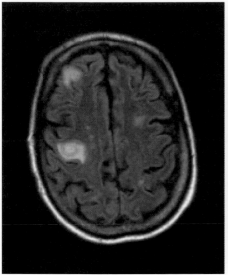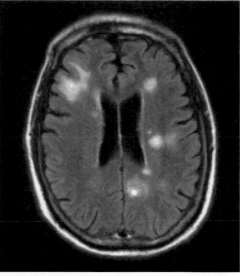

FIG. 5.5 Glioblastoma multiforme magnetic resonance imaging "butterfly" lesion. (From Wikimedia Commons. https://commons.wikimedia.org/wiki/Glioblastoma#/media/File:Glioblastoma_-_MR_coronal_ with_contrast.jpg. By Christaras A from anonymized patient MR. [GFDL (http://www.gnu.org/copyleft/ fdl.html), CC-BY-SA-3.0 (http://creativecommons.org/licenses/by-sa/3.0/) or CC BY 2.5 (http://creative commons.org/licenses/by/2.5)].)

Clinical Presentation: Pilocytic—meaning "fiber-like cells" under the microscope; pilocytic astrocytoma often forms cyst component in the tumor. It can occur in any region of the brain. However, when it occurs in the posterior fossa in children, it will need to be differentiated from medulloblastoma.

PPx: None

MoD: Arises from astrocytes (grade I astrocytoma)

Dx:
1. Head MRI/CT
2. Brain biopsy (Eosinophilic & corkscrew fibers)

Tx:
1. Surgery
2. Chemoradiation

Medulloblastoma

Buzz Words: (Most commonly growing in the posterior fossa!) Cerebellar mass + hydrocephalus + drop metastases to spinal cord + most common malignant brain tumor in children and adolescents

Clinical Presentation: Children and adolescents presenting with headache, signs/symptoms of elevated ICP, and ataxia

PPx: None

MoD: Arises from neuroectodermal cells → grows rapidly → compresses 4th ventricle → hydrocephalus

Dx:
1. Head MRI/CT
2. Brain biopsy (Homer-Wright rosettes)

Tx: Radiation, surgery, chemotherapy

Primary Central Nervous System Lymphoma

Buzz Words: Solitary ring-enhancing lesion + malignant + immunocompromised

Clinical Presentation: An immunocompromised patient aged 25–65 presents with focal neurologic deficits, a change in personality, or signs of elevated ICP

PPx: Optimize immune response

MoD: High-grade non-Hodgkin B-cell lymphoma in immunocompromised patients; EBV may be the cause of oncogenesis

Dx:
1. Brain MRI/CT
2. Brain biopsy

Tx: Chemoradiation

Metastatic

Buzz Words: Cancer cells first reside at gray/white junction of the cortices then they grow larger in size + headache + cancer risk factors

Clinical Presentation: Patients with a history of cancer, particularly lung, melanoma (high risk of bleeding), renal clear cell carcinoma, breast, or colon. Present with signs/symptoms of elevated ICP, focal neurologic deficits, headache, and/or seizures.

PPx: N/A

MoD: Malignant cells cross the blood-brain barrier → grow in the gray/white junction (Fig. 5.6)

Dx:
1. MRI with contrast
2. Brain biopsy

Tx: Radiation, surgery, chemotherapy

Benign

Differentiating between benign and malignant brain tumors is very high yield for the medicine shelf. For the benign tumors, recognize the buzz words and clinical presentation, and be familiar with the diagnostic steps, although most diagnoses are made through imaging.

Meningioma

Buzz Words: Symptoms depend on location of lesion; headache, focal weakness, Babinski sign + streak and

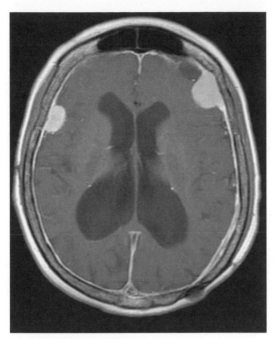

FIG. 5.6 Magnetic resonance imaging metastatic brain tumors at the gray–white junction. (From http://www.radiologytoday.net/onthecase/images/case/january_2011_fig4.jpg.)

tail (dural attachment) of the enhanced mass on MRI or CT+ seizure (Fig. 5.7)

Clinical Presentation: A 65-year-old patient (female > male) with a history of radiation exposure or NF2 presents with focal neurologic deficits.

PPx: Avoid ionizing radiation

MoD: Derived from meningothelial cells of dura matter; extracranial

Dx:

1. Brain MRI
2. Biopsy (psammoma bodies)

Tx/Mgmt: Surgery ± radiation

Pituitary Adenoma

Buzz Words: Bilateral temporal hemianopsia (no peripheral vision OR car accident because patient didn't see oncoming car)

Clinical Presentation: A patient presents with a chief complaint of a headache and difficulty with peripheral vision (bilateral hemianopsia).

Pituitary adenomas cause effects due to increased levels or decreased levels of hormones. Most commonly, pituitary adenomas secrete excess levels of

Cortical vascular territories

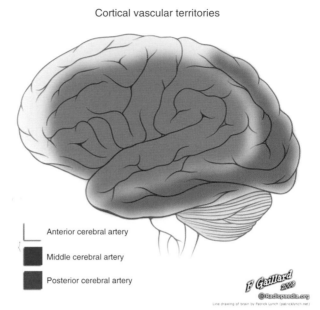

Anterior cerebral artery

Middle cerebral artery

Posterior cerebral artery

FIG. 5.7 Magnetic resonance imaging of radiation-induced meningioma. (From http://radiopaedia.org/cases/meningpostrtx2. Case courtesy of A. Prof Frank Gaillard, Radiopaedia.org, rID: 2629.)

prolactin. For example, galactorrhea may occur with prolactinomas due to elevated prolactin. Be aware that craniopharyngiomas may present in a similar manner with compressive symptoms but craniopharyngiomas are derived from embryonic tissues. Craniopharyngiomas have the additional finding of calcifications within the lesion.

If the adenoma actively secretes prolactin then the patient may have hypogonadism or lactation. If adenoma secretes growth hormone the patient will have signs/symptoms of acromegaly (i.e., deepening of voice, enlargement of body parts). MEN1 syndrome.

PPx: None

MoD: Tumor cells from pituitary cells (prolactin, growth hormone, etc.) may compress the optic chiasm causing bilateral hemianopsia.

Dx:

1. Head MRI/CT
2. Elevated serum prolactin level

Tx/Mgmt: Trans-sphenoidal surgery if lesion is large enough to cause visual symptoms ± radiation

Cerebrovascular Disease

Cerebrovascular disease is a broad term that describes diseases of the arteries or veins that affect the brain. The highest yield topic within cerebrovascular disease is acute stroke. In the hospital localization of lesions is important, whereas the shelf exam stresses the cause of stroke and management. It is still vital to understand general neuroanatomy when considering cerebrovascular disease. Understand that language is localized to the dominant hemisphere (usually the left) and that certain clinical syndromes can occur depending upon vascular lesions localized in specific brain regions. For instance, Wernicke aphasia is an aphasia syndrome caused by left-side middle cerebral artery (MCA) occlusion cutting off blood supply to the posterior portion of the superior temporal gyrus. Broca aphasia, on the other hand, is an aphasia due to left-side MCA occlusion cutting off blood supply to the posterior part of the inferior frontal gyrus. Understand the general neuroanatomy but do not get too caught up with the details.

Stroke symptoms by location

Cerebral Artery Occlusion/Infarction

Ischemic stroke can be further subdivided into different categories: large vessel, small vessel, and embolic. Large vessel strokes are usually due to a thrombus forming in a major artery (carotid arteries, vertebral arteries, basilar arteries, and their main branches—MCA, anterior cerebral artery [ACA], or posterior cerebral artery [PCA]). These cause local damage within areas of the brain, ultimately causing major neurologic deficits (e.g., aphasia, hemiparesis, visual field cut). Large vessel disease can be treated with the thrombolytic procedure, and/or anti-thrombolytic therapies.

Small vessel (lacunar) strokes are due to lipohyalinosis of penetrating arterioles of the brain. The risk factors of the lacunar ischemic stroke include longstanding hypertension, diabetes, smoking, and hyperlipidemia. Small vessel strokes often present with hemiparesis, sensory abnormalities, but lack major cortical signs, such as aphasia and neglect. Treating these underlying risk factors prevents further small vessel disease from evolving. Finally, embolic strokes are due to a clot traveling most commonly from the cardiac source, such as thrombi forming in left atrium due to AF or in the left ventricle due to acute cardiac infarction. Emboli can cause symptoms similar to that of a large vessel stroke, but the etiology of the stroke is different from large vessel disease. The embolic strokes are often treated by an anticoagulation drug, such as warfarin.

Buzz Words:

Large vessel
- **MCA:** Contralateral upper limb/facial paralysis/ sensory loss + Wernicke/Broca aphasia (left hemisphere) or hemineglect (right hemisphere)
- **ACA:** Contralateral leg paralysis/sensory loss+ abulia
- **PCA:** Homonymous hemianopia (c/l to lesion) ± thalamic aphasia/hemiparesis/sensory loss (Fig. 5.8)

Small vessel (lacunar stroke)
- **Pure motor hemiparesis:** contralateral face, arm, leg weakness *without* sensory deficits → infarct of internal capsule, corona radiata OR ventral pons OR cerebral peduncle
- **Pure sensory:** Contralateral sensory of body, face, limbs *without* motor symptoms→ VPL nucleus of thalamus infarct
- **Mixed motor + sensory**: Combination of the previous two clinical presentations
- **Ataxic hemiparesis:** Contralateral leg >arm weakness + ataxia → infarct of posterior limb internal capsule and thalamus OR ventral pons (Fig. 5.9)
- **Clumsy hand dysarthria:** Contralateral hand weakness + dysarthria

PPx:
1. Control hypertension and diabetes.
2. Smoking cessation.
3. Statins for hyperlipidemia.
4. Regular exercise and weight control.
5. Antiplatelet agents

MoD:
- Thrombotic: clot forms at the site of infarction due to vessel damage (usually 2/2 to atherosclerosis)
- Embolic: Embolus from a distal site travels to the brain (such as from atrial fibrillation)
- Hypoxic: global hypoxia due to hypoperfusion (such as shock caused by a myocardial infarction)
- Small vessel: lipohyalinosis of small vessels (such as lenticulostriates) → lacunar strokes

Dx:
1. Non-contrast CT to rule out hemorrhagic stroke
2. MRI

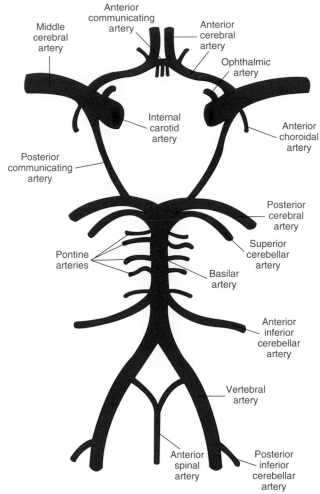

FIG. 5.8 Anterior cerebral artery, middle cerebral artery, posterior cerebral artery territories. (From https://radiopaedia.org/articles/cerebral-vascular-territories.)

3. Carotid duplex scan/ultrasound
4. Echo to look for cardiac thrombus
5. Electrocardiogram (EKG) to rule out atrial fibrillation as the cause

Tx/Mgmt:
- If less than 4.5 hours since symptom onset → tissue plasminogen activator (tPA)
- If less than 6–8 hours = interventional thrombectomy procedures
- For acute ischemic stroke or TIA, start aspirin within 48 hours. If the patient had IV or intra-arterial thrombolytic therapy start aspirin 24 hours after thrombolytic therapy

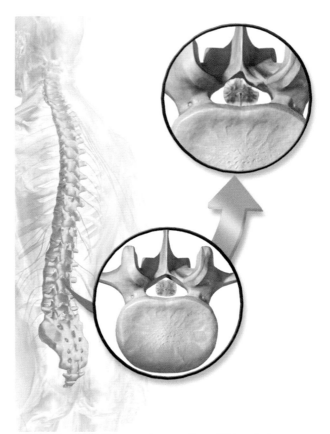

FIG. 5.9 Circle of Willis on angiogram. (From Wikimedia Commons. https://commons.wikimedia.org/wiki/File:Circle_of_Willis_en.svg. Public Domain.)

- For AF, start anticoagulation if it is safe to do so
- Secondary prevention of modifiable risk factors

Transient Ischemic Attack

Buzz Words: Sudden onset "curtain falling down" monocular vision loss = amaurosis fugax

Clinical Presentation: A 50-year-old man, with a history of smoking, atrial fibrillation, hypertension, and diabetes, complains of a sudden onset of left-sided weakness, which completely resolved spontaneously after 30 minutes.

PPx: Manage modifiable risk factors.

MoD: Usually embolic, but may also be thrombotic or due to transient hypotension→ block in cerebral blood flow resolves before the onset of permanent infarction. Amaurosis fugax is due to internal carotid artery (ICA) thrombosis or embolism.

Dx:
1. Non-contrast CT to rule out hemorrhagic stroke
2. MRI
3. Carotid duplex scan/ultrasound or CT angiography (CTA) or MRI of head/neck
4. Echo to look for cardiac thrombus
5. Holter EKG monitoring to investigate atrial fibrillation as the cause

Tx/Mgmt:
1. Antiplatelets (aspirin or clopidogrel) or anticoagulants (warfarin)
2. Secondary prevention of modifiable risk factors

Subarachnoid Hemorrhage (Non-Traumatic)

Buzz Words: "Worst headache of my life" + CSF with (w/) xanthochromia

Clinical Presentation: A 40-year-old woman presents with a onset "thunderclap" headache described as the "worst headache of my life." May have meningismus or lower back pain. Risk factors include: history of an aneurysm, trauma, tobacco use, hypertension, arteriovenous malformations (AVMs), amyloid angiopathy, recreational drug use (cocaine). Complications from the bleed include **rebleed**, seizures, increased ICP, and hydrocephalus.

PPx: HTN management

MoD: Rupture of berry aneurysm usually at bifurcation points within Circle of Willis

Dx:
1. Non-contrast CT (blood in basal cisterns)
2. LP w/ xanthochromia (especially if CT scan is negative but still suspecting subarachnoid hemorrhage (SAH)
3. Cerebral four-vessel angiogram to localize aneurysm

Tx/Mgmt:
1. Control blood pressure (BP)
2. Surgical intervention of aneurysm (clipping or coiling)
3. Nimodipine (calcium channel blocker) to prevent future vascular spasm
4. Ventriculostomy for developing hydrocephalus

Major Artery Stenosis/Dissection

Atherosclerosis is a major risk factor for arterial stenosis due to long-term inflammation and thrombus formation. Eventually, atherosclerosis can cause arterial stenosis, compromising blood flow to a certain area.

MNEMONIC

WHOML - "Worst headache of my life" = SAH

QUICK TIPS

Complications of SAH: Rebleed, vasospasm, elevated ICP, seizures, hyponatremia

QUICK TIPS

Vertebral artery dissection similar to carotid artery plus posterior circulation symptoms such as vertigo but with severe pain in the back of neck.

Carotid Artery Dissection

Buzz Words: Unilateral Horner syndrome + severe one-side head and neck radiating pain

Clinical Presentation: A 30-year-old man with Marfan's is playing football when he suddenly gets severe one-sided pain radiating across his head and neck on the right. His right eyelid is drooping and his right pupil is unusually constricted.

PPx: None

MoD: Trauma → intima tear → hemorrhage between intima and media → blockage and narrowing of lumen

Dx:

1. CT/MRI (rule out stroke) and CTA/MR angiography (MRA) (visualize vessels)
2. Carotid duplex good for screening but not as sensitive/specific as vascular imaging

Tx/Mgmt: Heparin bridge to warfarin and IR intervention

Subclavian Steal Syndrome

Buzz Words: Exercise-induced pain in arm + >15 mm Hg difference in systolic BP between the affected arm and the unaffected arm

Clinical Presentation: This is low yield for the medicine shelf, but is very much related to many of the cerebrovascular pathologies. Recognize that here the patient will have symptoms in one arm when exercising, which will be associated with headache or vertigo. Risk factors include: atherosclerosis (most common comorbidity), Takayasu arteritis, and thoracic outlet compression syndrome. Patients may present with arm claudication (paresthesia, cold, pale, pain) and vertebrobasilar symptoms (vertigo, dysphagia, headache, diplopia).

PPx: None

MoD: Stenosis of one-side subclavian artery → blood is "stolen" (shunting) from the ipsilateral vertebral artery to supply the arm when exercising → decreased perfusion to posterior fossa + claudication symptoms

Dx:

1. Clinical presentation
2. BP difference between arms

Tx/Mgmt: Surgical bypass

99 AR

Mechanism of subclavian steal syndrome

Vascular Dementia

Buzz Words: Stepwise decline in cognitive function; memory loss + focal deficits over time

Clinical Presentation: The patient has usually experienced multiple ischemic strokes affecting both hemispheres over the years. As a result, the cognitive function is "step-wisely" impaired by each stroke, and eventually the ability to handle daily living activities gradually declines.

PPx: Control stroke risk factors

MoD: Most commonly thrombosis or embolism of large or small arteries

Dx:

1. MRI
2. CT
3. Neuropsychological assessment

Tx/Mgmt:

1. Stroke prevention
2. Anticholinesterase inhibitor therapy

Venous Sinus Thrombosis

Buzz Words: Hypercoagulable state (pregnancy, hormone supplements, malignancy, polycythemia) + woman taking OCPs + focal neurologic sign → venous sinus thrombosis

Clinical Presentation: A 30- to 50-year-old patient (female > male) presents with headache, seizures, and left hemiparesis. Risk factors include oral contraceptives, pregnancy, hormone replacement therapy, malignancy (with hypercoagulable state), and the post-partum period.

PPx: Anticoagulation

MoD: Thrombosis → increased venous pressure → ruptured veins causing hemorrhage in brain.

Dx:

1. MR-venogram
2. Hypercoagulable work-up

Tx/Mgmt: Heparin bridge to warfarin

Arterio-Venous Malformation

Buzz Words: Headache + seizure + intracranial hypertension + focal deficit → AVM rupture

PPx: None

MoD: Congenital development of direct arterial to venous connection without capillaries

Dx:

1. Noncontrast CT for acute bleed
2. MRI with contrast to visualize AVM

Tx/Mgmt:

1. Surgery depending on location and vascular complexity
2. Symptomatic treatments, such as anti-seizure treatment

99 AR

Cerebral AV malformations overview

Disorders Relating to Spine, Spinal Cord, Spinal Nerve Roots

Spinal cord lesions cause lower motor neuron (LMN) symptoms (weakness, hyporeflexia, fasciculation) due to damage to motor neurons in the anterior horn. Injury to the pyramidal tract in the brain stem and motor cortex can cause upper motor neuron symptoms (hyperreflexia, Positive Babinski reflex, spasticity).

Both spinal cord and peripheral nerve lesions can cause weakness; but the sensory deficits are different between cord lesions and peripheral nerve lesions. So neurologic signs and symptoms can help guide your diagnosis. Many spinal cord injuries and conditions, such as cauda equine and conus medullaris syndrome, are emergencies so have a low threshold to send these patients for surgical evaluation.

Cauda Equina Syndrome

Buzz Words: Decreased patellar and Achilles reflex + bladder dysfunction + saddle anesthesia

Clinical Presentation: A 60-year-old patient with a history of prostate cancer presents with severe lower back pain radiating down only the left leg, and left leg weakness.

PPx: None

MoD: Trauma, compression by mass or abscess, stenosis, disc herniation → compression of lumbosacral spinal nerve roots.

Dx: MRI

Tx/Mgmt: Neurosurgical **emergency** → decompression

Conus Medullaris Syndrome

Buzz Words: Impotence + sudden onset low back pain and NOT legs + urinary retention + Babinski + sensory loss in S3-S5 distribution→ pure Conus medullaris syndrome does not cause any leg weakness and has preserved ankle jerks (Table 5.2).

Clinical Presentation:
- Sudden onset of symmetric low back pain + urinary retention + hyperreflexia
- Risk factors: intervertebral disc herniation, IV drug user (abscess formation), lumbar spondylosis

PPx: None

MoD: Spinal fracture, mass, disc herniation at L2 vertebral level.

Dx: MRI

Tx/Mgmt: Neurosurgical EMERGENCY → decompression

TABLE 5.2 Difference Between Cauda Equine and Conus Medullaris Syndrome

	Cauda Equina	Conus Medullaris
Vertebral Level	L2–S3 roots	L1–L2 cord & roots
Presentation	Gradual pain usually unilateral	Sudden bilateral pain
Motor	Asymmetric prominent weakness	Symmetric weakness
Reflexes	Areflexic	Hyperreflexic or normal
Sensory	Saddle anesthesia	Perineal anesthesia
Impotence	Less often	Often

Spinal Cord Compression

Buzz Words:
- Lower back pain + pain at night + weight loss → malignancy of back
- Lower back pain + pain at night + fever + IVDA → epidural abscess usually at T7–T10

Clinical Presentation: There are many processes that can cause compression of the spinal cord. On the medicine shelf, they will integrate both medicine and neurology by giving the presentation of a patient with neurologic symptoms secondary to a metastatic lesion. Be familiar with the types of cancer that spread to the vertebrae, which can cause focal findings. Additionally, IV drug use is a commonly tested topic, so if a patient has a history of IV drug use and has focal findings, then immediately consider using antibiotics and taking the patient to surgery to debride the abscess. For visualization, epidural spinal abscesses are best seen using MRI.

PPx: None

MoD: Tumors metastasize to the vertebra.
- Prostate cancer → osteoblastic metastases
- Multiple myeloma → osteolytic lesions
- Breast cancer → osteoblastic or osteolytic lesions
- IV drug abuse → introduction of bacteria into blood → hematogenous spread of bacteria to epidural space → abscess

Dx:
1. X-ray
2. MRI

Tx/Mgmt:
1. Prednisone to relieve swelling
2. Treat if primary cancer (surgery, chemoradiation)
3. If infectious, steroids + antibiotics + surgery for debridement of abscess

Spinal Stenosis (Lumbar)

Buzz Words: Pain improves by flexing at the hips and leaning forward (pushing a grocery cart) + weakness/numbness of legs → lumbar stenosis

Clinical Presentation: Spinal stenosis commonly presents with lower back and leg pain with walking, hence the term "pseudoclaudication" (Fig. 5.10). This may be confused with (vascular) claudication of the lower legs because vascular disease will also cause leg pain with exercise. The key distinguishing feature is that spinal stenosis resolves with flexion of the back. So, if a patient has less pain walking uphill or pushing a shopping cart, this condition should be high on your differential.

A typical patient may be an 80-year-old man with degenerative arthritis (or a 50-year-old obese patient) who complains of lower back pain that worsens with activity and radiates down bilateral legs.

PPx: None

MoD: Degeneration of joints with age → narrowing of spinal canal → compression of nerve roots

Dx: MRI of spine

Tx/Mgmt:
1. Nonsteroidal antiinflammatory drugs (NSAIDs)
2. Cortisone injections
3. Surgical laminectomy

Spinal Artery Thrombosis/Embolus/Infarct

Buzz Words: Weakness in legs, loss of pain/temp bilaterally below lesion + **preserved** proprioception/vibration (spare dorsal column) ± incontinence → Anterior cord syndrome.

Clinical Presentation: Vascular compromise of the spine presents with different symptoms depending on the region within the spine that is compromised. Anterior spinal artery occlusion causes ischemia of the anterior horn (motor), and the lateral spinothalamic tract (pain/temperature), but spares the dorsal column (vibration, touch, proprioception). Posterior spinal artery occlusion leads to posterior cord syndrome, which is very rare compared to anterior cord syndrome. Deficits include vibration, loss of proprioception, and fine touch due to damage to the dorsal column.

Central cord syndrome is usually not due to a vascular compromise but rather a hyperextension injury, such as an elderly person in a car accident or from syringomyelia. Damage to the central part of the spinal cord affects the bilateral spinothalamic tract fibers, which causes pain and temperature sensation deficits bilaterally in the distribution of the cord level that is affected. Syringomyelia classically causes "cape-like"

QUICK TIPS

Note that cervical spine stenosis will NOT present with these same symptoms.

sensory deficits, meaning loss of pain and temperature around the shoulders and upper arms (cervical cord syringomyelia).

   One risk factor to remember: surgery to fix aortic aneurysm (specifically if the patient gets hypotensive during surgery, experiences excessive bleeding, or is elderly).

PPx: None

MoD: Atherosclerosis, vasculitis, compression, hypotension, or injury of the artery (usually during AAA repair)

Dx: MRI (rule out cauda equina syndrome, compression, transverse myelitis)

Tx/Mgmt:

- If compressive, surgery to decompress
- If infectious → antibiotics, surgery, steroids to reduce inflammation

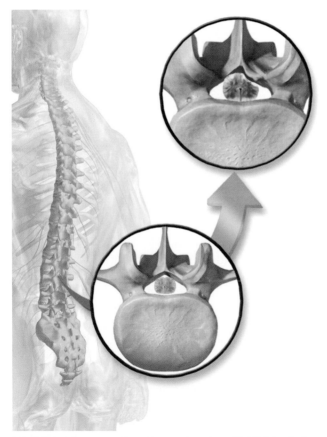

FIG. 5.10 Lumbar magnetic resonance imaging with L3–L4 spinal stenosis 2/2 disc herniation. (From Wikimedia Commons. By Blausen.com staff. "Blausen gallery 2014". Wikiversity Journal of Medicine. http://dx.doi.org/10.15347/wjm/2014.010. ISSN 20018762. [Own work.] Used under the Creative Commons Attribution 3.0 Unported License.)

Cranial and Peripheral Nerve Disorders

As discussed previously in the spinal cord disorders section, it is important to differentiate upper motor neuron symptoms from LMN symptoms. Peripheral nerve disorders fall in the category of LMN disorders, which presents as weakness, fasciculations, and areflexia. In order to understand the disease processes, one must first remember the normal anatomy of peripheral nerves and their functions. For instance, knowing that the ulnar nerve supplies sensory innervation to the 4th and 5th digits, whereas the median nerve supplies the 1st, 2nd, and 3rd digits, will help you recognize where the lesion is when a patient presents with sensory abnormalities of the hand. Try to focus on the buzz words in this section and how to manage common disorders, such as carpal tunnel syndrome.

Cranial Nerve Injuries/Disorders

Cranial nerve findings may be seen in both stroke (due to damage to the nerve fibers still traveling in the brain stem [intra-axial lesion]) and discrete injury to nerves outside of the brain stem (extra-axial lesion). In order to differentiate the etiology of cranial nerve findings, pay attention to the rest of the clinical presentation. For example, to differentiate the central type of facial palsy from the peripheral type facial palsy, the accompanying symptoms and signs are crucial clues.

Facial Nerve Palsy (Peripheral Type)

Buzz Words:
- **Bell palsy**: Acute onset paralysis of face (Fig. 5.11)
- **LMN lesion** (destruction of CN VII nucleus or CN VII): gradual paralysis of face + hyperacusis + **loss of taste to anterior 2/3 of tongue**
- Upper motor neuron (UMN) lesion (lesion of face in the cortex or fibers leading to the facial nucleus in the pons): lower facial weakness + sparing of forehead

Clinical Presentation: Bell palsy is the peripheral type of facial nerve palsy that usually resolves within weeks depending on the etiology. Patients present with gradual or acute paralysis of upper and lower muscles of facial expression. Risk factors include: a history of infection (Lyme, herpes, HIV, sarcoidosis), pregnancy (increased risk), diabetes (increased risk)

PPx: None

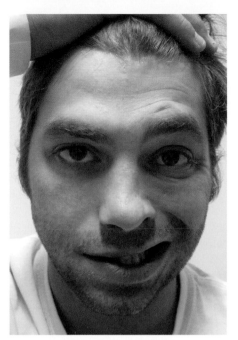

FIG. 5.11 Bell palsy versus supranuclear lesion. (From Wikimedia Commons. https://commons.wikimedia.org/wiki/File:Bellspalsy.J PG By James Heilman, MD. Used under the Creative Commons Attribution Share Alike 3.0 Unported license.)

MoD:
- Lyme disease, HSV, herpes zoster, HIV/AIDS, sarcoidosis, tumors, diabetes → Bell palsy
- Tumor (e.g., parotid) compressing CNII → LMN facial palsy
- Stroke in the cortex or subcortical region that involves fibers innervating the face → UMN lesion

Dx: Clinical diagnosis, but etiology can be distinguished by Lyme titer, CXR and serum angiotensin-converting enzyme (ACE) levels to rule out sarcoidosis, HIV testing

Tx/Mgmt:
1. Steroids (for all causes except for Lyme)
2. Acyclovir (80% patients have a full recovery)
3. Antibiotics for Lyme disease
4. Eye drops and eye patch to prevent corneal abrasions

Vestibular Neuritis (CN VIII Disease)

Buzz Words: Acute onset vertigo + **no hearing deficits** + nystagmus

Clinical Presentation: An adult with a recent viral infection presents with acute onset vertigo + nausea, vomiting, gait instability that lasts less than 1 week

PPx: None

MoD: Acute viral or post-viral inflammatory disorder of CN VIII

Dx:

1. History/Physical (nystagmus on physical exam)
2. MRI to rule out stroke

Tx/Mgmt:

1. Supportive care (fluids, antiemetics)
2. Corticosteroids

Peripheral Nerve/Plexus Disorders

Klumpke's Palsy (Brachial Plexus Lower Trunk injury)

Buzz Words (Fig. 5.12):

- Adult + grabbed branch during fall + atrophy of hypothenar muscles + sensory loss of pinky and lateral ring finger
- Newborn subjected to upward force on arm during delivery.

PPx: Avoid mechanical stress.

MoD: Traction on lower trunk (C8–T1) of brachial plexus → weakness of intrinsic hand muscles: lumbricals, interossei, thenar, hypothenar, sensory loss of ulnar distribution

Dx: Clinical presentation

Tx/Mgmt: Conservative, self-resolving

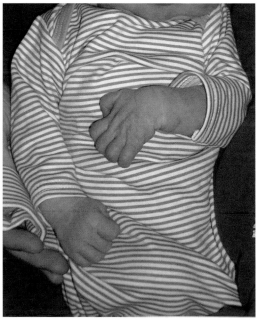

FIG. 5.12 Klumpke palsy. (From Buchanan E, Richardson R, Tse R: Isolated lower Brachial plexus (Klumpke) palsy with compound arm presentation: case report. *J Hand Surgery* 38(8):1567–1570, 2013.)

Thoracic Outlet Syndrome

Buzz Words: Klumpke palsy ± Horner syndrome + hoarseness → thoracic outlet syndrome caused by pancoast tumor

Clinical Presentation: Neurovascular bundle (lower brachial plexus + subclavian vessels) compressed between rib and clavicle

PPx: None

MoD: Mass compressing lower trunk of brachial plexus between clavicle/first rib or due to trauma. Apical lung tumor most common → compresses sympathetic chain (Horner's) + recurrent laryngeal nerve (hoarseness) + lower trunk of brachial plexus (Klumpke palsy).

Dx:
1. EMG
2. X-ray to rule out (r/o) lung tumor
3. Vascular imaging

Tx/Mgmt:
1. Surgical decompression
2. Removal of tumor

Axillary Neuropathy

Buzz Words: Fracture neck of the humerus, inability to abduct shoulder + loss of sensation on lateral shoulder

PPx: None

MoD: Fracture of neck of humerus or anterior dislocation of humerus

Dx: XR of the proximal humerus

Tx/Mgmt:
1. Immobilization with sling and analgesics
2. Orthopedic surgery in complicated cases

> **MNEMONIC**
> Mnemonic for nerves affected by humerus fractures: The order of nerves from superior to inferior = A.R.M. (axillary = humeral neck, radial = humeral shaft, median = Supracondylar fracture)

Musculocutaneous Neuropathy

Buzz Words:
Loss of sensation on lateral forearm + weakness of biceps and supination

PPx: None

MoD: Upper trunk compression

Dx: X-ray of the cervical spine

Tx/Mgmt:
1. Supportive
2. Orthopedic surgery in complicated cases

Radial Neuropathy ("Saturday Night Palsy")

Buzz Words: Using crutches/fell asleep with arm over chair/fracture of spiral groove of humerus → + wrist drop + sensory loss of dorsolateral hand (Fig. 5.13)

PPx: Avoid compression of axilla.

> **QUICK TIPS**
> Sensory loss of dorsolateral hand due to handcuffs = cheiralgia paresthetic (handcuff neuropathy)

Radial Nerve Compression

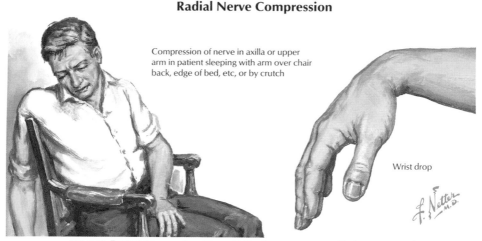

Compression of nerve in axilla or upper arm in patient sleeping with arm over chair back, edge of bed, etc, or by crutch

Wrist drop

FIG. 5.13 Radial nerve palsy. (From Netter Images. www.netterimages.com.)

MoD: Compression of axilla or fracture of spiral groove of humerus → radial nerve damage

Dx: Humeral or cervical x-ray

Tx/Mgmt:

1. Supportive care if no fracture is present
2. If fractured, cast the arm

Median Neuropathy

Buzz Words: Fracture of distal humerus (supracondylar fracture) or distal radius + weakness of wrist flexion, abduction, opposition of thumb (Fig. 5.14) + "Ape hand" + "Pope's blessing."

PPx: None

MoD: Lesion of median nerve as it crosses distal humerus and distal radius

Dx: X-ray of humerus and forearm

Tx/Mgmt:

1. Reduce fracture and cast
2. Supportive care

Carpal Tunnel

Buzz Words: Repetitive hand work (i.e., typing) + pregnancy + shakes hand during sleep to alleviate paresthesia/pain → carpal tunnel syndrome (Figs. 5.15 and 5.16)

Clinical Presentation: A 30-year-old pregnant female with a history of hypothyroidism, diabetes, and obesity presents with numbness and tingling of the thumb, index, and middle finger. On physical exam, she has atrophy of the thenar muscles.

PPx: Avoid repetitive wrist flexion/extension.

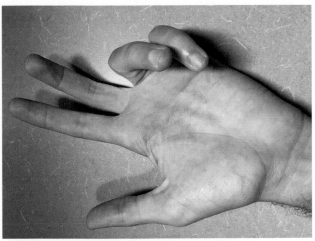

FIG. 5.14 Median neuropathy. (Courtesy Cody Nathan.)

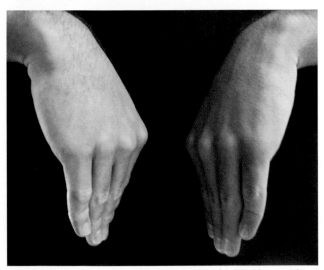

FIG. 5.15 Phalen Test = forced flexion of wrists for 30–60 seconds causes paresthesia in median nerve distribution. (Courtesy Cody Nathan.)

MoD: Compression of the median nerve within the carpal tunnel 2/2 swelling (due to diabetes mellitus, pregnancy, hypo/hypothyroidism, dialysis-related amyloidosis)

Dx:

1. Clinical presentation
2. Nerve conduction studies
3. EMG to rule out other conditions (radiculopathy or polyneuropathy) and when evaluating for surgery

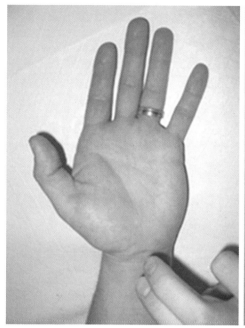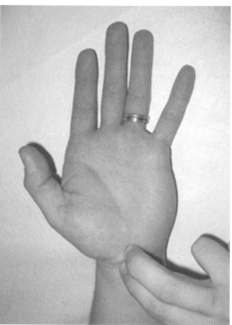

FIG. 5.16 Tinel test = tingling when tapping the median nerve at the wrist. (From: Bellaplanta J, Lavelle W, et al: Hand pain. In: Smith H, ed. *Current Therapy in Pain,* Philadelphia. 2009, Elsevier, pp. 156–167.)

Tx/Mgmt:
1. Rest, splint, NSAIDs
2. Corticosteroid injections (no more than three per year)
3. Surgery with carpal tunnel release as last resort

Guillain-Barré Syndrome (Acute Inflammatory Demyelinating Polyneuropathy)

Buzz Words: Areflexia + CSF with elevated protein (normal glucose/white blood cells [WBCs]) ± autonomic dysfunction (orthostatic hypotension, arrhythmias, etc.)

Clinical Presentation: In adults, the etiology is most often infectious, and symptoms may be preceded by a viral infection or bloody diarrhea (*Campylobacter jejuni*). Patients may present with ascending paralysis (weakness developing in legs first; then weakness developing in the arms).

PPx: None

MoD: Viral or bacterial infection → autoimmune destruction of Schwann cells and peripheral myelin due to molecular mimicry

Dx:
1. Clinical diagnosis
2. LP w/ CSF showing elevated protein

3. Nerve conduction study and EMG (for diagnosis and prognosis)

Tx/Mgmt:
1. Supportive care (intubation if FVC <15 mL/kg, monitor changes in BP, heart rate [HR], heart rhythm)
2. IVIG or plasmapheresis (equal efficacy)

Herpes Zoster (Shingles)

Buzz Words: Burning pain + rash does **not** cross the midline

Clinical Presentation: The location of the pain depends on the nerve (i.e., cranial nerve [CN] V or spinal nerves) that is affected, but the clinical presentation is similar regardless of the location of the pain. Note that the pain may occur **before** the rash ever appears. Risk factors: history of immunosuppression, trauma, HIV, organ transplant, or malignancy.

A classic patient: 60-year-old man presents with burning pain followed by vesicular rash within a dermatomal distribution.

PPx:
- Herpes zoster vaccine >60 years old
- Avoid contact with persons who have open shingles rash

MoD: Reactivation of varicella zoster (dormant in dorsal root ganglion)

Dx: Clinical presentation (pain followed by vesicular rash)

Tx/Mgmt:
1. Antiviral medications (acyclovir, valacyclovir, famciclovir) best within 72 hours of symptom onset
2. Analgesics
3. Management of post-herpetic neuropathic pain

Neurologic Pain Syndromes

These are not very high yield for the medicine shelf, although there are a few questions that commonly come up on the test. Understand the classic presentation of trigeminal neuralgia and that it can be treated with carbamazepine (high yield). Fibromyalgia may show up as a distractor in the answer choices, but make sure you have ruled out every other disease process before picking this option.

Trigeminal Neuralgia

Buzz Words: Facial pain triggered by **brushing teeth, talking, chewing.**

> **QUICK TIPS**
>
> Chronic inflammatory demyelinating polyneuropathy is similar to GBS except it is developing more slowly (evolving more than (>2 months) and it responds to steroids (GBS does **not** respond to steroids)

Clinical Presentation:
- Age: Older adults (usually >40 years old but may occur in 20s–30s)
- Gender: Female > male
- Chief complaint: Brief unilateral shooting/electrical face pain (CN V distribution)
- PMH: diagnosed with compressive lesion such as a schwannoma or meningioma

PPx: None
MoD: Compression of CN V nerve root
Dx:
1. Clinical presentation
2. MRI (r/o structural lesions near CN V)

Tx/Mgmt:
1. Carbamazepine, oxcarbazepine
2. Lamotrigine
3. Surgery (last resort for those who fail medical therapy)

Global Cerebral Dysfunction

Global cerebral disorders affect the cerebrum and can cause altered mental status. It is important to recognize the underlying cause of delirium in the patient because it may be treatable. The most commonly tested form of delirium is in an elderly person from a nursing home who presents with acute onset delirium due to a urinary tract infection (UTI). Keep in mind, though, that the differential for etiology of delirium is incredibly long, so focus on the clinical history to help narrow your differential diagnosis (Table 5.3).

TABLE 5.3 Delirium Versus Dementia

	Delirium	Dementia
Timing	Acute	Insidious
Course	Waxing/waning	Gradual
Hallucinations	Common	Less common (paranoia late)
Attention	Impaired	Preserved (affected late)
Duration	Hours/days	Month/years

Delirium (State of Acute Confusion)

Buzz Words: ± Visual hallucinations + disrupted sleep cycle + UTI + medications affecting cognition (especially benzodiazepines).

Clinical Presentation: Elderly, hospitalized patients who present with acute onset **waxing/waning** consciousness and cognitive dysfunction. Elderly patients who have UTIs or other infections, electrolyte disturbances, or liver or renal failure are at increased risk.

PPx: Keep patient oriented and allow the patient to sleep + prevent underlying cause (alcohol withdrawal, remove Foley if unnecessary to prevent UTI).

MoD: Caused by a variety of metabolic (alcohol, hypoxia), infectious (UTI, sepsis), or iatrogenic causes (medications including anticholinergics, benzodiazepines).

Dx:
1. Clinical diagnosis
2. CT/MRI to rule out structural abnormalities
3. EEG to rule out seizure
4. Culture (urine, blood) to rule out infection

Tx/Mgmt: Treat underlying causes

Alzheimer Disease

Buzz Words: <24 on Mini Mental-State Examination (MMSE) + neuritic plaques and tangles + getting lost in familiar places + preserved remote memories + difficulty forming new memories + aggression and paranoia late in the course.

Clinical Presentation: An elderly patient presents with progressive forgetfulness and impairment of activities of daily life. Risk factors include: family history of Alzheimer disease, cerebrovascular disease, brain trauma, diabetes, obesity, long-term use of anticholinergic medications.

PPx: None

MoD:
- Extracellular plaques composed of amyloid beta plaques and intracellular neurofibrillary tangles → neuronal degeneration and atrophy
- Familial-type Alzheimer disease (early onset) is due to mutations in genes coding for amyloid precursor protein and presenilin-1 protein (PSEN-1) and presenilin-2 protein (PSEN-2) → amyloid peptide accumulation

Dx:
1. Clinical history and MMSE
2. R/o reversible causes of dementia by checking thyroid-stimulating hormone, T3/T4, B12, RPR for syphilis
3. MRI head to r/o structural lesions (shows diffuse atrophy/enlarged ventricles with disproportionate atrophy of the hippocampus)
4. Definitive diagnosis is by autopsy

QUICK TIPS

Elderly patient with acute onset waxing/waning alertness + hallucinations + cognitive dysfunction = think delirium in the setting of **UTI**

QUICK TIPS

Dementia must be distinguished from age-associated cognitive decline (such as forgetting car keys, having trouble finding words occasionally)

QUICK TIPS

Down syndrome (Trisomy 21) increases the risk of developing Alzheimer's due to amyloid beta protein precursor located on chromosome 21.

Tx/Mgmt:

1. Donepezil, galantamine, rivastigmine (all acetylcholinesterase inhibitors)
2. For moderate or severe stage of Alzheimer disease → add memantine (*N*-methyl-D-aspartate [NMDA] antagonist)
3. Antipsychotics, such as quetiapine, sometimes are used to manage psychotic behaviors

Frontotemporal Dementia (aka Pick Disease)

Buzz Words: Inappropriate behavior/poor judgment + disinhibition + hypersexuality + **intraneuronal silver staining inclusions** (tau bodies aka Pick bodies) or TDP-43 inclusions + degeneration of frontal lobes and temporal lobes

Clinical Presentation: Pick disease is manifested by the lobar atrophy of frontal and temporal lobes; on brain examination, the remaining neurons often display a specific type of inclusion body (Pick body) under the microscope, formed by the abnormally aggregated tau protein. These patients often first present with behavioral and personality changes, usually starting before the age of 65.

PPx: None

MoD: Severe atrophy of the frontal and temporal lobes secondary to tau protein inclusions or TDP-43 protein inclusions.

Dx:

1. Clinical history and MMSE
2. CT/MRI (disproportionate atrophy of frontal/temporal lobes)
3. R/o reversible dementia (hypothyroid, B12, syphilis, normal pressure hydrocephalus [NPH])
4. Definitive diagnosis with autopsy

Tx/Mgmt: Symptomatic management

Lewy Body Dementia

Buzz Words: Episodic confusion + impaired visuospatial function + **alpha synuclein**

Clinical Presentation: A 70-year-old male with a history of depression presents with new onset visual hallucinations. He exhibits dementia symptoms less than 12 months after onset of bradykinesia, tremor, abnormal posture, rigidity (vs. Parkinson disease shows dementia late in the course).

PPx: None

MNEMONIC

HaLewcinations in **Lew**y body dementia

MoD: Intra cytoplasmic alpha-synuclein inclusions distributed throughout the cortex and substantia nigra → degeneration of dopaminergic neurons and cortical/subcortical neurons

Dx: Clinical history and exam (Parkinsonian syndrome, hallucinations, rapid eye movement (REM) sleep behavior disorders, and dementia)

Tx/Mgmt:

1. Treat Parkinsonian features with levodopa-carbidopa
2. Treat cognitive symptoms with acetylcholinesterase inhibitors (rivastigmine or donepezil)
3. Dopaminergic agonists often trigger visual hallucinations and psychotic behaviors.

Amyotrophic Lateral Sclerosis and Muscle Diseases

Amyotrophic Lateral Sclerosis (Motor Neuron Disease)

Buzz Words: UMN and LMN symptoms + muscle atrophy + fasciculations + hyperreflexia + difficulty breathing/swallowing (Table 5.4)

Clinical Presentation: Amyotrophic lateral sclerosis (ALS), also known as Lou Gehrig disease in the United States, presents with various UMN and LMN signs. The incidence of ALS is highest in people starting around age 70, but may present as early as the 20s. The majority of cases are sporadic but about less than 10% are inherited. There is no cure for this disease. A typical patient may be a 60-year-old male with a chief complaint of progressive asymmetric weakness.

PPx: None (10% familial)

MoD: Loss of motor neurons in the anterior horn of the spinal cord, brainstem motor nuclei, motor cortex. Some cases caused by mutation of superoxide dismutase.

99 AR

ALS and upper and lower motor neurons

QUICK TIPS

Sensory, cognition, bladder/bowel control are preserved in ALS

TABLE 5.4 Upper Motor Neuron Versus Lower Motor Neuron Signs

UMN	LMN
Spastic	Flacid
Hyperreflxia	Hyporeflexia
No atrophy	Atrophy

LMN, Lower motor neuron; *UMN*, upper motor neuron.

Dx:
1. Clinical presentation
2. EMG (denervation + fibrillation potentials)
3. CT/MRI to rule out structural lesion
4. Genetic testing

Tx/Mgmt: Riluzole

Muscular Dystrophy (Duchenne Versus Becker)

This more commonly shows up on pediatric shelf exams, but it is still fair game for the medicine shelf because some patients with certain types of muscular dystrophy can live until their 30s and 40s with complications of the illness. Pay close attention to the buzz words and how to diagnose the disease. Additionally, it is important to know the major complications of the illness, such as dilated cardiomyopathy, respiratory compromise, and scoliosis, so these issues can be addressed early. Treatment is mainly supportive, so you will not be tested on this in detail.

Buzz Words: Gower's sign + pseudohypertrophy of calves + elevated CK + dystrophin mutation + intellectual disability + waddling gait

Clinical Presentation: Presents with proximal muscle weakness (usually lower extremities before upper) demonstrated by difficulty walking up steps, running, jumping, etc. around age 2–3 years old in Duchenne's, present with symptoms in teenage years for Becker's. Primarily male due to X-linked inheritance.

PPx: None

MoD: X-linked frameshift mutation → truncated dystrophin protein → inability to anchor muscle fibers → muscle necrosis

Dx:
1. Clinical and family history
2. Elevated CK
3. Muscle biopsy
4. Genetic testing (*dystrophin* mutation)

Tx:
1. Supportive (physical therapy, respiratory support)
2. Glucocorticoids to improve motor strength and pulmonary function and delay onset of cardiomyopathy

Movement Disorders

Movement disorders are characterized by too much (hyperkinetic) or too little (hypokinetic) movement. The most commonly tested hypokinetic disorder is Parkinson disease, discussed below. Hyperkinetic disorders such

MNEMONIC

Common cause of **D**eath in **D**ystrophy = **D**ilated cardiomyopathy

QUICK TIPS

Becker's Dystrophy = **non-**frameshift mutation, later onset, less severe than Duchenne

as Huntington disease and dystonia also appear on the exam and it is important to recognize their clinical picture. It is important to recognize which medications can cause movement disorders because cessation of medication could be a way to reverse the current symptoms. The pathophysiology of these disorders can be complicated and involves interactions between the basal ganglia and the thalamus.

Acute Dystonia

Buzz Words: Neuroleptic exposure + torticollis (sustained contraction of neck muscle) + blepharospasm (focal dystonia of eye muscles).

Clinical Presentation: Dystonia is an involuntary sustained muscle contraction within one or multiple muscles. The most common dystonias are those involving the neck (torticollis), orbicularis oculi (blepharospasm), and hand (writer's cramp, or in musicians). Recognize which medications are prone to causing dystonia and how to treat acute dystonia.

A patient may present with a chief complaint of posturing exacerbated by movement. Risk factors include a history of conditions that expose individuals to anti-dopaminergic medications (i.e., schizophrenia or gastroparesis) and a family history of dystonia.

PPx: Avoid medications causing dystonia.

MoD: Neuroleptic induced caused by antagonism of D2 receptor

Dx: Clinical exam w/ spastic muscle contraction (dystonia of neck [torticollis], tongue, and mouth are common).

Tx/Mgmt:
1. Stop neuroleptics
2. Diphenhydramine or benztropine (anticholinergics)
3. Botox injection therapy

Essential Tremor

Buzz Words: Tremor improves w/ alcohol + tremor worse with action

Clinical Presentation: A 22-year-old man presents with fine symmetric tremor worse with **action.** He notes that his father had a quivering voice and his grandfather had a head tremor.

Essential tremor is the most common type of tremor and may occur in various parts of the body (e.g., head or hands). The key feature is that it is an **action** tremor, which helps to differentiate it from other types of tremors, such as intention tremor, which is more indicative

QUICK TIPS

Common medications causing dystonia: 1st generation antipsychotics (haloperidol, fluphenazine) and metoclopramide

gg AR

Essential tremor video

TABLE 5.5 Differentiating Tremors

	Essential Tremor	Parkinson Tremor	Cerebellar Tremor
Voluntary action	Worsens	Improves	Increases when arriving at target
At rest	None	Pill rolling	Rare

of cerebellar dysfunction. Essential tremor often runs in families and is very common. The clinical scenario may include that a person's tremor improves after a glass of wine because alcohol improves this tremor disorder (Table 5.5).

PPx: None

MoD: Common within families but no specific gene has been identified for all cases

Dx: Clinical exam showing action tremor

Tx/Mgmt:

1. Propranolol
2. Primidone

Huntington Disease

Buzz Words: A male family member who went "crazy" and had odd movements + caudate nucleus atrophy + **anticipation** (increased number of trinucleotide repeats with successive generations → earlier onset of symptoms in following generations) + increased risk of suicide

Clinical Presentation: Huntington disease is an autosomal dominant condition caused by CAG repeat expansions (repeats). It is characterized by chorea (dancing like movements) and personality change. It is a devastating disease in that it affects people at a relatively young age and there is no cure. A classic patient is a 50-year-old male with chorea movements (involuntary irregular movements), personality changes (depression, impulsive), and dementia.

PPx: Genetic counseling

MoD: Genetic mutation on HD gene on Chr4 → expansion of CAG repeats → gain of function mutation + aggregation of mutant huntingtin protein in neuronal nuclei → loss of GABA and ACh neurons in basal ganglia → atrophy of caudate/putamen

Dx:

1. Family history + clinical signs
2. MRI (caudate atrophy)
3. Genetic testing (CAG repeats on Chromosome 4)

QUICK TIPS

Anticipation = increasing length of CAG repeats with each generation causing earlier onset disease as generations progress

Tx/Mgmt:
1. Movement control (atypical antipsychotics, tetrabenazine/reserpine)
2. Mood control (selective serotonin reuptake inhibitors [SSRIs])

Parkinson Disease

Buzz Words: Resting "pill-rolling" tremor + Cogwheel rigidity + shuffling gait + masked facies (expressionless face) + hypophonia (low voice volume).

Clinical Presentation: A 60-year-old male has a resting tremor, slowed movements, stiffness, and rigidity, and falls down easily during the pull test.

PPx: None

MoD: Aggregation of alpha-synuclein bodies within the neurons of substantia nigra of the midbrain → death of dopaminergic neurons → decreased activation of direct pathway of basal ganglia → difficulty initiating movement

Dx:
1. Clinical exam (tremor, bradykinesia, rigidity, shuffling gait)
2. MRI/CT to rule out mimics (NPH, Progressive supranuclear palsy)
3. Improved symptoms w/ levodopa-carbidopa

Tx/Mgmt:
- Levodopa-carbidopa = decarboxylase inhibitor that prevents degradation of levodopa in periphery
- Catechol-O-methyltransferase (COMT) inhibitors = prevents degradation of levodopa
- Monoamine Oxidase B (MAO-B) inhibitors (rasagiline, selegline) = prevent the breakdown of DA in CNS
- Dopamine agonists (bromocriptine, pramipexole) = directly act on striatal neurons
- May cause hypotension or hallucinations
- Anticholinergic agents (benztropine) = reduce tremor
- Deep brain stimulation = electrodes inhibit subthalamic nucleus (indirect pathway) as last resort

Headache

Pay close attention to the buzz words here because the diagnosis for migraine, tension, and cluster headaches is primarily based on the clinical picture. Tension headaches are bilateral and usually due to stress, whereas migraine

99 AR

Shuffling gait in Parkinson disease

and cluster headaches are usually unilateral. Migraine headaches tend to run in families, although this is not always the case. Imaging becomes necessary if there are red flag signs associated with the headache. For instance, new onset headaches in adults accompanied by focal findings warrants imaging. Additionally, early morning headaches, or headaches associated with increased ICP, which can present with nausea and vomiting, warrants imaging. Finally, if the patient is having the "worst headache of my life" then be suspicious for subarachnoid hemorrhage.

Migraine

Buzz Words: Pulsating pain + nausea/vomiting + photophobia + phonophobia

Clinical Presentation: A 30-year-old woman presents with unilateral headaches lasting between 5 hours to 3 days preceded by nausea and photophobia. Her mother had similar headaches.

PPx: Taking NSAIDs during the aura prior to the onset of pain.

MoD: "Cortical spreading depression" = hyperpolarization followed by depolarization across cortex → release of substrates that cause irritation of CN V (substance P, CGRP, potassium)→ pain

Dx:
1. Clinical diagnosis of two or more headaches for 4–72 hours
2. MRI or CT (r/o structural lesion or SAH)

Tx/Mgmt:
1. Abortive therapy (NSAIDs, triptans, ergotamine)
2. Prophylactic therapy if >6 per month (propranolol, topiramate, amitriptyline, valproate, calcium channel blocker)
3. Supportive therapy (anti-emetics such as metoclopramide, ondansetron)
4. Avoid triggers (e.g., caffeine, chocolate, wine, overuse of NSAIDs to prevent rebound headache)
5. Lifestyle change (adequate sleep, balanced diet, exercise).

Tension

Buzz Words: Stress-induced headache + constant bilateral "band-like" pressure

Clinical Presentation: A 40-year-old female under stress about her new job and recently ended relationship complains of bilateral headaches lasting 30 minutes to hours or days. She denies nausea, vomiting, photophobia, or phonophobia.

PPx: None
MoD: Unclear, possibly due to muscle contraction.
Dx: Clinical presentation
Tx/Mgmt:
1. Lifestyle changes
2. NSAIDs or acetaminophen
3. Amitriptyline for chronic pain

Cluster

Buzz Words: Periorbital pain + conjunctival injection + lacrimation + rhinorrhea ± Horner syndrome
Clinical Presentation: A 40-year-old male with a history of smoking presents with episodic, left-sided headaches around his eye lasting 15 minutes to 3 hours. His left eye becomes red and teary. He previously experienced this for several weeks last year, but they disappeared and did not come back until recently.
PPx: None
MoD: Dilation of blood vessels → pressure on CN V
Dx: Clinical presentation
Tx/Mgmt:
1. Abortive (sumatriptan and 100% O_2). Use steroids as second-line
2. Prophylactic (verapamil)

Epilepsy

Generalized Clonic-Tonic Seizure

Buzz Words: Impaired consciousness ± postictal confusion; usually genetic in origin
  Subtypes
  - **Absence epilepsy**: Blank staring and blinking with altered consciousness + can be **induced by hyperventilation** + loss of memory for seconds; common in children (Fig. 5.17)
  - **Juvenile Myoclonic Epilepsy**: Quick myoclonic jerks + in the morning (e.g., drops toothbrush or comb) + may lead to generalized tonic clonic seizure; common in teenagers
  - **Idiopathic generalized epilepsy**: tonic-clonic seizures (whole body stiffening then twitching) + postictal confusion + sore muscles afterwards
Clinical Presentation: Seizure originates in an epileptogenic focus, which leads to rapid synchronous firing of the entire brain.
PPx: None

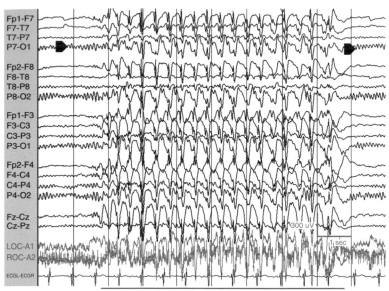

FIG. 5.17 Blue line indicates area of three spike and wave complexes per second (3Hz). (From Marcuse LV, Fields MC, Yoo J. [2016]. Epileptiform discharges, periodic or rhythmic patterns. *Rowan's primer of EEG* [2nd ed., pp. 98] Elsevier.)

MoD:
- Absence = genetic mutation in T-type Ca channels
- Juvenile myoclonic epilepsy (JME) and idiopathic epilepsy = synchronized neuronal discharge

Dx:
1. Clinical presentation
2. EEG findings (absence seizure = 3 Hz spike)

Tx/Mgmt:
- Absence:
  1. Ethoduximide
  2. Valproic acid
- JME
  1. Valproic acid
  2. Lamotrigine, levetiracetam, or topiramate
- Idiopathic generalized epilepsy
  1. Phenytoin
  2. Valproic acid

Partial Seizures

Buzz Words: Twitching of face or extremities lasting seconds to minutes + **no** postictal confusion + aura (e.g., smelling burning rubber, déjà vu, fear, jamais vu)

Clinical Presentation: Focal seizures with synchronous firing of neurons in one region of the brain, such as marching along the motor cortex

PPx: None

MoD: Synchronized neuronal discharge; may be 2/2 a lesion in the brain (stroke, tumor, blood, mesial temporal sclerosis).

Dx: Clinical findings and localized spike and wave on EEG.

Tx/Mgmt:

1. Carbamazepine
2. Valproic acid
3. Lamotrigine

Sleep Disorders

Sleep is divided into four discrete stages, which cycle throughout sleeping.

- Stage 1 (non-REM—N1): Theta waves, muscle tone relaxed, slow eye movements
- Stage 2 (non-REM—N2): K complexes and sleep spindles with no eye movements and little muscle movement
- Stage 3 (non-REM—N3): **Delta** sleep, low frequency, slow wave sleep, deep sleep, most restful sleep
- Stage REM (R): Slow, fast voltage on the EEG, **no muscle tone** and **rapid eye movements,** vivid dream recall

Cataplexy and Narcolepsy

Buzz Words: Excessive daytime sleepiness + **loss of muscle tone w/ laughter or extreme emotion (cataplexy)** + hallucinations prior to sleep + sleep paralysis when waking + fast onset REM

Clinical Presentation: A 23-year-old medical student is excessively sleepy during the day and frequently falls asleep suddenly in class and in church, despite sleeping 9 hours a night. When his friend scares him, he often drops whatever he is holding.

PPx: None

MoD: Loss of neuropeptides orexin A/B (hypocretin1/2) in the hypothalamus

Dx:

1. Sleep diary
2. Multiple sleep latency test
3. Polysomnography (rules out other sleep disorders)

Tx/Mgmt:

1. Modafinil
2. Amphetamine
3. Methylphenidate
4. Cataplexy treated with venlafaxine, fluoxetine, atomoxetine. Sodium oxybate if refractory.

Insomnia

Buzz Words: Fatigue + anxious about sleep

Clinical Presentation: A 45-year-old man with a history of drug abuse and schizophrenia who is stressed out about a new job is unable to fall asleep at night despite lying in bed for hours. When he does fall asleep, he wakes easily. He is exhausted and sleepy all day and dreads nighttime when he must unsuccessfully try to fall asleep.

PPx: Proper sleep hygiene

MoD: Likely multifactorial, exact etiology unknown

Dx:

1. Sleep diary
2. Rule out other causes (e.g., medication, substance abuse)

Tx/Mgmt:

1. Educate on proper sleep hygiene, relaxation techniques
2. If stress/anxiety related, treat with cognitive behavioral therapy, SSRIs
3. Benzodiazepines **short** term (reduce sleep latency, can cause dependence)
4. Non-benzo hypnotics: zolpidem, esZopiclone, Zaleplon (ZZZ for sleep)
5. Ramelteon (melatonin agonist)

Sleep Terrors

Buzz Words: NO memory of the event in morning (vs. nightmares which patients remember) + stage 3 sleep

Clinical Presentation: A 9-year-old boy occasionally wakes up from sleep screaming. When his parents ask him what happened, he does not recall screaming nor what prompted it. As he grows up, these events stop completely.

PPx: None

MoD: Sympathetic hyperactivation

Dx: Clinical presentation

Tx/Mgmt:

1. Supportive/reassurance
2. Benzodiazepines if injuring self during episodes or if they are bothersome for patient/sleeping partner

Rapid Eye Movement Sleep Behavior Disorders

Buzz Words: Loss of muscle atonia in REM → kicking sleeping partner, yelling in sleep

Clinical Presentation: A 60-year-old male (may rarely occur in children) is brought in by his wife because he acts out his dreams almost every night, yelling and thrashing in bed.

PPx: None

MoD: Dysfunction of REM nuclei within the pons → loss of muscle atonia in REM. **Highly** predictable of developing neurodegenerative diseases (Parkinson disease and Lewy Body disease).

Dx:
1. Clinical history
2. Polysomnography (lack of atonia during REM)

Tx/Mgmt:
1. Establish safe sleep environment
2. Melatonin
3. Clonazepam

Restless Leg Syndrome

Buzz Words: Impaired sleep + nocturnal awakenings + feeling of something "crawling" on legs + leg "tingling," "itching"

Clinical Presentation: A 40-year-old female has an irresistible urge to move her legs as she is trying to fall asleep every night. The urge is alleviated by moving her legs, but then the urge reappears again. Risk factors include iron deficient anemia, uremia, neuropathy, and pregnancy.

PPx: None

MoD: Unknown, though postulated to be 2/2 low central iron stores and dopamine dysfunction

Dx:
1. Clinical history
2. Polysomnography (r/o periodic limb movement disorder, a REM behavior disorder characterized by repetitive twitching of legs/arms during sleep)

Tx/Mgmt:
1. Check iron studies
2. Pramipexole, ropinirole (dopamine agonists)
3. Gabapentin

Traumatic and Mechanical Disorders of Increased Intracranial Pressure

The first part of this section deals with acute emergencies related to head trauma, which is high yield not only for the medicine shelf exam but also for the neurology exam, emergency medicine, surgery, and ultimately Step 2 CK. Be aware of how to recognize subdural hematoma versus epidural hematoma because management and prognosis can be different.

The second part of this section deals with a chronic rise in ICP, which is commonly tested on many shelf exams. The important point here is that these can be devastating illnesses, but they are treatable, so being able to recognize their clinical picture is vital to the patient's wellbeing.

QUICK TIPS

Patients with this disorder are at risk for developing Parkinson's or Lewy body dementia

Elevated Intracranial Pressure

Management of elevated ICP (brain edema) is a critical part of treating patients with head injury. Being able to treat patients quickly can help prevent brain herniation. Below, you will find the steps for decreasing ICP, which has been organized by the fastest to the slowest method.

1. Elevate head 30 degrees above the bed → improves venous drainage to reduce ICP.
2. Hyperventilation and intubation → protects the airway and also decreases ICP by removing CO_2, which normally causes dilation of the vessels (helps within 30 seconds, but is not a long-term therapy).
3. IV mannitol or hypertonic saline → helps decrease pressure within 5 minutes by drawing fluid out of the cells.
4. External ventricular drain → both diagnostic and therapeutic in that you can monitor ICP and also adjust the ICP using the drain (helps within minutes).
5. Medically induced coma → decreases metabolic demand and causes vasoconstriction (helps within hours).
6. Steroids → useful if there is a space-occupying lesion such as a neoplasm. This decreases inflammation within the brain and should be done **first** if a lesion is causing neurologic issues.

Epidural Hematoma

Buzz Words: Head trauma + lens shaped/biconvex hematoma + hematoma does **not** cross suture lines + lucid interval (mental status improves briefly after insult then deteriorates later) + fixed dilated pupil (if uncal herniation occurs)

PPx: None

MoD: Traumatic injury → fracture of temporal bone → rupture of middle meningeal artery

Dx: Non-contrast CT w/ biconcave hematoma limited by suture line (Fig. 5.18)

Tx/Mgmt: Emergent craniotomy, ventriculostomy for ICP monitoring and adjustment

Subdural Hematoma

Buzz Words: Trauma (in elderly may be as simple as bumping head) + obtunded + concave/semilunar hematoma + chronic subdurals common in alcoholics

PPx: None

MoD: Traumatic injury → tearing of bridging veins within the subdural space

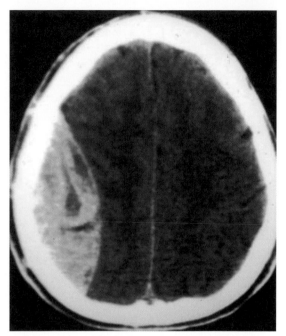

FIG. 5.18 Non-contrast computed tomography head of epidural hematoma. (From Wikimedia Commons. https://en.wikipedia.org/wiki/Epidural_hematoma. Used under [WP:NFCC#4], Fair use, https://en.wikipedia.org/w/index.php?curid=36208911.)

Dx: Non-contrast CT scan shows crescent shaped hematoma (may cross suture lines; Fig. 5.19)

Tx/Mgmt:

1. Decrease ICP (elevate head of bed to 30 degrees, hyperventilate, mannitol)
2. Craniotomy or ventriculostomy (especially if midline is deviated)

Intraparenchymal Hemorrhage

Buzz Words: Hypertension + exertion + headache, nausea, vomiting ± focal deficits

PPx: None

MoD:

- Long standing hypertension → rupture of small penetrating arteries
- Cerebral amyloid angiopathy (usually in the elderly) → blood vessel damage
- Brain tumors → neovascularization → new blood vessels prone to rupture
- Trauma → rupture of cerebral blood vessels

"Many Cancerous Tumors Love Bleeding"

MNEMONIC

Common metastatic brain tumors causing hemorrhage: **M**elanoma, **R**enal clear cell carcinoma, **C**horiocarcinoma, **T**hyroid, **B**reast, **L**ung

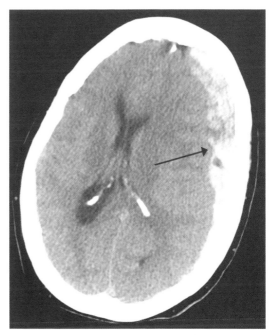

FIG. 5.19 Non-contrast computed tomography head of subdural hematoma *(arrow)*. (From Wikimedia Commons: https://commons .wikimedia.org/w/index.php?curid=19364350. By James Heilman, MD—Own work, CC BY-SA 3.0. Used under the Creative Commons Attribution Share Alike 3.0 Unported license.)

Dx:
1. Non-contrast CT to visualize hemorrhage
2. MRI to visualize underlying structural lesions

Tx/Mgmt:
1. Lower BP (labetalol, hydralazine, nicardipine, or nitroprusside)
2. Decrease ICP (elevate head of bed, mannitol)
3. Anti-epileptics if the patient is seizing

TBI (Contusion, Concussion, Post-Concussion Syndrome)

Buzz Words:
- Within 30 minutes of head injury; confusion + normal neuroimaging + memory impairment + headache ± loss of consciousness → concussion
- Headache + lethargy + mental slowing + dizziness; months after trauma → post-concussive syndrome
- Focal neurologic deficits → contusion (focal brain damage) and diffuse axonal injury

PPx: None

MoD: Trauma → axonal rupture/shear stress and ultimately damage (if the brain parenchyma is already damaged—contusion); diffuse axonal injury

Dx:

1. Clinical presentation
2. CT/MRI to rule out hematoma
3. X-ray of C-spine to rule out spinal cord injury

Tx/Mgmt:

1. Neuro exam to check the signs of brain edema
2. Refrain from contact sports until symptoms resolve

Idiopathic Intracranial Hypertension (Pseudotumor Cerebri)

Buzz Words: ± Papilledema (not necessary for the diagnosis but suggestive of ICH when present) + tinnitus + visual disturbance

Clinical Presentation: A 22-year-old recently obese female on isotretinoin for acne presents with new-onset headache and blurry vision.

PPx: Avoid oral contraceptive pills, maintain normal body mass index, avoid excessive vitamin A intake.

MoD: Unknown

Dx:

1. Clinical signs of increase ICP (headache, visual disturbance) + fundoscopic exam to observe papilledema (Fig. 5.20)
2. MRI (r/o space occupying lesion as the cause of elevated ICP)
3. LP **after** imaging (to avoid herniation) demonstrates elevated opening pressure

Tx/Mgmt:

1. Weight loss if obese
2. Acetazolamide to reduce CSF
3. Furosemide
4. Serial LPs as a bridge prior to surgery
5. Optic nerve fenestration if vision loss is progressing
6. Ventriculo-peritoneal shunting (V-P) or spinal-peritoneal shunting (last resort)

Normal Pressure Hydrocephalus

Buzz Words: Enlarged ventricles + wet, wobbly, whacky

Clinical Presentation: An elderly patient presenting with: urinary incontinence (wet), gait disturbance (wobbly), and memory impairment (whacky). The patient may have had a history of subarachnoid hemorrhage, meningitis, or Paget disease (which can cause inflammation of arachnoid granulations).

PPx: None

QUICK TIPS

The most devastating effect of idiopathic intracranial hypertension is **vision loss.**

Wet, wild, and wacky comic

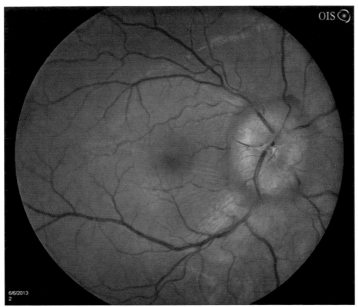

FIG. 5.20 Opthalmoscopic image showing papilledema in a patient with pseudotumor cerebri. (From Calhoun JS. (2013, June 30). *Papilledema Probable to Pseudo Tumor Cerebri.* [Photograph]. Retrieved from http://imagebank.asrs.org/file/7278/papilledema-probable-to-pseudo-tumor-cerebri.)

MoD: Impaired absorption of CSF by the arachnoid granulations without evidence of obstruction of flow

Dx:

1. Clinical presentation
2. MRI (ventriculomegaly; Fig. 5.21)
3. LP to see if it alleviates symptoms (checking gait improvement)

Tx/Mgmt: Ventricular shunting

Congenital/Genetic Disorders

This section is higher yield for the pediatric and neurology shelf exam, although it still is testable material on the medicine shelf exam. Many of these disorders are associated with compilations outside of the nervous system (such as hypertrophic cardiomyopathy with Friedreich ataxia) so it is worth knowing these diseases. Focus predominantly on the **buzz words** in this section. For instance, if the stem mentions that a patient has a cutaneous lesion best identified with a Wood lamp then immediately you should think of a Shagreen patch on a patient with tuberous sclerosis. These disorders are easily confused, but if you know the clinical pictures these questions will be easy points on the exam.

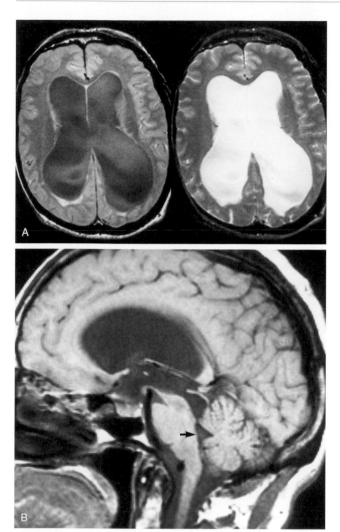

FIG. 5.21 Magnetic resonance imaging brain demonstrating normal versus normal pressure hydrocephalus; notice enlarged ventricles. (From Grainger RG, Allison DJ, Adam A, Dixon AK, editors: *Grainger and Allison's Diagnostic Radiology: A Textbook of Medical Imaging,* 4th ed, London, 2001, Harcourt.)

Friedreich Ataxia

Buzz Words: Frequent falls + dysarthria + diabetes + **hypertrophic cardiomyopathy** (most common cause of death) + areflexia + scoliosis + loss of position/vibration

Clinical Presentation: A 17-year-old boy with a family history of weakness and gait ataxia presents with those same symptoms.

PPx: Genetic counseling

MoD: Autosomal recessive GAA repeat on Chr9 → abnormal frataxin iron binding protein → mitochondrial dysfunction → degeneration of posterior column spinal cord.

Dx:
1. Clinical presentation
2. Genetic testing
3. Echocardiogram for HCM

Tx/Mgmt:
1. Supportive
2. HCM treatment

Neural Tube Defects

- **Spina bifida** = failure of posterior vertebral arch closure.
- **Meningocele** = protrusion of meninges through vertebral defect.
- **Meningomyelocele** = meninges and neural tissue protrude through vertebral defect.
- **Holoprosencephaly** = forebrain fails to develop two hemispheres (not sustainable for life).
- **Anencephaly** = failure of cranial end of neural tube to form causing absence of skull/brain.

PPx: Adequate maternal folate intake

Sturge-Weber

Buzz Words: Port wine stain in CNV1, V2 distribution + seizures + intellectual disability + intracranial calcifications + glaucoma

PPx: None

MoD: Congenital somatic mutation in GNAQ gene → dysfunctional neural crest cells

Dx:
1. MRI to visualize leptomeningeal venous malformation
2. EEG for seizure monitoring

Tx/Mgmt:
1. Argon laser therapy for port wine stain
2. Antiepileptic drugs for generalized seizures
3. Reduce intraocular pressure for glaucoma

Tuberous Sclerosis

Buzz Words: Hamartomas in CNS and skin + Ash leaf spots (hypopigmented macule) + Shagreen patches + cardiac rhabdomyoma + intellectual disability + mitral regurgitation + seizures (infantile spasms common in infancy; Fig. 5.22). None

gg AR
Sturge Weber port wine stain

gg AR
Tuberous sclerosis mnemonic

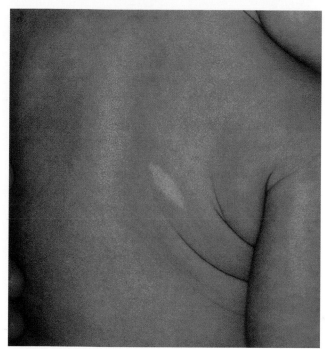

FIG. 5.22 Ash-leaf spot and Shagreen patch. (From Tsao H, Luo S: Neurofibromatosis and tuberous sclerosis. *Dermatology.* 61: 925–941, 2012.)

MoD: TSC1 (hamartin on Chr 9) and TSC2 (tuberin on Chr 16) → impaired the mTOR (mammalian target of rapamycin) pathway

Dx:
1. Clinical findings (e.g., cardiac rhabdomyosarcoma, angiolypomas, retinal hamartomas, shagreen patch, cortical dysplasia)
2. Genetic testing
3. EEG for seizure management

Tx/Mgmt:
1. Symptom control (e.g., controlling seizures with ACTH for infantile spasms and carbamzepime for partial seizures)
2. MRI to look for subependymal giant cell tumors
3. Echo to look for cardiac rhabdomyoma

Von Hippel Lindau syndrome

Buzz Words: Hemangioblastomas in retina, cerebellum, CNS + cavernous hemangiomas + bilateral renal cell carcinoma + pheochromocytoma

PPx: Genetic counseling
MoD: Autosomal dominant deletion mutation of *VHL* tumor suppressor gene on Chr3
Dx:
1. Genetic testing
2. HVA/VMA in urine or blood to rule out pheochromocytoma

Tx/Mgmt:
1. Resection of pheochromocytoma
2. Surveillance imaging CT or MRI for RCC

Neurofibromatosis I (Von Recklinghausen Disease)

Buzz Words: Café au lait spots, iris hamartomas (Lisch nodules), optic nerve glioma, pheochromocytoma, dermal neurofibroma, axillary freckling, bone abnormalities → NF1 (Fig. 5.23)
PPx: None
MoD: Mutated NF1 tumor suppressor gene on chromosome 17 → development of nerve sheath tumors derived from neural crest cells

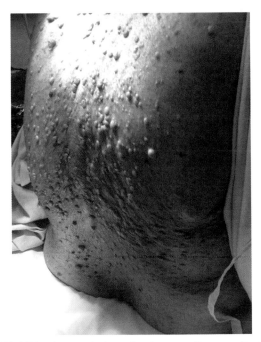

FIG. 5.23 NF1 cutaneous lesions showing neurofibromas. (From Wikimedia Commons. https://commons.wikimedia.org/wiki/File·Neu rofibromatosis.jpg. Public Domain.)

Dx:
1. Diagnostic criteria include two of the following:
   - ≥6 café au lait spots
   - ≥2 neurofibroma
   - Axillary/inguinal freckling
   - Optic glioma
   - ≥2 Lisch nodules
   - Bony lesions
   - 1st degree relative with NF1
2. MRI for optic glioma
3. Urine metanephrines for pheochromocytoma

Tx/Mgmt: Surgical removal of lesions

Adverse Effects of Drugs on the Nervous System

This topic is lower yield compared to others for the medicine shelf exam, yet it is still important to recognize the negative effects of these medications because toxicity of the drugs still may show up on the test. In particular, be able to recognize the main drugs that cause meningitis, the drugs that cause neuropathy, and the timeline for neuroleptic toxicity. Finally, be able to differentiate serotonin syndrome for neuroleptic malignant syndrome because both can be caused by psychiatric medications and they can present similarly, yet treatment is different for these two pathologic states.

Drug-Induced Meningitis

Buzz Words: Fever + neck stiffness in association w/ starting new medications

PPx: Avoid offending agents

MoD: Delayed hypersensitivity reaction or direct irritation of meninges

Dx:
1. Clinical findings of meningismus in setting of offending medication
2. LP (neutrophilic pleocytosis)

Tx/Mgmt: Remove offending drug

Drug-Induced Neuropathy

Buzz Words:
- **Vincristine** → peripheral neuropathy 2/2 microtubule inhibition in axons
- **Isoniazid** → peripheral neuropathy + hepatotoxicity 2/2 INH competing with B6
  - TB patient with neuropathy, think INH toxicity

Tx/Mgmt: Pyridoxine supplements for INH toxicity

Extrapyramidal Adverse Effects

Buzz Words:

- **Acute Dystonia** (4 hours–4 days after medication): sustained muscle contraction or spasm; neck contraction (torticollis), tongue protrusions, or oculogyric crises (forced, sustained eye elevation)
- **Akathisia** (4 days after medication): Motor restlessness
- **Parkinsonism** (4 weeks after medication): Bradykinesia, shuffling gait, resting hand tremor, masked facies

Multiple examples of tardive dyskinesia

- **Tardive Dyskinesia** (4 months–4 years after medication): Involuntary movements of tongue, face, and extremities (**irreversible**)

PPx: Avoid antipsychotics (e.g., haloperidol)

MoD: Inhibition of dopamine at the D2 receptor in the nigrostriatal pathway → extrapyramidal symptoms

Dx: Clinical presentation (pay attention to timing of onset after medication initiation)

Tx/Mgmt:

- **Acute Dystonic Reaction:** anticholinergics (diphenhydramine or benztropine)
- **Akathisia:** decrease drug, add propanolol or benzodiazepeines
- **Parkinsonism:** anticholinergics (benztropine or dopamine agonist amantadine)
- **Tardive Dyskinesia:** If caused by neuroleptic, change the medication (preferably to 2nd generation). If caused by metoclopramide, stop the medication. May also add anticholinergics, benzodiazepines, or botox injections

Neuroleptic Malignant Syndrome

Buzz Words: Autonomic instability + elevated creatine kinase

Clinical Presentation: Neuroleptic malignant syndrome (NMS) occurs when patients are taking antipsychotic medications. It causes extremely high temperatures, muscle rigidity, and autonomic instability. Do not confuse this with serotonin syndrome, which is caused by psychiatric medications that increase serotonin (serotonin norepinephrine reuptake inhibitors [SNRIs], tricyclic antidepressants [TCAs], and monoamine oxidase [MAO] inhibitors). Both syndromes may cause elevated temperature, but the temperature in serotonin syndrome is not as high as in neuroleptic malignant syndrome. Also, serotonin syndrome can cause increased tone, yet it differs from NMS because it also causes clonus, hyperreflexia, and diarrhea. Serotonin syndrome is treated with serotonin antagonist cyproheptadine, whereas NMS is treated with dantrolene and supportive therapy.

A classic patient is a 40-year-old male with a history of schizophrenia on an antipsychotic (e.g., risperidone, olanzapine) with acute onset of altered mental status, a temperature of 105, and extreme rigidity.

PPx: Avoid offending agent

MoD: Unknown

Dx:

1. Clinical signs
2. Elevated CK
3. MRI to rule out stroke
4. LP to rule out meningitis

Tx/Mgmt:

1. Stop causative agent
2. Supportive therapy
3. Dantrolene
4. Bromocriptine

> **QUICK TIPS**
>
> Serotonin syndrome is caused by MAO inhibitors, SNRIs, and TCAs and causes clonus (spasms), hyperreflexia, hyperthermia, and altered mental state; it is treated with the serotonin antagonist cyproheptadine. Neuroleptic malignant syndrome is caused by antipsychotics and causes muscle rigidity, autonomic instability, and hyperthermia; it is treated with dantrolene.

GUNNER PRACTICE

1. A 27-year-old woman presents to the emergency room with tingling in her right hand. Her symptoms started 3 days prior to admission and have progressively worsened. A year ago she presented with an unsteady gait and tingling in her left foot. The FLAIR MRI of her head shows hyperintense lesions oriented perpendicular to the lateral ventricles. What CSF findings are most consistent with her disease process?
   A. WBC 15; PMN 5%; Glucose 70; Protein 75
   B. WBC 200; PMN 90%; Glucose 30; Protein 80
   C. WBC 300; PMN 10%; Glucose 70; Protein 90
   D. WBC 5; PMN 10%; Glucose 60; Protein 250

2. A 72-year-old man presents to the emergency room complaining of left-sided weakness. While eating breakfast this morning, his wife noticed his left face looked asymmetric and he dropped his fork while eating. On physical exam, his left arm is weaker than his left leg. He also has notable left nasolabial fold flattening. He is unable to speak or repeat phrases, but is able to follow one step commands. His medical history is significant for hypertension, smoking, and diabetes. Which of the following is the next best step in management?
   A. MRI of the head
   B. Non-contrast CT head

C. LP

D. EEG

3. A 32-year-old pregnant woman presents to the clinic complaining of intermittent numbness and tingling in her right hand for the past 3 months. The tingling is localized to the thumb, index, and part of the middle finger. It has progressed to the point where it wakes her up from sleep in the middle of the night. She has taken ibuprofen, which slightly alleviates the symptoms. The tingling is exacerbated when she is typing at work. On physical exam, she has normal muscle bulk and tone in both arms. There is decreased sensation to pinprick along her right thumb, palm, and index finger. Her reflexes are +2 bilaterally in her biceps and brachioradialis. What is the next best step in management?

A. Corticosteroid injection

B. Acetaminophen as needed

C. Surgical evaluation

D. Wrist splinting

E. Oral steroids

Notes

ANSWERS: What Would Gunner Jess/Jim Do?

1. WWGJD? A 27-year-old woman presents to the emergency room with tingling in her right hand. Her symptoms started 3 days prior to admission and have progressively worsened. A year ago she presented with an unsteady gait and tingling in her left foot. The FLAIR MRI of her head shows hyperintense lesions oriented perpendicular to the lateral ventricles. What CSF findings are most consistent with her disease process?

Answer: A. WBC 15; PMN 5%; Glucose 70; Protein 75

Explanation: The clinical scenario of a young female with focal symptoms separated by space and time is suggestive of MS. The additional MRI finding of "Dawson fingers," which are periventricular hyperintense signals, represents demyelinated plaques. The CSF findings associated with MS include mildly elevated WBCs, normal PMNs, normal glucose, and elevated protein (pleocytosis). Additionally, the CSF will show elevated IgG and oligoclonal bands, which is suggestive of MS, although these findings may be seen in other neurologic disorders.

B. WBC 200; PMN 90%; Glucose 30; Protein 80 → Incorrect. Elevated WBCs with predominance of PMNs, low glucose, and elevated protein is indicative of bacterial meningitis. Key distinguishing features of this CSF analysis include the low glucose due to bacterial consumption and predominance of PMNs versus viral meningitis, which would show lymphocytosis. The clinical scenario presented lacks symptoms of meningitis, which would include fever, stiff neck, plus positive Kernig and Brudzinski signs. Other symptoms that may be present in bacterial meningitis include encephalopathy, headache, and maculopapular rash (for *N. meningitides*).

C. WBC 300; PMN 10%; Glucose 70; Protein 90 → Incorrect. Elevated WBCs in the setting of a normal glucose, slightly elevated PMNs, and elevated proteins may be suggestive of viral meningitis. Not noted in the answer choice, but another important feature to distinguish bacterial from viral meningitis, is the presence of lymphocytosis in viral meningitis. Another important feature is that viral meningitis is not associated with low glucose.

D. WBC 5; PMN 10%; Glucose 60; Protein 250 → Incorrect. Normal WBCs in the presence of elevated protein with normal glucose and PMNs is indicative of GBS. Although this patient had difficulty walking a year ago, which may occur with GBS, these symptoms resolved and she has new symptoms that include tingling in her hand. Other clinical features to be aware of in GBS are ascending weakness, dysautonomia (tachycardia, hypertension, arrhythmias), and respiratory distress as an uncommon but severe complication.

2. **WWGJD?** A 72-year-old man presents to the emergency room complaining of left sided weakness. While eating breakfast this morning his wife noticed his left face looked asymmetric and he dropped his fork while eating. On physical exam his left arm is weaker than his left leg. He also has notable left nasolabial fold flattening. He is unable to speak or repeat phrases, but is able to follow one step commands. His medical history is significant for hypertension, smoking, and diabetes. Which of the following is the next best step in management?

Answer: B. Non-contrast CT head

   Explanation: The patient presents with symptoms suggestive of a right middle cerebral artery stroke. He has contralateral face, arm, and leg hemiparesis plus a Broca aphasia (unable to speak spontaneously or repeat words). His ability to follow verbal commands indicates that his comprehension is intact and thus he is not suffering from Wernicke aphasia. The next best step in management is to get a non-contrast CT of the head to rule out a hemorrhagic stroke. Although the majority of strokes (around 85%) are ischemic, it is critical to rule out a hemorrhagic stroke before proceeding with management. If there is no evidence of a hemorrhagic stroke on CT, then it may be possible to proceed with intravenous thrombolytics such as tPA.

   A. MRI of the head → Incorrect. An MRI is a useful tool in terms of characterizing lesions within the brain, such as tumors or strokes. In the acute setting though, the non-contrast CT is the first step because you must rule out a hemorrhagic cause of stroke in order to guide management. MRI would be a useful next step for characterizing the stroke because certain findings on MRI can help differentiate where the stroke is and also when the stroke occurred (acute vs. chronic).

   C. LP → Incorrect. LP would not help in terms of diagnosing a stroke. LP would be useful in the setting of high clinical suspicion for subarachnoid hemorrhage that had indeterminate CT scan results. Subarachnoid hemorrhage may present with focal findings but the presentation almost always includes the "worst headache of my life" or "thunderclap" headache. A non-contrast CT scan would be the best first choice in terms of diagnosing subarachnoid hemorrhage, but, if this test is negative and clinical suspicion is high, an LP showing xanthochromia would be diagnostic for subarachnoid hemorrhage.

D. EEG → Incorrect. An EEG will show abnormalities in a patient with stroke, but this is not the best initial test for diagnosis. EEG may show signs such as focal slowing in the region of the stroke. Strokes also increase the risk for seizures, and in such a case where a patient has signs of seizures who has a history of stroke then EEG is a good test to characterize the seizures.

3. **WWGJD?** A 32-year-old pregnant woman presents to the clinic complaining of intermittent numbness and tingling in her right hand for the past 3 months. The tingling is localized to the thumb, index, and part of the middle finger. It has progressed to the point where it wakes her up from sleep in the middle of the night. She has taken ibuprofen, which slightly alleviates the symptoms. The tingling is exacerbated when she is typing at work. On physical exam she has normal muscle bulk and tone in both arms. There is decreased sensation to pinprick along her right thumb, palm, and index finger. Her reflexes are +2 bilaterally in her biceps and brachioradialis. What is the next best step in management?

Answer: D. Wrist splinting

Explanation: The paresthesias in the distribution of the median nerve highly suggests carpal tunnel syndrome. Risk factors for carpal tunnel syndrome include pregnancy, diabetes, female gender, and connective tissue disease. The best initial step for treatment includes wrist splinting. It is best to start with conservative treatment before moving to more aggressive treatment modalities. It is best to do wrist splinting throughout the night (and day if possible) as well as avoiding activities that exacerbate symptoms, such as typing.

A. Corticosteroid injection → Incorrect. Corticosteroid injection is a viable treatment option for carpal tunnel syndrome, but only after more conservative measures have been attempted. If a patient has tried wrist splinting and NSAIDs for about 3 months without relief then an injection with methylprednisone is recommended.

B. Acetaminophen as needed → Incorrect. Acetaminophen is not proven to improve symptoms of carpal tunnel syndrome. Recent studies have also shown that NSAIDs show little benefit compared to placebo for treatment of carpal tunnel syndrome. The best initial step is to splint the wrist in a neutral position.

C. Surgical evaluation → Incorrect. Surgery is advisable in patients with severe carpal tunnel syndrome who have failed conservative treatment options. Evidence of axonal damage by nerve conduction studies or EMG is recommended prior to utilizing surgery as a treatment option. Carpal tunnel release surgery involves cutting the flexor retinaculum in order to decompress the median nerve.

E. Oral steroids → Incorrect. Oral steroids have been shown to be effective for short-term control of carpal tunnel syndrome symptoms. These are not the first-line therapy due to numerous side effects, and should be utilized after wrist splinting and steroid injections have failed. If there is evidence of ongoing nerve damage, surgery is a more effective means of treatment than long-term oral steroid use.

Suggested Readings

1. Uptodate.com.
2. Drislane F. *Blueprints Neurology.* 4th ed. Philadelphia: Wolters Kluwer Health/ Lippincott Williams & Wilkins; 2014.
3. Agabegi SS, Derby EA. *Step-up to Medicine.* Philadelphia: Lippincott Williams & Wilkins; 2005.
4. Le T. *First Aid for the USMLE Step 2 CK.* New York: McGraw-Hill, Medical Pub. Div; 2006.

Cardiovascular Disease

Junqian Zhang, Jacques Greenberg, Leo Wang,
Hao-Hua Wu, Rebecca Gao, and Nadia Bennett

GUNNER COLUMN

Introduction

The heart is one of the most dynamic organs in the human body. It provides the driving force of the circulatory system and can adapt to a wide range of hemodynamic conditions. Dysfunction of the cardiovascular system can occur in many acute and chronic contexts and has both local and systemic manifestations.

This chapter is divided into sections based on pathology within the cardiovascular system. For example, the heart itself can be afflicted by disease including ischemia, valvular dysfunction, infection, and arrhythmias. In addition, the vascular system may have pathologies that may be independent of cardiac disease.

The medicine shelf exam will assess both factual knowledge as well as application of principles in the context of the cardiovascular system. First, it ensures a solid foundation of knowledge about etiologies, risk factors, diagnostic criteria, and treatment for specific cardiac pathologies. Second, it associates buzz words with specific diseases. Finally, and most importantly, it conceptualizes the cardiovascular system (pump + pipes analogy works well) and works through different scenarios on how the heart (heart rate, stroke volume) and vasculature (systemic vascular resistance, mixed venous oxygen saturation) is expected to respond to changing conditions in the circulatory system.

The Heart and Great Vessels

- Left anterior descending artery (LAD) supplies the left ventricle (LV) (Fig. 6.1)
- Right coronary artery (RCA) supplies the right ventricle (RV) and both the sinoatrial (SA) and atrioventricular (AV) nodes
- The majority of individuals have a right-dominant circulation: this means that the posterior descending artery (PDA) comes off of the RCA (and not the left circumflex artery).

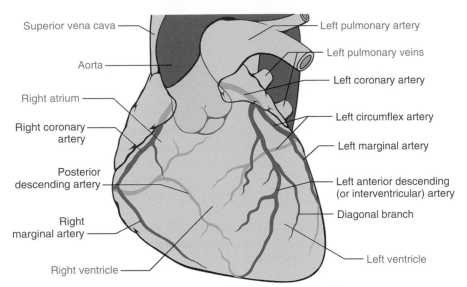

FIG. 6.1 Coronary circulation. (From Wikimedia Commons. https://commons.wikimedia.org/wiki/File:Coronary_arteries.svg. By Patrick J. Lynch, medical illustrator derivative work: Fred the Oyster [talk] adaption and further labeling: Mikael Häggström. Used under the Creative Commons Attribution-Share Alike 3.0 Unported License.)

Ischemic Heart Disease

Stable Angina

Buzz Words: Sub-sternal chest pressure or pain on EXER-TION that goes away with rest

Clinical Presentation: Sub-sternal chest pressure or pain that may radiate to the arm, shoulder, neck, or jaw. The pain may be accompanied by diaphoresis and shortness of breath. Women and the elderly may have atypical symptoms, including epigastric pain or nausea. No elevation in cardiac enzymes (troponin, creatine kinase).

PPx: Exercise, appropriate healthy diet.

MoD: Chronic atherosclerotic disease of coronary vessels prevents adequate delivery of blood to the myocardium during periods of high oxygen demand

Dx:

1. Baseline electrocardiogram (EKG)
2. Exercise EKG
   - Exercise EKG is only indicated if baseline EKG is normal
   - For patients with abnormal baseline EKG or who cannot tolerate exercise → pharmacologic stress (with coronary vasodilators—dipyridamole, regadenoson) echocardiography

3. Cardiac enzymes (no elevation in troponin or creatine kinase)
4. Coronary angiogram (if EKG or echo abnormal)

Tx/Mgmt:
1. Treat modifiable risk factors—obesity, diabetes mellitus, cholesterol
2. Sublingual nitroglycerin for acute exacerbations
3. **β-blockers, calcium channel blockers** (CCBs), or **long-acting nitrates** (isosorbide mononitrate) for chronic stable angina

Unstable Angina

Buzz Words: Sub-sternal chest pressure or pain with exertion that occurs at rest

Clinical Presentation: Sub-sternal chest pressure or pain that may radiate to the arm, shoulder, neck, or jaw **at rest** even without exertion. Other features may include diaphoresis and shortness of breath. No elevation in cardiac enzymes (troponin, creatine kinase).

PPx: Control risk factors including atherosclerosis, hyperlipidemia, DM, smoking.

MoD: Atherosclerotic plaque instability that leads to temporary partial occlusion of coronary artery with subsequent resolution—note that the distinction between stable and unstable angina is based on clinical findings.

Dx:

NSTEMI and unstable angina

1. EKG (transient ST-segment depression or T wave inversions during acute symptoms)
2. Cardiac enzymes (no elevation in troponin or creatine kinase)

Tx/Mgmt:
1. **Sublingual nitroglycerin** for acute symptoms
2. Aspirin, β-blockers, heparin 3. Coronary angiography ± angioplasty or CABG

Non-ST-Elevation Myocardial Infarction

Buzz Words: ST-depressions or T wave inversions + chest pain ± radiation to the arm and jaw

Clinical Presentation: Non-ST-elevation myocardial infarction (NSTEMI). A patient may have typical anginal chest pain (crushing substernal chest pressure is classic) ± radiation to jaw, shoulder, or arm ± diaphoresis, nausea, or vomiting and a sense of impending doom.

PPx: Control risk factors including atherosclerosis, hyperlipidemia, and DM.

MoD:
Acute plaque rupture within coronary circulation with partial occlusion or transient total occlusion that leads to partial-thickness myocardial infarction

Dx:
1. EKG—ST-depressions or T-wave inversions in contiguous leads
2. Cardiac enzymes—elevation of troponin and creatine kinase

Tx/Mgmt:
1. OH BATMAN—oxygen, heparin, β-blockers, aspirin, thrombolysis, morphine, ACE inhibitors, nitroglycerine.
   - Give aspirin and typically heparin prior to coronary catheterization.
2. Secondary prevention of future acute coronary syndrome with the following: aspirin, β-blocker, ACE inhibitors or angiotensin receptor blockers (ARBs), statin, spironolactone
   - Avoid β-blockers in patients with bradycardia, decompensated heart failure with low ejection fraction, heart block, asthma, and chronic obstructive pulmonary disease (COPD).
   - ARBs can be used in patients who are allergic to ACE inhibitors.

ST-Elevation Myocardial Infarction

ST-elevation myocardial infarction (STEMI). Note the ST-elevations in contiguous leads V_1–V_4 (Fig. 6.2).
Buzz Words: ST-elevation in contiguous leads + crushing substernal chest pressure ± radiation to jaw, shoulder, or arm ± diaphoresis, nausea, or vomiting

gg AR
STEMI ECG

MNEMONIC
OH BATMAN for the treatment of NSTEMI (oxygen, heparin, β-blockers, aspirin, thrombolysis, morphine, ACE inhibitors, nitroglycerine)

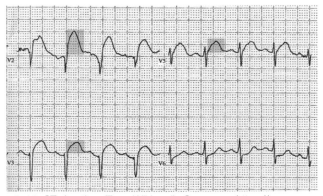

FIG. 6.2 ST elevation. (From Wikimedia Commons. https://commons.wikimedia.org/wiki/File:12_Lead_EKG_ST_Elevation_tracing_color_coded.jpg. Public Domain.)

Clinical Presentation: Typical anginal chest pain (crushing substernal chest pressure is classic) ± radiation to jaw, shoulder, or arm ± diaphoresis, nausea, or vomiting. Women and the elderly may have atypical symptoms, including epigastric pain.

PPx: Control risk factors include atherosclerosis, hyperlipidemia, and DM.

MoD: Acute plaque rupture within coronary circulation with complete occlusion leading to full-thickness myocardial infarction

Dx:
1. EKG—ST-elevations >1 mm in contiguous leads
2. Cardiac enzymes—elevation of troponin and creatine kinase
   - Troponin is more sensitive but stays elevated for up to 2 weeks after MI → use CK-MB if suspicious for repeat-MI

Tx/Mgmt:
1. **OH BATMAN**—oxygen, heparin, β-blockers, aspirin, thrombolysis, morphine, ACE inhibitors, nitroglycerine
   - Give aspirin and typically heparin prior to coronary catheterization
2. Coronary catheterization (door-to-balloon time < 90 minutes is ideal)Secondary prevention of future acute coronary syndrome with: aspirin, β-blocker, ACE inhibitors or ARBs, statin, spironolactone
   - Avoid β-blockers in patients with bradycardia, decompensated heart failure with low ejection fraction, heart block, asthma, and COPD.
   - ARBs can be used in patients who are allergic to ACE inhibitors.
3. Ventricular arrhythmias are common after MI and are the most common cause of cardiac failure and death in the immediate post-MI period.
4. Ventricular free-wall rupture, septal rupture, and papillary muscle rupture most commonly occur during the first 7–10 days after MI.
   - Posteromedial papillary muscle is most prone to rupture due to single blood supply from the RCA.
5. Ventricular aneurysms tend to occur months after MI.

QUICK TIPS
Localization of Infarct Based on EKG Changes

Location	ST-elevations	ST-depressions
Left Lateral	I, aVL, V_5–V_6	aVR
Right	Use right-sided leads	I, aVL, V_5–V_6
Anterior	V_1–V_3	None
Posterior	None	V_1–V_3

Prinzmetal Angina (Variant Angina)

Buzz Words: Young, female smokers + anginal chest pain + nighttime

Clinical Presentation: Young and **middle-aged female smokers** who present with typical chest pain, especially at night. This is associated with **migraines** and Raynaud phenomenon (i.e., other vasospasm-related disorders); this can also occur secondary to cocaine use.

MoD: Coronary artery vasospasm leading to tissue ischemia/infarction

Dx:
1. EKG—typically normal but may show ST-segment abnormalities during episodes of vasospasm
2. **Coronary angiography** with provocation testing with **ergonovine** or **acetylcholine** is the gold standard.

Tx/Mgmt: **CCBs** or **nitrates. β-blockers are contraindicated,** as they can lead to exacerbation of vasospasm (i.e., unopposed α-adrenergic stimulation).

Arrhythmias

Premature Atrial Contractions/Premature Ventricular Contractions

Buzz Words: Asymptomatic or mild discomfort + premature contraction of the atria or ventricles (Figs. 6.3 and 6.4)

Clinical Presentation: Patients are typically asymptomatic. Patients with frequent premature atrial contractions (PACs) or premature ventricular contractions (PVCs) may have mild chest discomfort or palpitations.

MoD: Premature atrial or ventricular electrical activity that interrupts normal sinus rhythm

Dx:
1. EKG—premature P-wave and subsequent QRS complex interrupting the expected progression of beats (PAC), wide-complex, bizarre QRS interrupting the expected progression of beats (PVC)
2. Holter monitor—for patients who are intermittently symptomatic

Tx/Mgmt:
1. Asymptomatic PACs/PVCs—no treatment
2. Symptomatic PACs/PVCs—**β-blockers**

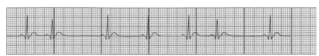

FIG. 6.3 Premature atrial contraction. (From Wikimedia Commons. https://commons.wikimedia.org/wiki/File:PAC.png. Public Domain.)

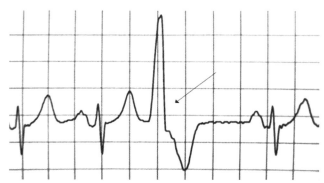

FIG. 6.4 Premature ventricular contraction. (From Wikimedia Commons. https://commons.wikimedia.org/wiki/File:PVC10.JPG. By James Heilman, MD. Used under the Creative Commons Attribution Share-Alike 3.0 Unported license.)

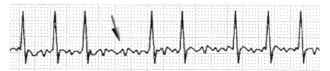

FIG. 6.5 Atrial fibrillation. (From Wikimedia Commons. https://commons.wikimedia.org/wiki/File:Afib_ecg.jpg. By J. Heuser (Own work) Used under the Creative Commons Attribution Share-Alike 3.0 Unported license.)

Atrial Arrhythmia

Atrial Fibrillation

Buzz Words (Fig. 6.5): Irregular rhythm, absence of P-waves

Clinical Presentation: Can be paroxysmal or chronic. Patients can be asymptomatic or have symptoms ranging from palpitations, chest discomfort, lightheadedness, and syncope to hemodynamic instability.

- Atrial fibrillation with rapid ventricular response indicates rapid conduction through the AV node and ↑ventricular rate.
- Long-standing tachycardia can lead to dilated cardiomyopathy.

MoD: Ectopic atrial conduction usually originating from around the pulmonary veins

- Causes of atrial fibrillation include but are not limited to structural heart disease, valvular heart disease (mitral regurgitation, mitral stenosis), asthma and COPD, hyperthyroidism, hypertension, obstructive sleep apnea, and alcohol consumption.

Dx:

1. EKG showing absence of P-waves and irregularly irregular rhythm
2. Holter monitor for paroxysmal atrial fibrillation

Tx/Mgmt:

1. Hemodynamically unstable → **synchronized cardioversion**
2. Hemodynamically stable
   - Onset less than 48 hours
     - Rate control—**β-blockers** (metoprolol), **non-dihydropyridine CCBs** (verapamil, diltiazem)
   - Onset greater than 48 hours
     - Use CHA_2DS_2-VASc
     - Score of 0 in males or 1 in females → no anticoagulation needed
     - Score of 1 in males → consider anticoagulation
     - Score ≥2 → anticoagulate
   - Consider rate control, rhythm control (Class I & III antiarrhythmics), synchronized cardioversion, or catheter ablation (of the electrical pathways near the pulmonary veins)

CHA2DS2-VASc calculator

QUICK TIPS

CHA_2DS_2-VASc—Risk of Stroke in Patients with Atrial Fibrillation

	Condition	Points
C	Congestive heart failure	1
H	Hypertension > 140/90 mm Hg	1
A_2	Age ≥75	2
D	Diabetes mellitus	1
S_2	Prior stroke or transient ischemic attack	2
V	Prior vascular disease (MI, peripheral vascular disease)	1
A	Age 65–74	1
Sc	Female sex	1

Atrial Flutter

Buzz Words: **Sawtooth** waves on EKG

Clinical Presentation: Patients can be asymptomatic or have symptoms ranging from palpitations, chest discomfort, lightheadedness, and syncope to hemodynamic instability.

MoD: Ectopic atrial conduction originating from around the tricuspid annulus. Causes of atrial flutter include, but are not limited to, structural heart disease, valvular heart disease (mitral regurgitation, mitral stenosis), asthma and COPD, hyperthyroidism, hypertension, and obstructive sleep apnea.

Dx: EKG showing sawtooth pattern between 250 and 300 bpm with no discernable P-waves (Fig. 6.6)

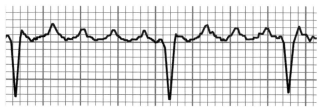

FIG. 6.6 Atrial flutter. (From Wikimedia Commons. https://commons. wikimedia.org/wiki/File:Atrial_flutter34.svg. By Atrial_flutter34.JPG: James Heilman, MD derivative work: Mysid (using Perl and Inkscape) [This file was derived from Atrial flutter34.JPG:]. Used under the Creative Commons Attribution Share-Alike 3.0 Unported License.)

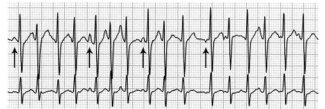

FIG. 6.7 Multifocal atrial tachycardia. (From Wikimedia Commons. https://commons.wikimedia.org/wiki/File%3AMultifocal_atrial_tachycardia_-_MAT.png. By Jer5150 [Own work]. Used under the Creative Commons Attribution Share-Alike 3.0 Unported license.)

Tx/Mgmt:
1. Hemodynamically unstable
   - Synchronized cardioversion
2. Hemodynamically stable
   - β-blockers, CCBs + anticoagulation for at least 4 weeks
   - Anticoagulation for at least 4 weeks and then cardioversion
   - Ablation

Multifocal Atrial Tachycardia

Buzz Words (Fig. 6.7): Irregularly irregular supraventricular tachycardia with at least three different P-wave morphologies

Clinical Presentation: Patients can be asymptomatic or have symptoms ranging from palpitations, chest discomfort, lightheadedness, and syncope to hemodynamic instability. Particularly common in older people with COPD

MoD: Multiple atrial foci (≥3) of electrical activity

Dx:
1. Tachycardia with at least three different P-wave morphologies
2. Irregularly irregular rhythm

Tx/Mgmt:
1. Treatment of underlying cause

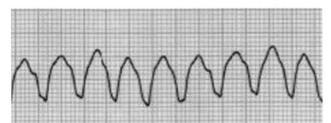

FIG. 6.8 Ventricular tachycardia. (From Wikimedia Commons. https://commons.wikimedia.org/wiki/File:Lead_II_rhythm_ventricular_tachycardia_Vtach_VT_(cropped).JPG. Public Domain.)

2. Vagal maneuvers and adenosine can break reentrant supraventricular tachycardias but are not as useful for multifocal atrial tachycardia
3. **β-blockers** and **CCBs** can be used for rate control

Reentrant Tachycardia

Buzz Words: Narrow-complex tachycardia which may be asymptomatic or present with palpitations, chest discomfort, and lightheadedness

Clinical Presentation: A patient may be asymptomatic or present with palpitations, chest pain, SOB, lightheadedness, or syncope.

MoD: Rapid electrical conduction with reentrant conduction through an accessory pathway between the atria and ventricles (most commonly seen in Wolf-Parkinson-White [WPW] syndrome) or within the AV node itself (AV nodal reentrant tachycardia)

Dx:
1. AV reentry → see section on WPW syndrome
2. AV nodal reentry → EKG with narrow complex tachycardia and retrograde P-waves

Tx/Mgmt: AV nodal reentry → vagal maneuvers; medications that slow conduction through the AV node include the following: adenosine, CCBs, β-blockers

Re-entrant tachycardia

Ventricular Arrhythmia

Ventricular Tachycardia

Buzz Words (Fig. 6.8): Wide-complex monomorphic tachycardia

Clinical Presentation: A patient may present with palpitations, lightheadedness, SOB, or syncope. This is a serious condition that can lead to cardiac arrest.

MoD:
- Ectopic pacemaker in the ventricles or reentrant circuit around area of infarcted myocardium → monomorphic ventricular tachycardia (VT)

Ventricular tachycardia

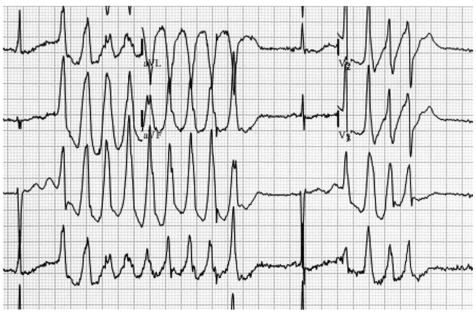

FIG. 6.9 Torsades de pointes. (From Wikimedia Commons. https://commons.wikimedia.org/wiki/File:Torsades_de_Pointes_TdP.png. By Jer5150 [Own work]. Used under the Creative Commons Attribution Share-Alike 3.0 Unported License.)

- Torsades de pointes is a polymorphic VT that is associated with prolonged QT interval (Fig. 6.9).
  - Common causes of torsades de pointes include the following: hypokalemia, hypomagnesemia, drugs (fluoroquinolones, erythromycin, typical antipsychotics).
  - Treat with magnesium sulfate.

Dx:
1. EKG with wide-complex tachycardia
   - Must distinguish from SVT with aberrancy (meaning a supraventricular tachycardia that excites the ventricles too quickly, leading to bundle branch blocks and wide-complex tachycardia presentation)

Tx/Mgmt:
1. Hemodynamically unstable → cardioversion
   - Pulseless VT → defibrillation
2. Hemodynamically stable
   - Procainamide, sotalol, amiodarone

Ventricular Fibrillation
Buzz Words: Low-amplitude undulating EKG without QRS complexes

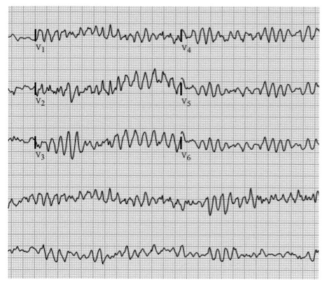

FIG. 6.10 Ventricular fibrillation. (From Wikimedia Commons. https://commons.wikimedia.org/wiki/File:Ventricular_fibrillation.png. By Jer5150 [Own work]. Used under the Creative Commons Attribution Share-Alike 3.0 Unported License.)

Clinical Presentation: Ventricular fibrillation (VF) may occur following cardiac arrest and lead to hypotension, syncope, and/or sudden death.

MoD: Uncoordinated electrical activity in the ventricles leading to systolic dysfunction and collapse of the systemic circulation

Dx: EKG showing fine or coarse fibrillating line (Fig. 6.10)

Tx/Mgmt:

1. **Defibrillation** ± epinephrine, amiodarone
2. **Pulseless electrical activity** = cardiac rhythm on EKG that is expected to produce a pulse but does not.
   - Treat with **CPR** + epinephrine → defibrillation if reverts to pulseless VT or VF.
3. **Asystole** = absence of cardiac electrical activity (flat line on EKG)
   - Treat with **CPR** + epinephrine → defibrillation if reverts to pulseless VT or VF

Conduction Blocks

1st Degree Heart Block

Buzz Words: Prolonged PR interval ≥0.2 seconds + regular rhythm

Clinical Presentation: Patient is asymptomatic. Prolonged PR interval ≥0.2 seconds.

MoD: Delay of conduction in the AV node

Dx: EKG—PR prolongation ≥0.2 seconds

Tx/Mgmt: No treated needed.

2nd Degree Heart Block
Mobitz Type I (Wenckebach) (Fig. 6.11A)

Buzz Words: Prolonging of the PR interval followed by a dropped beat; grouped beating + abnormal rhythm

Clinical Presentation: Patient is often asymptomatic. Progressive **prolonging of PR interval** ending with a dropped beat → compare the PR intervals of the beats just before and just after the dropped beat. The QRS interval is normal.

MoD: Delay of conduction at the level of the AV node

Dx: EKG—progressive prolonging of the PR interval followed by a drop beat

Tx/Mgmt: No treatment needed

Mobitz Type II (see Fig. 6.11B)

Buzz Words: Constant PR interval followed by a dropped beat; grouped beating

Clinical Presentation: **PR interval is constant** prior to dropped beat. QRS interval is typically prolonged

MoD: Delay of conduction in the bundle of His

Intro to heart blocks

QUICK TIPS

Compare the PR interval of the last beat before the dropped beat with the first beat following the dropped beat

Mobitzl or Wenckebach

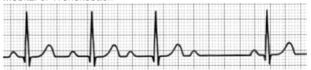

Mobitzl II

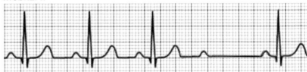

2:1 block

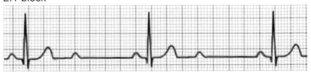

FIG. 6.11 Types of second-degree heart block. (A) Mobitz I or Wonckebach. (B) Mobitz II. (From Wikimedia Commons. https://commons.wikimedia.org/wiki/File:Second_degree_heart_block.png. By Npatchett [Own work]. Used under the Creative Commons Attribution-Share Alike 4.0 International license.)

Dx: EKG—constant PR interval before and after a dropped beat with prolongation of the QRS complex ≥0.12 seconds

Tx/Mgmt: Pacemaker insertion to prevent complete heart block

3rd Degree (Complete) Heart Block

Buzz Words (Fig. 6.12): Complete dissociation of the electrical activity between the atria and the ventricles

Clinical Presentation: Complete dissociation of the atria and ventricles. Spontaneous atrial and ventricular pacemakers are firing independently → no association between P-waves and QRS complexes

MoD: Damage to the AV node (most commonly by ischemia) leads to loss of conduction of atrial signals into the ventricles.

Dx: EKG showing dissociation between P-waves and QRS complexes (typically ≥0.1 seconds). The duration between successive P-waves is constant. The duration between successive QRS complexes is also constant.

Tx/Mgmt: Pacemaker insertion

QUICK TIPS
Look for buried P-waves presenting as weird blips in QRS or T-waves

Bundle Branch Blocks
Left Bundle Branch Block (LBBB)

Buzz Words (Fig. 6.13): Delay in electrical conduction system of the left heart with prolonged QRS, dominant S-wave in V_1, and notched R-wave in V_6

Clinical Presentation: Patients are typically asymptomatic. On auscultation, patients may have paradoxical splitting of S_2.

MoD: Disease of the conducting system of the left heart impedes conduction from the atria to the LV. Etiologies include myocardial infarction (look at left lateral leads I, V_5, V_6), aortic stenosis (AS), and dilated cardiomyopathy (think left heart pathology).

Dx: EKG—with prolonged QRS ≥0.12 seconds and prominent S-wave in V_1 and notched R-wave in V_6 (Fig. 6.14).

Tx/Mgmt: No specific treatment is necessary for isolated LBBB. New-onset LBBB can be a sign of myocardial ischemia, however, and should prompt further investigation (e.g., troponins).

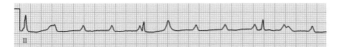

FIG. 6.12 Complete heart block. (From Wikimedia Commons. https://commons.wikimedia.org/wiki/File:Complete_A-V_block_with_resulting_junctional_escape.png. By Jer5150 [Own work]. Used under the Creative Commons Attribution Share-Alike 3.0 Unported License.)

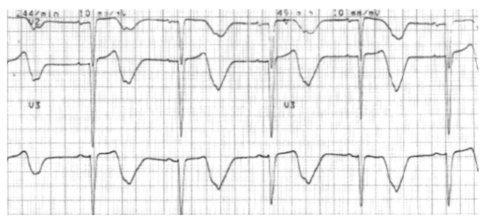

FIG. 6.13 Left bundle branch block. (From: http://www.elsevier.pt/en/revistas/revista-portuguesa-cardio-logia-334/artigo/left-bundle-branch-block-atrioventricular-block-torsade-pointes-S2174204913000846)

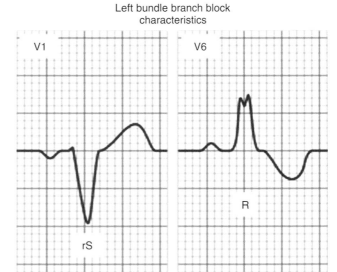

FIG. 6.14 Left bundle branch block. (From Wikimedia Commons. https://commons.wikimedia.org/wiki/File:Left_bundle_branch_block_ECG_characteristics.png. By A. Rad at the English language Wikipedia, CC BY-SA 3.0, https://commons.wikimedia.org/w/index. php?curid=2478480. Used under the Creative Commons Attribution Share-Alike 3.0 Unported License.)

Right Bundle Branch Block
Buzz Words:
Delay in electrical conduction system of the right heart with prolonged QRS, RSR' (rabbit ears pattern) in V_1–V_3, and wide slurred S-wave in V_6

Clinical Presentation: Typically asymptomatic

MoD: Disease of the conducting system of the right heart impedes conduction from the atria to the RV. Etiologies

Right bundle branch block
characteristics

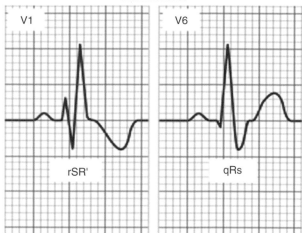

FIG. 6.15 Right bundle branch block. (From Wikimedia Commons. https://commons.wikimedia.org/wiki/File:Right_bundle_branch_block_ECG_characteristics.png. Used under the Creative Commons Attribution Share-Alike 3.0 Unported License.)

include myocardial infarction, pulmonic stenosis, massive PE (causing right heart strain), and dilated cardiomyopathy (think right heart pathology).

Dx: EKG—with prolonged QRS ≥0.12 seconds, RSR' (rabbit ears pattern) in V_1–V_3, and wide slurred S-wave in V6 (Fig. 6.15)

Tx/Mgmt: No specific treatment is necessary for isolated right bundle branch block (RBBB). New-onset RBBB can be a sign of myocardial ischemia, however, and should prompt further investigation (e.g., troponins).

Long-QT Syndromes

- **Romano-Ward syndrome** = autosomal dominant long-QT syndrome
- **Jervell and Lange-Nielsen syndrome** = autosomal recessive long-QT syndrome + sensorineural hearing loss

Sick Sinus Syndrome

Buzz Words: Impaired conduction from the sinus node that may cause periods of tachycardia and periods of conduction block/bradycardia

Clinical Presentation: May be asymptomatic or present with palpitations, chest pain, lightheadedness, and syncope
- **Tachy-Brady syndrome** = subset of sick sinus syndrome with periods of tachycardia and

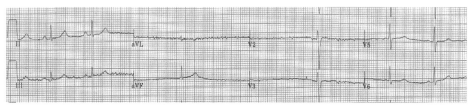

FIG. 6.16 Tachy-brady syndrome. Note the transition from tachycardia to bradycardia. (From ECGpedia. org. http://en.ecgpedia.org/images/7/79/E000167.jpg. Courtesy of Vincent de Rover. Used under the Creative Commons Attribution Share-Alike 3.0 Unported License.)

bradycardia often associated with ischemic or valvular heart disease (Fig. 6.16)

MoD: Scarring, degeneration, or damage to the conduction system that impairs conduction from the sinus node.

Dx:

1. EKG—showing periods of arrhythmia (e.g., sinus block, sinus bradycardia, and atrial fibrillation) during acute events
2. Holter monitor is often necessary, as conduction blocks may be transient

Tx/Mgmt:

1. Patients with bradyarrhythmias require pacemaker
2. Patients with isolated tachyarrhythmias may be managed medically with β-blockers and CCBs.

Wolf-Parkinson-White Syndrome

Buzz Words (Fig. 6.17): Up-sloping first segment of QRS (**delta wave**), prolonged QRS, decreased PR-interval

Clinical Presentation: Patients are typically asymptomatic when not in reentrant rhythm. When arrhythmic, patients may have palpitations, lightheadedness, and/or syncope.

MoD: Presence of an accessory conduction tract between the atria and ventricles (Bundle of Kent) that allows for bypass of the AV node. Reentrant rhythm can occur with retrograde conduction from the ventricles through the accessory tract and back into the atria.

Dx:

EKG shows:

- Decreased PR-interval
- Characteristic up-sloping first segment of QRS (**delta wave**)
- Prolonged QRS

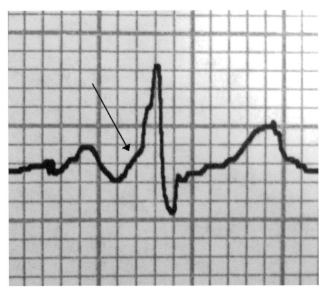

FIG. 6.17 Delta wave of Wolf-Parkinson-White syndrome (Wiki). Note the shortened PR-interval and upsloping R-wave in the QRS complex. (From Wikimedia Commons. https://commons.wikimedia.org/wiki/File:DeltaWave09.JPG. By James Heilman, MD [Own work]. Used under the Creative Commons Attribution Share-Alike 3.0 Unported License.)

Tx/Mgmt: **Procainamide** or amiodarone for tachyarrhythmias associated with WPW

Heart Failure

Congestive Heart Failure
Systolic Dysfunction (heart failure with reduced ejection fraction/HFrEF)

Buzz Words: Orthopnea, reduced ejection fraction (EF ≤ 55%), pulmonary edema

Clinical Presentation:
- Left-sided HF—SOB, pulmonary edema (rales, crackles), orthopnea, paroxysmal nocturnal dyspnea, decreased perfusion (e.g., cyanosis, AKI, and hepatic injury)
- Right-sided HF—edema, ascites, ↑JVP, liver enlargement (nutmeg liver), hepatojugular reflux, decreased perfusion (e.g., cyanosis, AKI, and hepatic injury)

PPx: Control of risk factors—HTN, EtOH, atherosclerosis/CAD risk factors

MoD: Variable but all lead to impaired ventricular contraction (↓ejection fraction)

Dx:
1. EKG (LVH/RVH → high amplitude QRS complex)
2. Echocardiogram showing reduced ejection fraction
3. Elevated levels of pro-brain natriuretic peptide (pro-BNP)

QUICK TIPS
Avoid adenosine, β-blockers, CCBs as they can increase conduction through the accessory pathway → ↑↑HR

99 AR
2013 ACCF/AHA guidelines for treatment of heart failure

QUICK TIPS
Nutmeg liver is caused by venous congestion of hepatic vessels (dark areas) and areas of uninvolved tissue.

QUICK TIPS
The only β-blockers shown to improve survival are metoprolol tartrate, carvedilol, and bisoprolol.

QUICK TIPS
Hydralazine can be of benefit in African Americans with NYHA class III-IV heart failure.

QUICK TIPS
New York Heart Association (NYHA) Heart Failure Classes

Tx/Mgmt:
1. Acute HF—diuretics (furosemide), noninvasive positive pressure ventilation
2. Chronic HF
   - Survival benefit: ACE inhibitors, ARBs, β-blockers, spironolactone
   - Symptom management without survival benefit: diuretics, digoxin, hydralazine

Class	Description
I	No limitation of physical activity
II	Slight limitation of physical activity—fatigue, SOB, or palpitations with ordinary physical activity Comfortable at rest
III	Marked limitation of physical activity—less than ordinary activity causes fatigue, SOB, or palpitations Comfortable at rest
IV	Unable to carry on any physical activity without discomfort Symptoms of heart failure at rest

Diastolic Dysfunction (heart failure with preserved ejection fraction/HFpEF)

Buzz Words: Preserved ejection fraction (EF ≥55%)

Clinical Presentation: Similar to systolic heart failure as described above

MoD: Impaired relaxation (diastolic dysfunction) of the ventricles → increased left ventricular end-diastolic pressure → back-up of pressure through the left heart, pulmonary circulation, and right heart

Dx:
1. EKG
2. Echocardiography showing preserved ejection fraction
3. Elevated levels of pro-BNP

Tx/Mgmt:
1. Current treatments do not improve survival
2. β-blockers, ACEIs, and diuretics for symptom management

High-Output Cardiac Failure

Buzz Words: Increased ejection fraction, hyper-dynamic circulation, bounding pulses with widened pulse pressure

Clinical Presentation: Patients may present with SOB, dyspnea, pulmonary edema, peripheral edema in the setting of increased EF (hyper-dynamic circulation). On exam, check for bounding pulse with widened pulse pressure.

MoD:
- Anemia—blood is unable to provide enough oxygen for tissues → requires faster circulation
- Arteriovenous fistulas (e.g., hereditary hemorrhagic telangiectasia, knife wound in the thigh causing a shunt)—shunting of blood from the arterial to venous system simulates anemia (tissues are not getting enough oxygen), so the heart must pump faster to deliver more blood
- Paget disease of the bone—increased vascularization of metabolically active bone
- Sepsis—dilation of peripheral vasculature
- Thyrotoxicosis
- Wet beriberi (vitamin B1 deficiency)

Dx:
1. EKG
2. Echocardiography—evidence of increased ejection fraction and hyperdynamic circulation
3. Pro-BNP levels can be used for evidence of ventricular strain

Tx/Mgmt:
1. Treatment of underlying etiology:
   - Anemia—blood transfusions or iron supplementation depending on the cause of anemia
   - AV-fistulas—surgical repair
   - Paget disease of the bone—bisphosphonates, calcitonin
   - Thyrotoxicosis—depends on the cause (radioactive iodine for Graves, surgical resection for hot thyroid nodule)
   - Wet beriberi—replete vitamin B1 (thiamine)

Valvular Heart Disease

Aortic Valve Disease
Aortic Stenosis
Buzz Words: Pulsus parvus et tardus (weak & late-arriving pulse), crescendo-decrescendo murmur at the right upper sternal border that radiates to carotids

Clinical Presentation:
- SAD—syncope, angina, dyspnea
- *Pulsus parvus et tardus*—weak & late arriving carotid pulse

> **QUICK TIPS**
> Recall that aortic stenosis and cardiac tamponade can lead to narrowed pulse pressures

> **QUICK TIPS**
> FAST B1P—fistula, anemia, sepsis, thyrotoxicosis, wet beriberi (B1), Paget disease of the bone

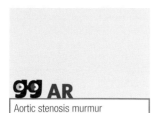

Aortic stenosis murmur

- Early **systolic** ejection murmur—crescendo-decrescendo murmur best heard at the right upper sternal border
  - Radiates to carotids
- Soft aortic component of the second heart sound

MoD:
- Narrowing of aortic valve increases afterload → LV strain, weak pulses, inadequate delivery of blood
- Typically occurs in older individuals → most commonly due to senile sclerocalcific changes of the aortic valve
- AS in younger individuals is often caused by bicuspid/unicuspid aortic valves or rheumatic fever (developing nations)

Dx: Echocardiography to visualize valve, measure flow, pressure gradient, and valve area

Tx/Mgmt:
1. Aortic valve replacement is indicated in the following:
   - Patients with symptomatic disease
   - Patients with severe AS (pressure gradient ≥40 mm Hg) with LVEF ≤40% or undergoing other cardiac surgery

Aortic Regurgitation

Buzz Words: Waterhammer pulse, decrescendo murmur at the right upper sternal border

Clinical Presentation: Dyspnea on exertion, orthopnea, chest pain

Early diastolic murmur—**decrescendo murmur** best heard at the right upper sternal border

Increased pulse pressure (difference between systolic and diastolic blood pressures) → bounding pulses

Austin Flint murmur = rumbling mid-diastolic murmur heard in severe aortic regurgitation (AR)

MoD: Most often caused by **dilation of the aortic root**—can occur with bicuspid aortic valve, collagen vascular diseases (Marfan syndrome, Ehlers-Danlos syndrome), rheumatic fever, ankylosing spondylitis, or idiopathic. Loss of adequate valve coaptation leads to backflow of blood into the LV after ventricular systole.

Dx: Echocardiography to visualize valve and measure flow

Tx/Mgmt:
1. **Aortic valve replacement** is the treatment of choice Indications include symptomatic disease or with EF ≤ 50%

2. ACEIs, ARBs, and CCBs may be useful in patients with AR and HTN to reduce afterload on the strained LV.

Mitral Valve Disease

Mitral Stenosis

Buzz Words: Opening snap with a mid-diastolic, low-pitched, rumbling murmur

Clinical Presentation: Mid-diastolic, low-pitched, rumbling murmur with opening snap

Dyspnea on exertion, orthopnea, chest pain

Secondary atrial fibrillation

PPx: Prevention of rheumatic heart disease

MoD: Thickened, fibrotic, calcified mitral valve → reduced diastolic flow through the mitral valve → ↑left atrial pressures → back up of pressure into the pulmonary circulation

Chronic increase in left atrial pressures leads to dilatation → disruption of electrical conduction system → atrial fibrillation

Dx:

1. EKG
2. **Echocardiography**—visualize valve, measure flow, pressure gradient, and valve area

Tx/Mgmt:

1. For patients with mild mitral stenosis:
   - Dietary sodium restriction
   - Careful titration of β-blockers while avoiding medications that reduce afterload (to prevent hypotension)
   - Rheumatic fever prophylaxis with penicillin or azithromycin
   - Monitor for sequelae of mitral stenosis → atrial fibrillation (anticoagulated as necessary)
2. **Mitral valve replacement** or balloon valvuloplasty for refractory disease or recurrent embolization due to atrial fibrillation

Mitral Valve Prolapse

Buzz Words: Mid-systolic click followed by a systolic decrescendo murmur

Clinical Presentation: Can be asymptomatic or present with palpitations, chest pain, or dyspnea on exertion

Mid-systolic click followed by decrescendo murmur (systolic)

   Murmur increases in duration with Valsalva or decreasing preload

99 AR

Mitral stenosis murmur

99 AR

Mitral prolapse and regurgitation

Risk factors include collagen vascular disorders (Marfan syndrome, Ehlers-Danlos syndrome), polycystic kidney disease, Graves disease

MoD: Myxomatous valve degeneration

Dx: Echocardiography showing variable prolapse of the mitral valve leaflets into the LA during ventricular systole

Tx/Mgmt:

1. Most patients require no treatment.
2. Those with symptomatic mitral valve prolapse (MVP) can be treated with β-blockers.
3. No antibiotic prophylaxis is needed for dental procedures in otherwise healthy patients with MVP.

Mitral Regurgitation

Buzz Words: Mid-systolic, blowing murmur that radiates to the axilla

Clinical Presentation: Signs of congestive heart failure—SOB, orthopnea, paroxysmal nocturnal dyspnea

Atrial fibrillation due to LA dilation → *P mitrale* = broad P-wave with two peaks

Initially see increased ejection fraction → decrease in EF suggests systolic heart failure

MoD: MVP is the most common predisposing factor.

Other causes include ischemic heart disease, rheumatic fever, and connective tissue disease.

Posterior MI can lead to ischemia of the posteromedial papillary muscle → acute mitral regurgitation (MR).

Dx: Echocardiography—measure degree of regurgitation

Tx/Mgmt:

1. Medical management is aimed at decreasing afterload with ACEIs or hydralazine to increase the forward ejection fraction while minimizing the regurgitant fraction
2. Surgical repair for ↓EF, severe pulmonary hypertension, or new onset atrial fibrillation

Tricuspid Valve Disease

Tricuspid Stenosis

Buzz Words: Mid-diastolic murmur that is best heard over the left sternal border

Clinical Presentation: Mid-diastolic murmur that is best heard over the left sternal border, which may increase with inspiration

Right-heart dysfunction with backup of pressure into the venous system

QUICK TIPS

For posterior MI, look for inverse changes (ST-depressions) in the anterior precordial leads V_1 and V_2.

May result in hepatic congestion and peripheral edema
Jugular venous pressure is increased

MoD: Almost always caused by rheumatic heart disease

Dx: Echocardiography

Tx/Mgmt:

1. Medical management with diuretics and salt restriction to decrease preload on right heart
2. Balloon valvuloplasty or surgical replacement for refractory symptomatic disease

Tricuspid Regurgitation

Buzz Words: Blowing systolic murmur best heard at the lower left sternal border that increases with inspiration, large C-V waves on jugular venous tracings

Clinical Presentation: Right-sided heart failure—ascites, peripheral edema
Pan-systolic murmur that increases with inspiration
Large C-V waves in the jugular venous pulse

MoD: Dilation of the tricuspid annulus—most commonly, 2/2 RV dilation
Rheumatic heart disease, myxomatous degeneration

Dx: Echocardiography

Tx/Mgmt:

1. For patients with left-sided heart failure leading to tricuspid regurgitation
   • Diuretics and ACE inhibitors
2. Tricuspid valve replacement for symptomatic patients or those with RV dysfunction

Pulmonic Valve Disease

Pulmonic Stenosis

Buzz Words: Systolic ejection murmur at the right upper sternal border, right-sided S_4, loud S_2

Clinical Presentation: Asymptomatic or dyspnea on exertion/signs of right heart failure
Systolic ejection murmur at the right upper sternal border
Loud S_2
RVH → may present with right-sided S_4

MoD: Congenital: Tetralogy of Fallot (ToF), Noonan syndrome, congenital rubella syndrome, Williams syndrome, Alagille syndrome
Acquired: carcinoid syndrome

Dx: Echocardiography showing reduced flow through the pulmonic valve

Tx/Mgmt: Balloon valvotomy is the preferred treatment.

gg AR
Tricuspid regurgitation murmur

gg AR
Heart murmurs

Pulmonic Regurgitation

Buzz Words: Diastolic murmur best heard at the right upper sternal border

Clinical Presentation: Patients are typically asymptomatic prior to right ventricular dysfunction.

Dyspnea on exertion, lightheadedness, syncope, peripheral edema, hepatic congestion

Graham-Steell murmur = early, diastolic murmur heard best at the left sternal edge with the patient in full inspiration

MoD: Etiologies include iatrogenic, endocarditis, rheumatic heart disease, carcinoid disease, and congenital (ToF)

Dx: Echocardiography showing retrograde flow through the pulmonic valve

Tx/Mgmt:

1. Mild pulmonic regurgitation typically does not require treatment as the right heart can adapt to the low-pressure volume overload
2. Surgical valve repair in cases of RV strain or failure

Pericardial Disease

Pericardial Effusion

Buzz Words: Water bottle heart, enlarged cardiac silhouette, low-voltage on EKG with electrical alternans, pulsus paradoxus

Clinical Presentation: Variable depending on rate of formation and volume of effusion

Large volumes can accumulate with long-standing, slow effusions.

Rapid effusions cause cardiac dysfunction almost immediately.

Cardiac tamponade = effusion that results in equalization of intracardiac pressures → bulging of interventricular septum into the LV → ↓stroke volume → cardiogenic shock

Pulsus paradoxus = drop of >10 mm Hg in systolic BP with inspiration

MoD:

Etiologies include the following:

Post-myocardial infarction or cardiac surgery

Autoimmune disease

Acute pericarditis

Malignancy

Uremia

Blunt cardiac trauma

Dx:
1. Chest X-ray (CXR) —enlarged cardiac silhouette (water bottle heart) (Fig. 6.18)
2. EKG

   Low voltage—low amplitude QRS

   Electrical alternans—alternating amplitude of QRS with each beat (heart is moving in sac of fluid so the major axis of EKG changes with each beat) (Fig. 6.19)
3. Echocardiography
4. Diagnostic and therapeutic pericardiocentesis—if the etiology of the effusion is not known

Tx/Mgmt:
1. Asymptomatic, small effusions can be monitored if the patient is hemodynamically stable
2. Hemodynamically unstable patients (i.e., tamponade) require pericardiocentesis

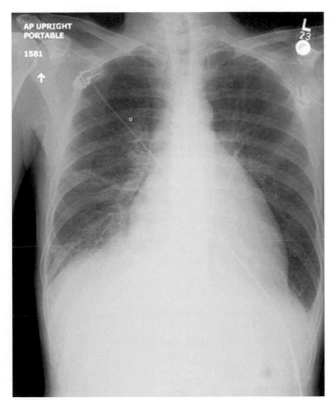

FIG. 6.18 Pericardial effusion. Note the enlarged cardiac silhouette. (From Wikimedia Commons. https://commons.wikimedia.org/wiki/File:Water_bottle.png. By Jer5150 [Own work]. Used under the Creative Commons Attribution Share-Alike 3.0 Unported License.)

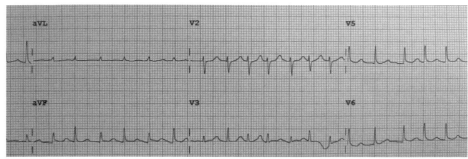

FIG. 6.19 Electrical alternans. Note the alternating amplitudes of the QRS complex as the heart swings in a pericardial effusion. (From Wikimedia Commons. https://commons.wikimedia.org/wiki/File:Electrical_Alternans.JPG. By James Heilman, MD [Own work]. Used under the Creative Commons Attribution Share-Alike 3.0 Unported License.)

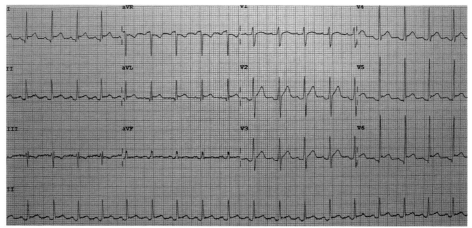

FIG. 6.20 Pericarditis. Note the diffuse ST-elevations with PR-depressions in all leads except aVR. (From Wikimedia Commons. https://commons.wikimedia.org/wiki/Category:Pericarditis#/media/File:Pericarditis2016.jpg. By James Heilman, MD [own work]. Used under the Creative Commons Attribution Share-Alike 3.0 Unported License.)

- Patients with large effusions typically require eventual treatment, even if they are asymptomatic

Pericarditis

Acute

Pericarditis (Wiki). Note the diffuse ST-elevations with PR-depressions in all leads except aVR (Fig. 6.20).

Buzz Words: Friction rub, diffuse ST-elevations with PR-depressions, improvement with sitting up and leaning forward

Clinical Presentation: Sharp chest pain that is classically improved while sitting up and leaning forward

Diffuse ST-elevations and **PR-depressions** in all leads except aVR on EKG

Pericardial **friction rub** on auscultation

MoD: Inflammation of the pericardium 2/2 **infection**, **uremia**, autoimmune (**Dressler syndrome**), or post-MI/pericardiotomy syndrome

Dx: Clinical presentation + EKG changes

Tx/Mgmt:

1. **Nonsteroidal antiinflammatory drugs (NSAIDs)** ± **colchicine** > steroids
2. Treatment of underlying cause in uremia or autoimmune disease

Constrictive

Buzz Words: Pericardial calcification

Clinical Presentation: Hypotension, syncope

Kussmaul sign = ↑ in JVD with inspiration

Pericardial calcification

Pericardial knock (early diastolic sound) on auscultation

MoD: Calcification and fibrosis of the pericardium leading to diastolic dysfunction and impaired filling

Developed countries—viral (coxsackievirus, echovirus adenovirus), radiation, cardiac surgery

Undeveloped countries—TB

Dx: Echocardiography showing calcifications and elevated diastolic pressures

Tx/Mgmt: Pericardiotomy

Endocarditis and Myocarditis

Endocarditis

Infectious

Buzz Words: Splinter hemorrhage, Roth spots, Janeway lesions, Osler nodes

Clinical Presentation: Fever, malaise

Splinter hemorrhage (Fig. 6.21), Roth spots (retinal hemorrhage with pale center), Janeway lesions (painless microabscess/embolus) (Fig. 6.22), Osler nodes (Osler = Ouch!; painful nodules in fingers—immune complex)

Embolic disease—stroke, arterial occlusion, seeding of bacteria causing local infection

MoD: Native valve—*Staphylococcus aureus*

Damaged valves— *Staphylococcus epidermidis*, *S. aureus*

Dental procedures—Viridans group streptococci (*Streptococcus mutans*, *Streptococcus mitis*, *Streptococcus sanguinis*)

IVDU—*S. aureus*, *Candida*, *Pseudomonas*

GU procedures—*Enterococci*

Colon cancer— *Streptococcus gallolyticus* (*Streptococcus bovis*), *Clostridium septicum*

99 AR

Duke criteria for endocarditis

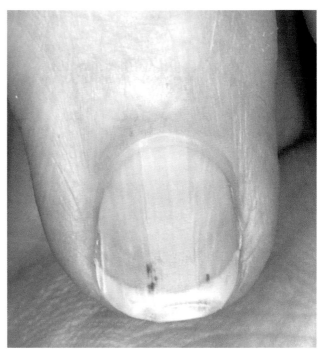

FIG. 6.21 Splinter hemorrhage. (From Wikimedia Commons. https://commons.wikimedia.org/wiki/File:Splinter_hemorrhage.jpg. By Splarka [Own work] [Public domain]. Used under the Creative Commons Attribution Share-Alike 3.0 Unported License.)

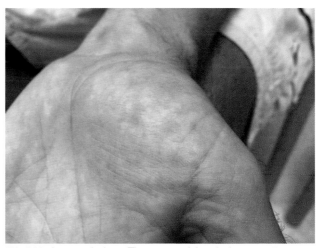

FIG. 6.22 Janeway lesions. These are painless lesions, most commonly seen on the acral extremities, that are caused by bacterial emboli. (From Wikimedia Commons. https://commons.wikimedia.org/wiki/File:Janeway_lesion.JPG. By Warfieldian [Own work]. Used under the Creative Commons Attribution Share-Alike 3.0 Unported License.)

Culture negative infectious endocarditis—HACEK organisms (although some are now able to be cultured), *Coxiella*, *Bartonella*, *Chlamydia*

Dx:
1. Large-volume blood cultures
2. Echocardiography

Tx/Mgmt: Antibiotics ± surgical debridement/valve replacement

Non-Infectious (marantic endocarditis)

Buzz Words: Sterile vegetations on cardiac valves associated with malignancy and autoimmune disease

Clinical Presentation: Sterile deposits on cardiac valves → can flick off and cause thrombotic disease

Libman-Sacks endocarditis is associated with systemic lupus erythematosus and presents with deposits on both the atrial and ventricular surfaces of cardiac valves

Most commonly causes valve dysfunction > embolic disease

Dx: Echocardiography

Tx/Mgmt:
1. Anticoagulation with warfarin
2. Treatment of underlying disease
3. Surgical valve repair/replacement

Myocarditis

Buzz Words: Acute-onset heart failure in a young or middle-aged, otherwise healthy individual

Clinical Presentation: May have viral prodrome—Upper respiratory infection (URI) symptoms, myalgias, fever

Cardiac manifestations are variable:
  Asymptomatic, chest pain, palpitations, arrhythmias, sudden cardiac death
  Signs of heart failure—SOB, orthopnea, paroxysmal nocturnal dyspnea

MoD: Viral infection is the most common cause: Coxsackie B, adenovirus, HCV, CMV, EBV, echovirus, parvovirus B19, influenza
  Initial viral infection and subsequent immune response cause damage to cardiac myocytes

Bacterial, fungal, and parasitic causes are also possible but are less common

Noninfectious etiologies include the following: giant cell myocarditis (rapidly progressive), alcohol, hypereosinophilic syndrome (Loeffler syndrome), sarcoidosis, thyrotoxicosis

Dx:
1. Endomyocardial biopsy is the gold standard but is not always required.
2. Echocardiography or other cardiac imaging to assess cardiac function

Tx/Mgmt:
1. Treat symptoms of heart failure—diuretics, ACEI, oxygen, ± β-blockers
2. Avoid NSAIDs, EtOH, and heavy exercise to prevent further cardiac stress.

Cardiac Trauma

Myocardial Contusion

Buzz Words: Sternal fracture + new-onset bundle branch block and ST-segment abnormalities

Clinical Presentation: New onset bundle branch block or arrhythmia (may be delayed up to 72 hours)

RV is the most commonly affected as it is the most anterior

Often associated with **sternal fracture**

MoD: Blunt chest trauma

Dx:
1. EKG—new-onset bundle branch block and/or ST-segment abnormalities
2. Echocardiography—wall-motion abnormalities
3. Cardiac enzymes—troponin and creatine kinase are typically elevated

Tx/Mgmt: Supportive care

Myocardial Free Wall Rupture

Buzz Words: Sudden-onset PEA arrest 3–7 days after MI

Clinical Presentation: Rapid onset cardiovascular collapse and death unless tamponade occurs

PEA arrest is common

Hypotension, tachycardia, ↑JVP, signs of cardiogenic shock

MoD: Typically occurs 3–7 days after MI or occasionally after myocardial trauma

Risk factors include the following: female gender, first ischemic event (i.e., scar tissue is tougher and less prone to rupture), low body mass index, and no myocardial hypertrophy

Dx: Clinical presentation (hypotension, PEA arrest) or at autopsy

Tx/Mgmt: Immediate surgical repair

Traumatic Aortic Rupture

Buzz Words: Acceleration-deceleration injury + tear at the attachment of the ligamentum arteriosum

Clinical Presentation: May be difficult to diagnose clinically because of other trauma that typically copresents.

Some patients may have differential blood pressures between upper and lower extremities.

Most commonly occurs just proximal to the attachment site of the ligamentum arteriosum (immobile part of the aorta)

Rupture occurs in the descending aorta, near the branch point of the left subclavian artery.

MoD: Acceleration-deceleration forces cause shearing of the aorta at places where the aorta is relatively immobile (i.e., tethered by the ligamentum arteriosum).

Dx:
1. CXR may show widened mediastinum
2. Computed tomography (CT) angiogram

Tx/Mgmt:
1. Blood pressure control with labetalol or nitroprusside to prevent complete tear
2. Immediate surgical or endovascular repair

Congenital Cardiac Malformations

Endocardial Cushion Defects
Ventricular Septal Defect

Buzz Words: Harsh, holosystolic blowing murmur along the left lower sternal border with palpable thrill

Clinical Presentation: Symptoms depend on size of the ventricular septal defect (VSD).

Small VSDs are typically asymptomatic and may close spontaneously.

Large VSDs allow passage of significant volume of blood from the LV to the RV → ↑RV pressures, ↑pulmonary blood flow.

Over time, the flow may reverse as pressures in the pulmonary and right heart increase (Eisenmenger syndrome) → late-onset cyanosis.

MoD: Communication between the LV and RV allows for blood flow from the high-pressure left-heart system into the low-pressure right heart.

Dx:
1. Auscultation with harsh, holosystolic blowing murmur along the left lower sternal border ± palpable thrill

QUICK TIPS

Small VSDs typically have louder murmurs due to increased turbulence.

- Large VSDs typically have very soft or no appreciable murmur.

2. Echocardiography

Tx/Mgmt:

1. No treatment for small VSDs
2. Surgical or catheter-based closures can be considered for symptomatic, large VSDs.

Atrial Septal Defect

Buzz Words: Fixed splitting of S_2, paradoxical embolization

Clinical Presentation: Typically asymptomatic into early adulthood

May eventually present with dyspnea on exertion, palpitations, and easily fatigued → Eisenmenger syndrome occurs late

May lead to paradoxical emboli—venous emboli that bypasses the lungs to cause obstruction in the arterial system

Patent foramen ovale = incomplete closure of the foramen ovale (fetal connection between the LA and RA)

MoD: Incomplete closure of the inter-atrial septum—most commonly due to ostium secundum defect. Associated diseases include Down syndrome, Ebstein anomaly, and fetal alcohol syndrome.

Dx:

1. Echocardiography
2. Doppler bubble study—inject air into the right atrium and look for bubbles in the left atrium

Tx/Mgmt: Percutaneous or surgical closure for symptomatic or large ASDs

Patent Foramen Ovale

Buzz Words: Incomplete closure of the foramen ovale from fetal circulation, paradoxical embolization

Clinical Presentation: Typically asymptomatic

May lead to paradoxical emboli—venous emboli that bypasses the lungs to cause obstruction in the arterial system.

MoD: Incomplete closure of the foramen ovale (between the LA and RA) from fetal circulation

Dx:

1. Echocardiography
2. Doppler bubble study—inject air into the right atrium and look for bubbles in the left atrium

Tx/Mgmt: No treatment for asymptomatic disease. Surgical closure if needed.

Patent Ductus Arteriosus

Buzz Words: Continuous machine-like murmur, widened pulse pressure and bounding pulse

Clinical Presentation: Affected infants are initially asymptomatic but may have increased work of breathing if patent ductus arteriosus (PDA) is large

Increased blood flow from the aorta into the pulmonary artery → widened pulse pressure / bounding pulse

Late cyanosis in lower extremities > upper extremities due to increased pressure in the pulmonary circulation

Continuous, machine-like murmur best heard at the right upper sternal border

May be associated with transposition of the great vessels → give prostaglandin E2 to keep the PDA open

Need to keep the ductus arteriosus open to have mixing of blood from the otherwise separate pulmonary and systemic circulations in transposition of the great vessels

MoD: Connection between the aorta and pulmonary trunk that persists after the immediate neonatal period

Blood flows from high-pressure systemic circulation (aorta) into the low-pressure pulmonary circulation

Associated with the following: congenital rubella syndrome, pre-term birth, and chromosomal abnormalities (Down syndrome)

Dx: Echocardiography

Tx/Mgmt:

1. NSAIDs (**indomethacin**) can be used to close PDA in the neonatal period
2. Surgical repair for later diagnosed lesions

Tetralogy of Fallot (Fig. 6.23)

Buzz Words: Boot-shaped heart, pulmonic stenosis, tet spells, overriding aorta, DiGeorge syndrome

Clinical Presentation: Major anomalies in ToF

Pulmonic stenosis—the most important factor in the degree of the cyanosis

VSD

RVH

Overriding aorta

Tet spells = acute-onset cyanotic spells in which affected children will often squat (↑SVR leads to ↑pulmonary blood flow)

99 AR

Patent ductus arteriosus

MNEMONIC

Prostaglandin E2 kEEps the ductus arteriosus open.

Normal heart   Tetralogy of Fallot

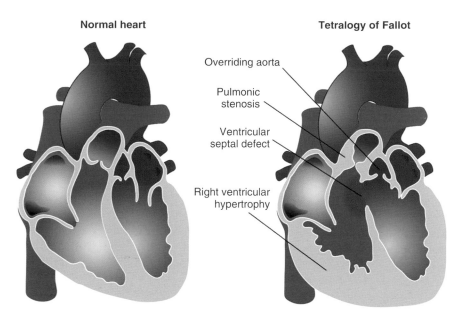

FIG. 6.23 Tetralogy of Fallot. (From Wikimedia Commons. https://commons.wikimedia.org/wiki/
File:Tetralogy_of_Fallot.svg. Public Domain. Used under the Creative Commons Attribution Share-Alike
3.0 Unported License.)

<table>
<tr><td>

MNEMONIC

PROVe—pulmonic stenosis, right
ventricular hypertrophy, overriding
aorta, ventricular septal defect

</td><td>

Most common cyanotic heart disease after the neonatal
period
Single S_2 (pulmonic stenosis)
MoD: Associated with DiGeorge syndrome (22q11
deletion)
Pulmonic stenosis reduces blood flow to lungs →
cyanosis
Dx:
1. CXR with boot-shaped heart (Fig. 6.24 and 6.26)
2. Echocardiography
Tx/Mgmt:
1. Surgical correction
2. β-blockers, morphine, intranasal fentanyl for tet spells

Transposition of the Great Vessels (Fig. 6.25)

Buzz Words: Egg-on-a-string heart (narrow mediastinum) +
single S_2 + cyanosis within the first 24 hours of life
Clinical Presentation: Cyanosis within the first 24 hours of life
Single S_2
ASD, VSD, or PDA is present.
MoD: Caused by failure of spiralization of the aorticopul-
monary septum
May be associated with maternal diabetes mellitus

</td></tr>
</table>

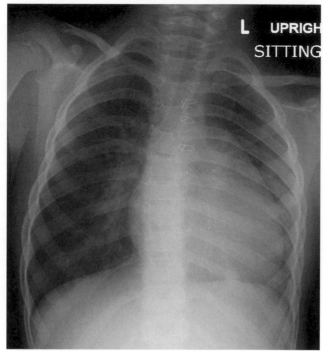

FIG. 6.24 Boot-shaped heart. Note the boot-shaped protrusion caused by right ventricular hypertrophy seen in tetralogy of Fallot. (From Wikimedia Commons. https://commons.wikimedia.org/wiki/File:HeartTOP. jpg. By James Heilman, MD. Public Domain. Used under the Creative Commons Attribution Share-Alike 3.0 Unported License.)

Dx:
1. Echocardiography
2. CXR with egg-on-a-string heart

Tx/Mgmt:
1. Prostaglandin E2 to keep PDA open
2. Surgical repair

Total Anomalous Pulmonary Venous Return

Buzz Words: Young baby with cyanosis, right ventricular hypertrophy

Clinical Presentation: RVH, right axis deviation
Cyanosis

MoD: Pulmonary veins empty into the RA instead of the LA

Dx: CXR with snowman sign/figure-of-8 sign

Tx/Mgmt: Surgical repair

Truncus Arteriosus

Buzz Words: Common arterial trunk for the aorta and the pulmonary artery

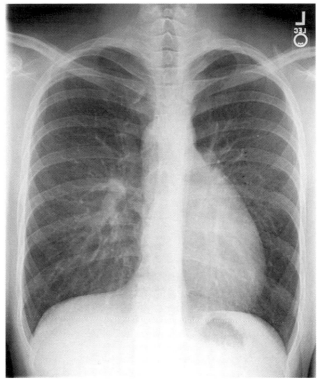

FIG. 6.25 Transposition of great vessels, looks like egg on its side. (From Wikimedia Commons. https://commons.wikimedia.org/wiki/File:Transposition-of-great-vessels.jpg. By Madhero88. Used under the Creative Commons Attribution Share-Alike 3.0 Unported License.)

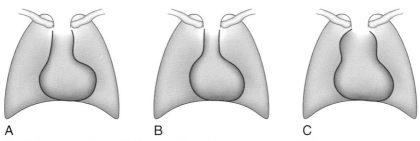

A   B   C

FIG. 6.26 (A) Tetralogy of Fallot. (B) Transposition of the great vessels. (C) Total anomalous pulmonary venous return. (From Park MK. *Pak's Pediatric Cardiology for Practitioners*. 6th ed. Philadelphia: Elsevier; 2014. Fig. 4.3.)

Clinical Presentation: Dyspnea

Pulmonary congestion and edema

MoD: Failure of septum formation in the common arterial trunk → increased flow through the pulmonary circulation

Associated with DiGeorge syndrome

Dx: Echocardiography

Tx/Mgmt: Surgical repair

Tricuspid Atresia

Buzz Words: Complete absence of the tricuspid valve with hypoplasia of the RV

Clinical Presentation: Progressive cyanosis

Left axis deviation with LVH

MoD: Complete absence of the tricuspid valve with RV hypoplasia → LV must function as the sole ventricle for pumping blood through the pulmonary and systemic circulations

Dx: Echocardiography

Tx/Mgmt: Surgical repair

Cardiac Neoplasms

Atrial Myxoma

Buzz Words: Ball valve-type obstruction, tumor plop, most common primary cardiac tumor in adults

Clinical Presentation: Shortness of breath, palpitations, dizziness, paroxysmal nocturnal dyspnea

Fever

Tumor emboli can cause arterial obstruction

MoD: Most common primary cardiac tumor (rhabdomyosarcoma is the most common in children). Overall, metastatic disease is much more common—**lung**, breast, esophagus, melanoma, lymphoma/leukemia

Most commonly located in the LA

Dx:

1. Echocardiography
2. Tumor plop heard on auscultation (mid-diastolic rumble that is similar to mitral stenosis)

Tx/Mgmt: Surgical removal

Hypertension and Hypotension

Hypotension

Orthostatic Hypotension

Buzz Words: Syncope + decrease in systolic BP of ≥ 20 mm Hg or diastolic BP of ≥ 10 mm Hg when moving from supine to sitting to standing position

Clinical Presentation: Patients may present dizziness, lightheadedness, syncope, temporary decrease in vision or hearing upon standing up.

MoD: Intravascular volume depletion, autonomic dysfunction (diabetes mellitus, multiple system atrophy), medication side effect (tricyclic antidepressants, α1-antagonists [doxazosin, prazosin, tamsulosin, terazosin])

Dx: Orthostatic vital signs—decrease in systolic BP of ≥ 20 mm Hg or diastolic BP of ≥ 10 mm Hg taken 3 minutes after moving from supine to sitting to standing position

Tx/Mgmt:

1. Increase fluid intake
2. Medications to increase blood pressure: midodrine (α1-agonist), dopamine antagonists, tyramine, indomethacin

Carotid Sinus Hypersensitivity

Buzz Words: Bradycardia, hypotension, or syncope with constriction of the neck (e.g., when wearing a tight-fitting collared shirt)

Clinical Presentation: Patients present with bradycardia and hypotension with light contact with the carotid area of the neck (e.g., when shaving or with a tight-fitting shirt collar)

MoD: Hypersensitivity of the carotid baroreceptor leads to increased vagal tone with light external compression of the carotid area

Dx:

1. Carotid sinus massage can reproduce symptoms
2. Rule out other common causes of syncope:
   Orthostatic syncope—orthostatic vital signs
   Vasovagal—tilt-table test
   Cardiogenic—EKG, echocardiogram

Tx/Mgmt:

1. Patient should not be allowed to drive until treatment
2. Maintain adequate hydration and increase electrolyte intake
3. Pacemaker insertion can be considered for patients with recurrent episodes associated with bradycardia

Hypertension

Buzz Words: Blood pressure ≥ 140/90 mm Hg

Clinical Presentation: Insidious and asymptomatic until secondary effects become evident. Patients are at increased risk for cardiovascular disease, renal disease, and stroke.

MoD: May be primary (idiopathic/essential) or secondary to other pathology.

Causes of secondary hypertension include the following:
  Chronic renal failure
  Renal artery stenosis—classically in older males with a history of atherosclerotic disease
  Fibromuscular dysplasia—classically in younger women

2017 ACC hypertension guidelines

Hyperaldosteronism—via increased sodium absorption in the distal convoluted tubule

Hyper- or hypothyroidism—via hyperdynamic circulation (hyperthyroidism) or vasoconstriction (hypothyroidism)

Obstructive sleep apnea

Others—scleroderma, pheochromocytoma

Dx:
1. Measurement of blood pressure ≥ 140/90 mm Hg on two separate occasions
2. Diagnosis of renal artery stenosis and fibromuscular dysplasia through CT angiogram

Tx/Mgmt:
1. Lifestyle modification—weight loss, reduce dietary sodium
2. Medication:
   - In patients with CKD → start with ACE inhibitor or ARB
   - In patients without CKD
     - If African-American → HCTZ or CCB
     - Otherwise → HCTZ or ACE inhibitor or ARB or CCB

Hypertensive Urgency

Buzz Words: Systolic BP ≥ 180 mm Hg or diastolic BP ≥ 110 mm Hg without evidence of end-organ dysfunction

Clinical Presentation: Systolic BP ≥ 180 mm Hg or diastolic BP ≥ 110 mm Hg without evidence of end-organ dysfunction

MoD: Depends on the underlying cause of hypertension. Etiologies include medication noncompliance, cocaine, MAOI with tyramine ingestion (from cured meats, wine, and cheese), and pheochromocytoma

Dx:
1. Systolic BP ≥ 180 mm Hg or diastolic BP ≥ 110 mm Hg without evidence of end-organ dysfunction
2. Neurologic exam, funduscopic exam, EKG, urinalysis

Tx/Mgmt: Gradual lowering of blood pressure with oral agents—HCTZ, CCBs. No need for intravenous medications for rapid lowering of blood pressure in asymptomatic patients

Hypertensive Emergency

Buzz Words: Systolic BP ≥ 180 mm Hg or diastolic BP ≥ 120 mm Hg in the setting of end-organ dysfunction

Clinical Presentation: Systolic BP ≥ 180 mm Hg or diastolic BP ≥ 120 mm Hg in the setting of end-organ dysfunction (e.g., headache, vision changes, oliguria, chest pain, and SOB). Complications include stroke, encephalopathy, subarachnoid hemorrhage, MI, renal damage, aortic dissection, and pulmonary edema.

MoD: Pressure-related damage to small blood vessels leading to end-organ dysfunction

Dx: Systolic BP ≥ 180 mm Hg or diastolic BP ≥ 120 mm Hg in the setting of end-organ dysfunction

Tx/Mgmt:

1. Rapid control of blood pressure with IV antihypertensive agents including labetalol, sodium nitroprusside, fenoldopam (dopamine-1-receptor agonist), or clevidipine (CCB)
2. In neurologic emergencies → aim to lower the MAP by 25% over 8 hours
   - Labetalol and nifedipine are the preferred medications for neurologic pathology associated with hypertensive emergency.

Vascular Disease

Arterial Disease

Peripheral Artery Disease

Buzz Words: Cool, pale extremities with weak or absent pulses; loss of hair, shiny skin

Clinical Presentation: Cool, pale extremities, weak/absent pulses, loss of hair, atrophy, necrosis, gangrene Intermittent limb claudication (pain with activity)

PPx: Management of risk factors—abstain from **smoking**, control of DM, HLD, and HTN

MoD: Destruction or chronic occlusive disease of peripheral vessels → ↓ perfusion of extremities Smoking damages the vascular endothelium and promotes atherosclerotic changes.

Dx:

1. Ankle brachial index (ABI) ≤ 0.9
2. Duplex ultrasound & Doppler studies

Tx/Mgmt:

1. Smoking cessation, management of comorbid conditions
   - Cessation of smoking prevents further accelerated vascular disease but does not necessarily significantly improve existing vascular pathology
2. Supervised exercise program
3. Medications—cilostazol (anti-platelet + vasodilator), pentoxifylline
4. Surgical intervention—angioplasty, stenting, bypass, thrombolysis

Thromboangiitis Obliterans (Buerger Disease)

Buzz Words: Corkscrew arteries on imaging, tobacco-associated vascular inflammation leading to thrombosis

Clinical Presentation:

Inflammation of the peripheral vasculature leading to the following:

Limb claudication

Decreased/absent peripheral pulses

Cyanosis

Hair loss and shiny skin

Ulcerations and gangrene

MoD: Unknown, but exposure to tobacco is a very strong risk factor

Dx:

1. Diagnosis of thromboangiitis obliterans often necessitates exclusion of other pathology:
   - Patients are usually males between 20 and 40 with a history of current or recent tobacco use
   - Presence of distal extremity ischemia, as evidenced by claudication, ulceration, or gangrene
   - Exclusion of vasculitis, embolic disease, diabetes mellitus, and hypercoagulable states
   - Arteriographic findings consistent with arterial occlusion

Tx/Mgmt:

1. Smoking cessation is key
2. Medical therapy:
   - Iloprost (prostaglandin) can be used for vasodilation and improves symptoms without changing the course of disease
   - Thrombolytic agents have been used as an experimental treatment
3. Hyperbaric oxygen may help with wound healing
4. Surgical revascularization can be attempted in select patients with suitable obstruction that can be bypassed

Embolic Disease

Buzz Words: Amaurosis fugax, livedo with blue toes, acute arterial thrombus

Clinical Presentation: Acute embolization causing end-organ dysfunction depending on the vessel that is occluded

Carotid plaque rupture → amaurosis fugax, Hollenhorst plaques in the retinal vasculature, transient ischemic attack, stroke

Cholesterol embolism classically presents after vascular manipulation in patients with underlying atherosclerotic disease.

Livedoid skin changes with blue toes is classic.

Variable organ dysfunction—renal, gastrointestinal, CNS—depending on the location of embolus

MoD: Unstable atherosclerotic plaques in the aorta, carotid, or heart can embolize.

Vegetations from endocarditis can also embolize.

Dx:

1. Echocardiogram
2. Carotid duplex ultrasound
3. Skin biopsy showing cholesterol clefts (in cholesterol embolism)

Tx/Mgmt:

1. Anticoagulation with warfarin for patients with cardiac thrombus
2. Carotid endarterectomy for patients with carotid stenosis ≥ 50% and history of TIA or stroke in the preceding 6 months
3. Statins for patients with cholesterol emboli

Compartment Syndrome

Buzz Words: Pain, pulselessness, paresthesias, paralysis, pallor, poikilothermia; compartment pressures ≥ 30 mm Hg

Clinical Presentation: 6Ps—**pain, pulselessness, paresthesias, paralysis, pallor, poikilothermia** (difference in temperature between affected segment and surrounding areas)

Complications include permanent muscle or nerve damage → rhabdomyolysis

MoD:

Etiologies include the following:

Bleeding into a limb

Crush injuries (tissue edema + bleeding)

Ischemic reperfusion injury

Tissue swelling after casting

Dx:

1. Diagnosis is typically by clinical presentation.
2. Intracompartmental pressure ≥ 30 mm Hg is suggestive.

Tx/Mgmt: Fasciotomy

Venous Disease

Deep Vein Thrombosis

Buzz Words: Swelling and pain of a limb with limb asymmetry, Homan sign

Clinical Presentation: Swelling, pain, redness of the affected limb ± engorgement of superficial veins

Homan **sign** = pain with dorsiflexion of the foot (this test is historical and is not sensitive or specific)

PPx: Ambulation, compression stockings, anticoagulation (heparin or enoxaparin)

MoD: Most commonly occurs in the proximal deep veins of the lower extremities (femoral veins, popliteal veins, iliac veins)

Risk factors include hypercoagulable state (factor V Leiden, malignancy, recent surgery, hormone replacement therapy), endothelial cell damage, and venous stasis.

Dx:
1. Duplex ultrasound
2. D-dimer—can be used to rule out deep vein thrombosis (DVT) if negative

Tx/Mgmt:
1. Provoked DVT—an underlying factor can be identified to explain the DVT (e.g., concurrent malignancy, prior immobilization, recent surgery)
   - Anticoagulation with warfarin or low-molecular weight heparin for 3 months
2. Unprovoked DVT—no underlying factor can be identified
   - Anticoagulation with warfarin for 3–6 months for first episode
   - Anticoagulation for 12 months to indefinite for second episode
3. IVC filter (if patient is unable to tolerate anticoagulation)

Venous Insufficiency

Buzz Words: Lower extremity edema with evidence of stasis dermatitis ± prominent varicose veins due to venous valvular insufficiency

Clinical Presentation: Lower extremity edema with hyperpigmentation, scaling, and shiny, indurated appearance of the skin (**stasis dermatitis**)

Prominent varicose veins

Lipodermatosclerosis = chronic panniculitis (inflammation of fat) with sclerosis and inverted champagne bottle appearance of the lower leg

MoD: Dysfunction or destruction of venous valves leads to backflow and pooling in the dependent veins of the body.

Dx: Based on history and clinical exam

Tx/Mgmt:
1. Compression stockings
2. Leg elevation

QUICK TIPS

Patients with connective tissue disease (Marfan syndrome, Ehlers-Danlos syndrome, Loeys-Dietz syndrome) as well as those with syphilitic aortitis are at increased risk for thoracic aortic aneurysms

AR

Aortic aneurysm management

Disorders of the Great Vessels

Aortic Aneurysm

Buzz Words: Widened mediastinum (thoracic aortic aneurysm), pulsatile abdominal mass (AAA)

Clinical Presentation: AAA—pulsatile abdominal mass
  Risk factors include atherosclerosis, smoking, and hypertension.
Thoracic aortic aneurysm—widened mediastinum on chest radiograph
  Risk factors include smoking, hypertension, and atherosclerosis.

MoD: Weakening of the vascular wall (through atherosclerosis or intrinsic defects in collagen and support proteins) leads to ballooning and formation of an aneurysm.

Dx:
1. Male smokers between 65 and 75 years old should be screened with a one-time abdominal ultrasound.
2. Echocardiogram or CT angiogram for thoracic aortic aneurysms
3. CT angiogram can also be used for accurate assessment of abdominal aortic aneurysms.

Tx/Mgmt:
1. Modification of risk factors—statins, smoking cessation, and control of blood pressure
2. Surgical treatment is indicated for those at higher risk for rupture
   • AAA—diameter > 5.5 cm, rate of growth > 1 cm per year, current smokers
   • Thoracic aortic aneurysm—aneurysms > 5–6 cm

Aortic Dissection

Buzz Words: Tearing chest pain that radiates to the back

Clinical Presentation: Acute onset, severe, tearing chest pain that radiates to the back
May be associated with hypertension or hypotension, aortic insufficiency, acute MI, or acute stroke depending on location and progression of dissection
Dissection of the subclavian artery may lead to different blood pressure readings between arms.

PPx: Blood pressure control

MoD: Tearing of the tunica intima of the aorta → blood flow between the layers of the aorta leading to dissection
Risk factors include **hypertension**, collagen vascular disease (Marfan syndrome, Ehlers-Danlos syndrome), bicuspid aortic valve, and tertiary syphilis

Dx:
1. **TEE** is the diagnostic test of choice because of speed.
2. **Magnetic resonance imaging** is the gold standard (more sensitive and equal specificity compared to CT angiography).
   Aortography is not typically used anymore.
3. **CT angiography** is often used in the emergent setting because of high sensitivity and speed.
4. CXR may show widened mediastinum (Fig. 6.27)

Tx/Mgmt:
1. Blood pressure control with β-blockers (**labetalol**) or **CCBs** ± nitroprusside
2. Dissection of the ascending aorta (Stanford type A) → **surgery**
3. Dissection of the descending aorta (Stanford type B) → **medical management**

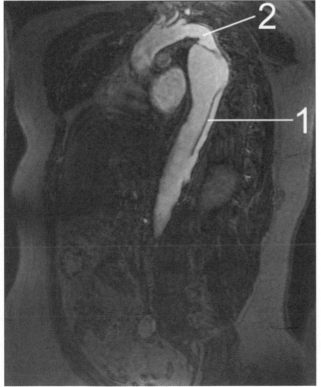

FIG. 6.27 Widened mediastinum on magnetic resonance imaging (1) Aorta descendens (2) Aorta isthmus. (From Wikimedia Commons. https://commons.wikimedia.org/wiki/File:AoDiss_MRT.jpg. By Dr. Lars Grenacher (www.grenacher.de), uploaded by J. Heuser JHeuser. Used under the Creative Commons Attribution Share-Alike 3.0 Unported License.)

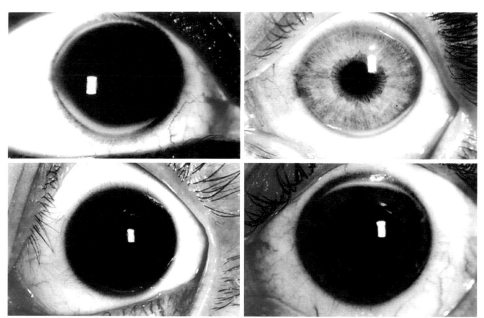

FIG. 6.28 Corneal arcus. Deposition of cholesterol in the limbic area of the pupil resulting in a white ring seen in hypercholesterolemia and in the elderly. (From Wikimedia Commons. https://commons.wikimedia.org/wiki/File:Four_representative_slides_of_corneal_arcus.jpg. © 2008 Zech and Hoeg; licensee BioMed Central Ltd. Used under the Creative Commons Attribution 2.0 Generic License.)

Dyslipidemia

Corneal arcus. Deposition of cholesterol in the limbic area of the pupil resulting in a white ring seen in hypercholesterolemia and in the elderly.

Familial Hypercholesterolemia

Buzz Words: Early atherosclerotic disease, tendon xanthoma, increased serum cholesterol

Clinical Presentation: Early atherosclerotic disease (CAD, MI, PAD), tendon xanthoma, corneal arcus (Fig. 6.28), xanthelasma (Fig. 6.29)

MoD: Mutation in the LDL receptor or ApoB that results in ability of the liver to clear cholesterol from the blood

Dx:

1. Total serum cholesterol:
   350–550 mg/dL is suggestive of heterozygous state
   650–1000 mg/dL is suggestive of homozygous state
2. Mutation analysis

Tx/Mgmt:

1. Homozygous mutants—high dose statins + lipid apheresis, liver transplant

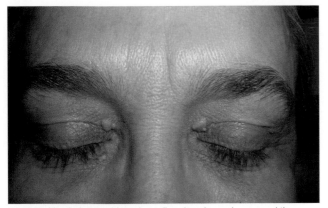

FIG. 6.29 Xanthelasma. Note the yellow-hued papules around the eyelids representing deposits of cholesterol. Xanthelasma may be seen in patients with hypercholesterolemia but may also be seen in normo-cholesterolemic patients. (From Wikimedia Commons. https://commons.wikimedia.org/wiki/File:Xanthelasma.jpg. By Klaus D. Peter. Used under the Creative Commons Attribution 3.0 Germany license.)

2. Heterozygous mutants—statins ± bile acid sequestrants (cholestyramine), niacin

Familial Hyperchylomicronemia (Lipoprotein Lipase Deficiency)

Buzz Words: Creamy layer in supernatant of blood sample, serum fasting triglycerides

Clinical Presentation: Eruptive xanthomas, acute pancreatitis (due to ↑↑ triglycerides)

No increased risk of atherosclerotic disease

MoD: Caused by deficiency in lipoprotein lipase

Dx:

1. Blood testing showing increased fasting triglycerides > 1000 mg/dL
2. Milky, creamy plasma with increased hyperchylomicronemia

Tx/Mgmt:

1. Low fat diet and avoidance of simple carbohydrates
2. Lipid lowering medications—omega-3-fatty acids, gemfibrozil

Familial Hypertriglyceridemia

Buzz Words: Triglycerides > 1000 mg/dL

Clinical Presentation: Xanthoma, corneal arcus, xanthelasma, acute pancreatitis (due to ↑↑ triglycerides). Increased risk of pancreatitis (triglycerides > 1000 mg/dL)/

MoD: Mutations in the ApoA5 and lipase I genes

Dx: Fasting serum triglycerides > 1000 mg/dL
Tx/Mgmt:
1. Low fat diet and avoidance of simple carbohydrates
2. Lipid lowering medications—omega-3-fatty acids, gemfibrozil

Medication Side Effects Involving the Heart

Cardiotoxic Drugs

Doxorubicin—causes dose-dependent cardiomyopathy;
    dexrazoxane can be used to mitigate cardiotoxicity
Traztuzumab (Herceptin)—cardiomyopathy → CHF

Cocaine—May Cause Coronary Artery Vasospasm and Typical ACS Chest Pain, Diaphoresis, HTN

Tx **CCBs** preferred; **avoid β-blockers** as they can cause
    unopposed α-adrenergic activity

QT-prolonging Medications

Antiemetics—ondansetron
Antipsychotics
TCA
Antiarrhythmics—amiodarone, sotalol, flecainide
Antibiotics—macrolides, fluoroquinolones, azole anti-
    fungals

Anti-hypertensives

CCBs can cause reflex tachycardia and peripheral edema.

GUNNER PRACTICE

1. A 30-year-old woman presents to her primary care physician for intermittent chest pain over the previous month. She endorses substernal pain and pressure after a smoke break at work and at night while in bed. Her past medical history is significant for acne vulgaris and irregular periods for which she takes an oral contraceptive. She endorses drinking alcohol in social situations but denies illicit drug use including marijuana, cocaine, and IV drugs. She is sexually active with one partner. Family history is significant for coronary artery disease in her father and ovarian cancer in her mother. Her pulse is 72/min, blood pressure is 142/92 mm Hg, respiratory rate is 12/min, and temperature is 99.1°F. Physical exam is unremarkable. EKG at the time of visit shows normal sinus rhythm without ST-segment abnormalities.

The acute management of future episodes of chest pain in this patient would be most similar to treatment of which of the following?

A. Acute myocardial infarction
B. Pheochromocytoma
C. Cocaine-induced vasospasm
D. Pericarditis
E. Pulmonary embolism

2. A 70-year-old man presents to the emergency room with crushing sub-sternal chest pain that radiates down his left arm. He has a history of diabetes mellitus, colon cancer, COPD, and coronary artery disease, for which he received a triple artery bypass 9 years prior. His home medications include metformin, insulin, budesonide/formoterol, aspirin, and atorvastatin. The patient's vital signs in the emergency room are temperature of 99.6°F, heart rate of 98/min, blood pressure of 110/73 mm Hg, respiratory rate of 20, and oxygen saturation of 91% on room air. He is given aspirin, clopidogrel, sublingual nitroglycerin, oxygen, heparin, and morphine. Soon after receiving his medications the patient becomes hypotensive, tachycardic, and is noted to have decreased peripheral perfusion. EKG shows ST-segmental elevations >1 mm in leads, II, III, and aVF. Which medication is the most likely cause of this patient's hypotension?

A. Clopidogrel
B. Nitroglycerin
C. Oxygen
D. Heparin
E. Aspirin

3. A 5-year-old boy is being seen by the pediatrician for shortness of breath and easy fatigability. His parents state that they have noticed that the patient's lips and acral extremities turn a blue hue during these episodes of shortness of breath. They have also noticed that the child tends to squat during these episodes. You suspect that the patient may have a congenital heart disease. Which of the following changes during squatting helps improve this patient's symptoms?

A. Increased SVR
B. Increased preload
C. Increased venous return
D. Decreased venous return
E. Decreased PCWP
F. Decreased SVR

ANSWERS: What Would Gunner Jess/Jim Do

1. WWGJD? A 30-year-old woman presents to her primary care physician for intermittent chest pain over last month. She endorses sub-sternal pain and pressure after a smoke break at work and also at night while in bed. Her past medical history is significant for acne vulgaris and irregular periods for which she takes an oral contraceptive. She endorses drinking alcohol in social situations but denies illicit drug use including marijuana, cocaine, and IV drugs. She is sexually active with one partner. Family history is significant for coronary artery disease in her father and ovarian cancer in her mother. Her pulse is 72/min, blood pressure is 142/92 mmHg, respiratory rate is 12/min, temperature 99.1°F. Physical exam is unremarkable. EKG at the time of visit shows normal sinus rhythm without ST-segment abnormalities. The acute management of future episodes of chest pain in this patient would be most similar to treatment of which of the following?

Answer: C, Cocaine-induced vasospasm

This patient is a young woman smoker with typical anginal chest pain—these symptoms are suggestive of **Prinzmetal variant angina.** Prinzmetal angina is caused by coronary artery vasospasm and classically occurs at night. Patients may have ST-segment changes on EKG and may also have positive cardiac enzyme markers. Treatment of acute episodes is with **CCBs** while **avoiding β-blockers**, as they can cause unopposed α-adrenergic stimulation and worsen vasospasm. The pathophysiology and treatment of Prinzmetal angina is very similar to that of cocaine-induced coronary artery vasospasm.

A. Acute myocardial infarction → Incorrect. Acute myocardial infarction presents with chest pain but is typically treated with oxygen, heparin, aspirin, clopidogrel, nitrates, morphine, and β-blockers.

B. Pheochromocytoma → Incorrect. Pheochromocytoma presents with paroxysmal hypertension, which may be complicated by chest pain, headache, and other end-organ dysfunctions. Treatment of pheochromocytoma is with α-blockers (phenoxybenzamine) and then β-blockers.

D. Pericarditis → Incorrect. Pericarditis presents with sharp chest pain that is relieved by sitting up and leaning forward. EKG findings include diffuse ST-elevations with PR-depressions with the exception of aVR. Pericarditis is treated with NSAIDs ± colchicine.

E. Pulmonary embolism → Incorrect. Pulmonary embolism can present with pleuritic chest pain but is also associated with shortness of breath and sometimes hemoptysis. EKG usually shows sinus tachycardia but may also show S1Q3T3. The treatment of acute PE is heparin.

2. WWGJD? A 70-year-old man presents to the emergency room with crushing sub-sternal chest pain that radiates down his left arm. He has a history of diabetes mellitus, colon cancer, COPD, and coronary artery disease for which he received a triple artery bypass 9 years prior. His home medications include metformin, insulin, budesonide/formoterol, aspirin, atorvastatin, and fish oil. The patient's vital signs in the emergency room are temperature 99.6°F, heart rate 98/min, blood pressure 105/72 mm Hg, respiratory rate 20, and oxygen saturation is 91% on room air. He is given aspirin, clopidogrel, sublingual nitroglycerin, oxygen, heparin, and morphine. Soon after receiving his medications the patient becomes hypotensive, tachycardic, and is noted to have decreased peripheral perfusion. EKG shows ST-segmental elevations >1 mm in leads, V1, V2, II, III, and aVF. Which medication is the most likely cause of this patient's new symptoms?

Answer: B, Nitroglycerin

This patient with cardiovascular risk factors presents with typical chest pain suggestive of acute coronary syndrome. His EKG findings of ST-segment elevations in V1, V2, II, III, and aVF are suggestive of inferior / anterior MI corresponding to ischemia in the right ventricle. Recall that patients with **right-sided MI** are very **preload sensitive** due to decreased RV contractility. Medications that decrease preload, such as **nitrates**, can lead to increased RV dysfunction and decreased cardiac output (recall that nitrates mostly function as venodilators to increase pooling of blood in the venous system → decreased preload → decreased myocardial wall stretch → decreased myocardial oxygen demand). In patients with suspected right-sided MI, **IV fluids** should be given for signs of hypotension. Morphine is another drug that can cause decreased preload.

A. Clopidogrel → Incorrect. Clopidogrel is an ADP receptor antagonist that works by inhibiting platelet aggregation. Clopidogrel has relatively few side effects (mainly thrombocytopenia/increased bleeding risk and rarely TTP) and does not cause acute hypotension in the setting of MI.

C. Oxygen → Incorrect. Oxygen does not cause hypotension in the setting of acute MI.

D. Heparin → Incorrect. Heparin can cause increased bleeding risk and heparin-induced thrombocytopenia ± thrombosis but does not cause acute hypotension in the setting of MI.

E. Aspirin → Incorrect. Aspirin does not cause hypotension in the setting of acute MI.

3. WWGJD? A 5-year-old boy is being seen by the pediatrician for shortness of breath and easy fatigability. His parents state that they have noticed that the patient's lips and acral extremities turn a blue hue during these episodes of shortness of breath. They have also noticed that the child tends to squat during these episodes. You suspect that the patient may have a congenital heart disease. Which of the following changes during squatting helps improve this patient's symptoms?

Answer: A, Increased SVR.

The child in this question likely has **tetralogy of Fallot**— the most common cyanotic heart disease to present after the neonatal period. Tetralogy of Fallot is characterized by **pulmonic stenosis**, **RVH**, **VSD**, and **overriding aorta. The degree of cyanosis is most dependent on the degree of pulmonic stenosis.** The presence of a stenotic pulmonic valve and a VSD means that blood in the RV preferentially leaves via the lower resistance of the VSD into the LV. Many patients with tetralogy of Fallot will squat during cyanotic (tet) spells to improve their oxygenation status. **Squatting increases the systemic vascular resistance** and decreases shunting of blood from the RV through the VSD. This means that more blood enters the pulmonary circulation, leading to improved oxygenation.

B. Increased preload → Incorrect. Squatting also increases preload by increasing venous return to the right heart, but this alone would only mildly improve hypoxia during a cyanotic spell.

C. Increased venous return → Incorrect. Squatting also increases venous return to the right heart, but this alone would only mildly improve hypoxia during a cyanotic spell (same principle as increased preload).

D. Decreased venous return → Incorrect. Squatting causes increased venous return.

E. Decreased PCWP → Incorrect. Squatting should theoretically cause an increase in pulmonary capillary wedge pressure. Regardless, mild-to-moderate fluctuations in the pulmonary capillary wedge pressure should not significantly influence the degree of hypoxia in tetralogy of Fallot.

F. Decreased SVR → Incorrect. Squatting increases the SVR to decrease the amount of blood shunted across the VSD.

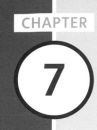
Diseases of the Respiratory System

William Plum, Lauren Briskie, Daniel Gromer, Leo Wang, Hao-Hua Wu, Rebecca Gao, and Nadia Bennett

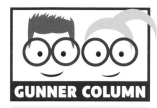

GUNNER COLUMN

Introduction

Diseases of the respiratory system may comprise 10%–15% of your exam. The respiratory system includes upper and lower airways, lungs, pleura, and the diaphragm. We will introduce and cover various pathologies in these categories. However, not all topics are covered equally. Some of the higher yield topics, on which we will focus with a heavier hand in this chapter, are worth giving your time to achieve mastery. These topics include chronic obstructive pulmonary disease (COPD), pneumonia, and cystic fibrosis (CF).

When a respiratory system question is presented, your first job as the acting clinician is to narrow down the diagnosis to either a respiratory, cardiovascular, or gastrointestinal pathology. Certain "Buzz Words" will be used for each of the different categories, which you must learn to quickly pick out from amidst the noise. After you narrow down the diagnosis to a specific organ system and pathology, you will need to decide the appropriate medical (or surgical management).

Disorders of the Lung Parenchyma

Alpha-1 Antitrypsin Deficiency

Buzz Words:

Emphysema/bronchiectasis + young adult + occasional smoker or nonsmoker + neonatal cholestatic jaundice + cirrhosis + liver cancer + panniculitis

Clinical Presentation:

99 AR

Antitrypsin deficiency pathology

Alpha-1 antitrypsin inhibits neutrophil elastase to protect the lung from protease-mediated destruction. When alpha-1 antitrypsin is deficient or its activity cannot keep up with the amount of damage done, neutrophil elastase activity is upregulated, leading to the destruction of lung tissue (e.g., early emphysema). In addition, defective alpha-1 antitrypsin may build up in the hepatocytes that they are made in, leading to jaundice, cirrhosis, and eventually liver cancer due to increased risk. Thus, suspect this disease in patients who develop emphysema/liver pathology at an early age.

PPx: Smoking cessation (avoiding any insult to lungs)

MoD: Alpha-1 antitrypsin can be deficient due to a decrease in production or abnormal protein.

Dx:

1. Chest x-ray (CXR)
2. Serum alpha1 antitrypsin levels
3. Genotyping (confirmation of diagnosis)

Tx/Mgmt:

1. Smoking cessation
2. Alpha1 antitrypsin replacement
3. Liver transplant

99 AR

A1AT deficiency overview

Cystic Fibrosis

Buzz Words: Bronchiectasis + pneumonia with staph/pseudo + hypoxia = barrel chest + clubbing + chronic rhinosinusitis + bilateral nasal polyps leading to nasal obstruction/chronic rhinosinusitis + foul smelling stool (failure to absorb ADEK) + failure to thrive (2/2 to know fat absorption)

99 AR

Cystic fibrosis video

Infertility!! (95% of males, 20% females) + osteopenia, kyphoscoliosis + digital clubbing + meconium ileus/ distal obstruction syndrome + exocrine pancreatic insufficiency + diabetes + recurrent pulmonary pathology

Clinical Presentation: CF is a congenital multiorgan disorder that primarily affects the lung and the pancreas. The chloride channels in CF are defective, so fluid cannot enter the respiratory or gastrointestinal lumen, and secretions that were meant to be cleared are stuck, leading to infection and digestive abnormalities. CF is one of the most high-yield diseases on the shelf, because it can present in many ways in different age groups (mostly peds, but now, patients are living into adulthood). Most notably, patients with CF frequently get pneumonia from organisms associated with immunocompromised patients, such as *Pneumocystis jirovecii*. Also, CF patients have difficulty with digestion owing to a lack of exocrine secretions from the pancreas. Importantly, the treatment for patients with CF is multifaceted. Chest PT, for instance, requires the patient's care provider to tap methodically on the patient's chest to loosen up secretions every single day. Lastly, for the purposes of the shelf, remember that CF is associated with infertility due to no semen production (male) or obstruction of semen entrance (female).

PPx: None (although avoid sick contacts if you have disease).

MoD: Mutation of the CFTR protein → defective chloride ion channels → increased loss of sodium in sweat

Congenital bilateral absence of vas deferens in males and thickened mucus in the fetal genital tract obstructs developing vas deferens → infertility

Even if the testes are descended and spermatogenesis is normal → sperm cannot be ejaculated, resulting in no semen production (obstructive azoospermia)

In females, viscous cervical mucus can obstruct sperm entry

Dx:

1. CXR
2. Spirometry
3. Quantitative pilocarpine iontophoresis for measurement of sweat chloride concentration; Pilocarpine = cholinergic drug that induces sweating; A chloride level >60 mmol/L on two occasions confirms diagnosis, DNA test to identify two CF mutations
4. F/u with DNA analysis
5. Nasal potential difference (defective nasal epithelial ion transport) test if sweat testing and DNA analysis equivocal
6. Sputum culture if pneumonia

Tx/Mgmt:

1. Supportive (steroids for rhinosinusitis or surgery for nasal polyps)
2. Antibiotics for infections (i.e., gentamicin)
3. Lung physiotherapy

Infectious, Immunologic, and Inflammatory Disorders of the Upper Airway

Upper respiratory infections (URI) are illnesses caused by infections of the upper respiratory tract, which include the nose, sinuses, pharynx, and larynx. Some terms to be familiar with are the following:

- **Rhinitis:** inflammation of the nasal mucosa
- **Rhinosinusitis:** inflammation of nasal mucosa + sinus mucosa
- **Nasopharyngitis:** inflammation of nasal mucosa + pharynx/uvula/tonsils, a.k.a. the common cold
- **Pharyngitis:** inflammation of pharynx/uvula/tonsils
- **Epiglottitis:** inflammation of the epiglottis
- **Laryngitis:** inflammation of the larynx
- **Laryngotracheitis:** inflammation of larynx, trachea
- **Tracheitis:** inflammation of trachea and subglottic area

Acute Nasopharyngitis ("The Common Cold")

Buzz Words: Daycare/childcare + sniffling + runny nose/congestion + sneezing + sore throat + winter + cough + no or low fever

Clinical Presentation: Whereas viral etiologies of the common cold will traditionally cause a nasopharyngitis, it can manifest with any of the pathologies above, including pharyngitis, rhinitis, or even sinusitis. The average adult gets up to 4–5 colds a year.

PPx: Adequate hand hygiene, reduce stress, stay away from the sick, and do not touch eyes/mouth/nose with bare hands. No vaccination exists.

MoD: Most common viral etiology is rhinovirus, which spread through air via close contacts with infected people and indirect contact with objects in environment → nose/mouth/eyes via droplets. Other causes of the common cold include adenovirus, coronavirus, coxsackievirus, parainfluenza, and RSV. RSV is very common in babies and can cause more severe symptoms. Parainfluenza is second most common in babies and children, and both RSV/parainfluenza can lead to hospitalization.

Dx:
1. Clinical presentation

Tx/Mgmt:
1. Nonsteroidal antiinflammatory drugs (NSAIDs)/acetaminophen
2. Antibiotics should **not** be prescribed
3. Ribavirin/corticosteroids in severe cases

Influenza ("The Flu")

Buzz Words: Lack of vaccinations + sniffling + runny nose/congestion + sneezing + sore throat + winter + muscle ache + fatigue + high fever + chest tightness

Clinical Presentation: The flu is caused by the influenza virus. Differentiate a cold from influenza by the presence of a high fever and myalgias (Fig. 7.1). In children, the flu can also cause nausea and vomiting. Some prominent complications include viral pneumonia, bacterial pneumonia, or superinfections leading to bacterial sinusitis. The flu causes around 500,000 deaths a year.

PPx: Frequent hand washing + annual influenza vaccine + surgical mask

MoD: Respiratory droplet transmission of influenza A, B, or C. Influenza A is most common and includes the H1N1 to H7N9 viruses. Viruses bind to hemagglutinin on epithelial cells → replication. Neuraminidase leads to the release of viral particles from host cells.

QUICK TIPS

Colds that do not resolve in 2 weeks or get better and then worse again should suspect **bacterial superinfection.**

QUICK TIPS

Coxsackievirus will also cause hand-foot-mouth disease (blisters and rash)

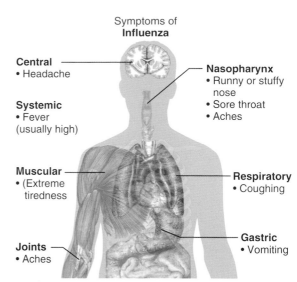

Symptoms of
Influenza

Central
• Headache

Systemic
• Fever
(usually high)

Muscular
• (Extreme
tiredness

Joints
• Aches

Nasopharynx
• Runny or stuffy
nose
• Sore throat
• Aches

Respiratory
• Coughing

Gastric
• Vomiting

FIG. 7.1 Symptoms of influenza. (From Wikimedia Commons. https://en.wikipedia.org/wiki/Influenza#/media/File:Symptoms_of_influenza.svg. From Häggström, Mikael. "Medical gallery of Mikael Häggström 2014." *WikiJournal of Medicine* 1(2). http://dx.doi.org/10.15347/wjm/2014.008. ISSN 20018762. Public Domain.)

Dx:
1. Clinical
2. Rapid influenza test only in severe cases (variable sensitivity)
3. Other tests exist (polymerase chain reaction [PCR], antigen detection, viral culture), but they are only used when it is absolutely critical to make influenza diagnosis (such as in a healthcare worker

Tx/Mgmt:
1. Tylenol/NSAIDs (avoid NSAIDs in children)
2. Neuraminidase inhibitors (oseltamivir, zanamivir)
   • Jury is still out on whether these are helpful in patients without other risk factors
   • AAFP states administration of antivirals based on clinical suspicion before waiting for test results and within 48 hours of symptoms
3. M2 inhibitors (amantadine, rimantadine). Infrequent.

Sinusitis

Buzz Words: Cold like symptoms + runny/stuffy noise + facial pain + tenderness over sinuses + nasal polyps
Chronic sinusitis: Halitosis
Maxillary sinusitis: Tooth pain
Frontal sinusitis: Forehead pain
Sphenoidal sinusitis: Eye pain

Ethmoidal sinusitis: Pain between eyes/upper nose

Clinical Presentation: Sinusitis occurs mostly due to infection but can also be caused by allergies and smoking; and in children, it can be caused by pacifier use or bottle drinking while supine. Untreated sinusitis can lead to meningitis or abscess formation.

PPx: Smoking cessation and frequent hand-washing

MoD: Viral or bacterial infection of sinuses, leading to swelling/congestion and blocked drainage ducts. Most commonly acute are viral causes, including rhinovirus, coronavirus, parainfluenza, RSV, enteroviruses, and metapneumovirus. Common bacterial causes include *Streptococcus pneumoniae*, *Haemophilus influenzae*, and *Moraxella catarrhalis*.

Dx:
1. Physical exam
2. Nasal cultures in chronic sinusitis
3. Endoscopy

Tx/Mgmt:
1. OTC decongestant
2. Saline flushes (e.g., Neti pot)
3. Antibiotic course
   - Amoxicillin first line, switch to Amox + Clavulanate if does not improve after 7 days
   - Clarithromycin/doxy for those with penicillin allergies
   - Typical Abx course = 7 days
4. Antihistamines if allergies are concomitant
5. If chronic and multiple failed antibiotic courses, consider sinus surgery: turbinectomy or balloon sinuplasty

QUICK TIPS

In diabetic with sinusitis, suspect mucormycosis

Epiglottitis

Buzz Words: Child + no HiB vaccination (or foreign immigrant) + difficulty swallowing, hoarse voice + stridor

Clinical Presentation: Typical patients are children with fever and difficulty swallowing. Stridor is caused by HiB or other bacterial infections of the epiglottis, and stridor is upper airway obstruction and is a **surgical emergency.** Since the advent of HiB vaccination, this now mostly occurs in older children and adults.

PPx: Vaccination against HiB can also use rifampin for people who may have been exposed.

MoD: Stridor is traditionally caused by HiB, but if immunized, suspect *S. pneumo*, *Streptococcus pyogenes*, *Staphylococcus aureus*. In addition, it is linked to cocaine usage.

99 AR

Epiglottitis vignette

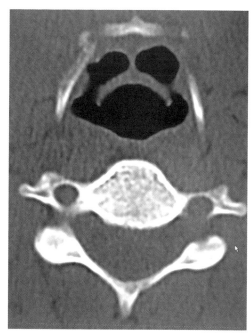

FIG. 7.2 Halloween sign on computed tomography. (From Wikimedia Commons. https://en.wikipedia.org/wiki/File:Halloweensign. jpg. Used under the Creative Commons Attribution-Share Alike 3.0 Unported License.)

Dx:

1. Laryngoscopy to rule out croup, peritonsillar abscess, retropharyngeal abscess
2. X-ray shows thumbprint sign
3. Computed tomography (CT) shows Halloween sign (Fig. 7.2)

Tx/Mgmt:

1. Endotracheal intubation
2. Ceftriaxone + vancomycin
3. Corticosteroids

Croup (Laryngotracheobronchitis)

Buzz Words: Barking cough, coryza, stridor, "steeple sign" on XR

Clinical Presentation: Most common in children 6 months to 3 years old. Peaks in fall and early winter. Onset is gradual and often begins with rhinorrhea, congestion, and coryza. Within the next 12–48 hours, the disease progresses to fever, barking cough, coryza, and inspiratory stridor. The patient then has increased difficulty breathing when lying down.

PPx: None

MoD: Most commonly caused by parainfluenza virus types 1 and 2. RSV second most common cause.
Dx: Clinical, may be assisted by finding of narrowed airway on anteroposterior neck radiograph.
Tx/Mgmt:
1. Supportive treatment and steroids in milder cases
2. Racemic epinephrine for moderate to severe cases

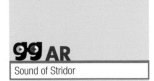

Sound of Stridor

Acute Laryngitis

Buzz Words: Hoarseness + URI symptoms
Clinical Presentation: Acute laryngitis is commonly seen in children from 5 years through adolescence and presents with hoarseness, sore throat, rhinorrhea, cough.
PPx: None
MoD: Acute infection causing inflammation of the mucosa of the larynx, most commonly due to viral respiratory tract infections
Dx: Clinical presentation
Tx/Mgmt: Usually self-limited. Treatment is supportive.

Bacterial Tracheitis

Buzz Words: Stridor + respiratory distress after viral URI/croup
Clinical Presentation: Bacterial tracheitis most commonly occurs following a viral URI or in a child with croup, and it presents with stridor, cough, respiratory distress, high fever, and rapid deterioration. Radiographic features include ragged and irregular tracheal border and a steeple sign.
PPx: None
MoD: Rare, but serious superinfection of the trachea; and it is most commonly caused by *S. aureus.*
Dx: Endoscopy for definitive diagnosis
Tx/Mgmt: In cases of severe obstruction or pending respiratory failure, airway management precedes diagnostic testing. Treat with antimicrobials.

Streptococcal pharyngitis

Buzz Words: Pharyngeal exudates + cervical adenopathy + fever in child
Clinical Presentation: The term tonsillitis may be used in cases when the involvement of the tonsils is prominent. Presents with pain on swallowing, pharyngeal exudates, cervical adenopathy, petechiae, and fever >104. Uncommon to have cough or hoarseness. Uncommon in children under 3 years of age.

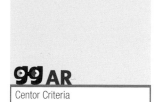

Centor Criteria

PPx: None

MoD: Inflammation of the pharynx and adjacent structures, which is most commonly caused by group A beta hemolytic strep

Dx: Rapid strep test. Throat culture is the gold standard for diagnosis.

Tx/Mgmt: Oral penicillin or amoxicillin x 10 days, and treatment is necessary to prevent acute rheumatic fever

Peritonsillar Abscess

Buzz Words: Muffled voice + severe sore throat + drooling + trismus + deviation of the uvula

Clinical Presentation: A peritonsillar abscess is most frequently seen in adolescents and young adults and presents with severe sore throat, drooling, trismus, and hot potato/muffled voice. It commonly presents with high fever.

PPx: Prompt treatment of strep infections.

MoD: Collection of pus located between the palatine tonsil and the pharyngeal muscles. Often polymicrobial, predominantly caused by Group A strep, Staph, and respiratory anaerobes.

Dx: Clinical. May see deviation of the uvula to the opposite side of abscess.

Tx/Mgmt: Drainage of abscess and antimicrobial therapy

Allergic Rhinitis

Buzz Words: Nasal itching, watery eyes, sneezing + runny nose + congestion

Clinical Presentation: Allergic rhinitis is concomitant with allergies and asthma and presents with nasal itching, itchy/watery eyes, watery rhinorrhea, nasal congestion, and sneezing. On exam, nasal turbinates are pale and edematous and may see allergic shiners—blue/gray discoloration under the eyes and a transverse nasal crease (allergic salute). Symptoms are usually intermittent in response to specific exposures such as cats and pollen.

PPx: Avoidance of allergens

MoD: Histamine release by mast cell degranulation in response to allergens

Dx: Clinical presentation

Tx/Mgmt: Symptomatic treatment with antihistamines, intranasal steroids

Infectious, Immunologic, and Inflammatory Disorders of the Lower Airway

Pneumonia

Buzz Words: Pleuritic chest pain + onset of fever/chills + crackles/rhonchi/wheezing + dyspnea

Clinical Presentation:

Two types of pneumonia:

- **Community Acquired Pneumonia (CAP):** most commonly caused by *S. pneumoniae* and occurs in community or <72 hours since start of hospitalization.
  - Typical
    - *S. pneumo* > *H. flu* > Aerobic GNRs (Klebsiella) > *S. aureus*
    - Pleuritic chest pain, thick, purulent sputum
    - Lobar consolidation on x-ray
  - Atypical
    - Mycoplasma > Chlamydia, coxiella, legionella
    - Influenza, adenovirus, parainfluenza, RSV
    - **Minimal sputum**
    - **Normal pulse + high fever (pulse-temperature dissociation)**
    - No consolidation on XR and reticulonodular infiltrates everywhere
- Nosocomial
  - > 72 hours after hospitalization
  - Most common is *Escherichia coli*, *Pseudomonas*, and *S. aureus*

PPx: Influenza vaccine and pneumococcus vaccine (>65 years old, patients at high risk, i.e., aseptic) (Table 7.1)

MoD: For bacterial pneumonia, the bacteria enter the airway through aspiration of organisms of the nose throat and upper esophagus. Some can also enter the airway through droplets (e.g., tuberculosis [TB] and Legionella). Bacteria then invade lung parenchyma, leading to inflammatory reaction that is seen clinically and on CXR.

Dx:

1. Complete blood count (CBC)
2. Blood cultures
3. PA/lateral x-Ray
4. Expectorated sputum culture and stain
5. Acid fast for TB, Silver Stain for pneumocystis pneumonia
6. Urinary antigen test for legionella

99 AR

Indications for pneumococcus vaccination

Tx/Mgmt:

1. Antimicrobial therapy <60 (Azithromycin, doxycycline)—outpatient
2. Antimicrobial > 60 (levofloxacin, moxifloxacin)—outpatient
3. Hospitalized patients: ceftriaxone + azithromycin
4. Hospital-acquired pneumonia Tx with Ceftazidime or imipenem or piperacillin/tazobactam

Cryptogenic Organizing Pneumonia (formerly bronchiolitis obliterans organizing pneumonia)

Buzz Words: Infectious pneumonia not responding to Abx with negative cultures

Clinical Presentation: Inflammation of bronchioles usually 2/2 chronic inflammatory process

PPx: N/A

TABLE 7.1 Centers for Disease Control and Prevention Recommendations for Pneumococcal Vaccination

Recommended Groups for Vaccination	Strength	Revaccination
Patients 65 and older	A	Second dose of vaccine if patient received vaccine 5 years or more earlier and was younger than 65 at the time of vaccination
Patients ages 2–64 with chronic cardiovascular disease, chronic pulmonary disease, tobacco use or diabetes mellitus (and patients ages 19–64 with asthma)	A	Not recommended
Patients ages 2–64 with alcoholism, chronic liver disease or cerebrospinal fluid leaks	B	Not recommended
Patients ages 2–64 with functional or anatomic asplenia	A	If patient is younger than 10, single revaccination 5 years or more after first dose. If patient is 10 or older, consider revaccination 3 years after previous dose.

TABLE 7.1 Centers for Disease Control and Prevention Recommendations for Pneumococcal Vaccination—cont'd

Recommended Groups for Vaccination	Strength	Revaccination
Patients ages 2–64 who live in special environments or social settings including Alaska Natives, American Indians, group homes, nursing homes, prisons or other institutional settings	C	Not recommended
Immunocompromised patients 2 years or older, including those with HIV infection, leukemia, lymphoma, Hodgkin disease, multiple myeloma, generalized malignancy, chronic renal failure, or nephrotic syndrome; those receiving immunosuppressive chemotherapy (including corticosteroids); and those who have received a transplant.	C	Single revaccination if 5 years or more have elapsed since the first dose. If patient is 10 years or younger, consider revaccination 3 years after previous dose.

The following categories reflect the strength of evidence supporting the recommendations for vaccination: A, Strong epidemiologic evidence and substantial clinical benefit support the recommendation for vaccine use. B, Moderate evidence supports the recommendation for vaccine use. C, Effectiveness of vaccination is not proven, but the high risk for disease and the potential benefits and safety of the vaccine justify vaccination. Strength of evidence for all revaccination recommendations is "C."

MoD: Recurrent pulmonary infections or autoimmune disease (rheumatoid arthritis [RA], lupus) or antineoplastic drugs or bronchial obstruction or ionizing radiation → chronic inflammation of bronchioles → organizing pneumonia

Dx:
1. Clinical presentation
2. CXR (3) Chest CT
3. Chest CT

Tx/Mgmt: Corticosteroids

Anthrax

Buzz Words: Myalgia, fever, malaise + severe dyspnea and shock leading to death

Clinical Presentation: Uncommonly seen in the United States, prodromal symptoms are nonspecific and variable. Early symptoms may mimic influenza and include myalgia, fever, and malaise. These symptoms last 4–5 days and are followed by a rapidly fulminant bacteremic phase with development of severe dyspnea, hypoxemia, and shock. Leads to death within days.

PPx:

For patients with a known exposure, post-exposure prophylaxis with antimicrobials and a vaccination series is available.

MoD: Anthrax results from inhalation of *Bacillus anthracis* spore-containing particles. It can occur when working with contaminated animal products such as wool or hides, but it can also occur because of bioterrorism. Spores release toxins causing hemorrhagic necrosis of thoracic lymph nodes, hemorrhagic mediastinitis, and in some cases, a necrotizing pneumonia.

Dx: Widening of the mediastinum is classic and should raise suspicion in combination with clinical symptoms. This can be diagnosed by PCR.

Tx/Mgmt:

1. IV antimicrobial therapy (Ciprofloxacin +Clindamycin)
2. Antitoxin
3. Supportive care

Bordetella pertussis (Whooping Cough)

Buzz Words: Inspiratory whoop + post-coughing emesis

Clinical Presentation: Classically seen in children 1–10 years old

- **Catarrhal stage:** severe congestion and rhinorrhea for 1–2 weeks
- **Paroxysmal stage:** severe coughing episodes with extreme gasp for air = inspiratory whoop and can have post-coughing emesis for 2–4 weeks
- **Convalescent stage:** decrease of frequency of coughing for 1–2 weeks

PPx: DTap vaccine

MoD: Caused by infection with *B. pertussis*

Dx: PCR of nasal secretions. Lymphocytosis is commonly present, but it is not diagnostic.

Tx/Mgmt:

1. Erythromycin or azithromycin for the catarrhal stage
2. Macrolides for close contacts

Aspiration Pneumonia/Lung Abscess

99 AR

Aspiration pneumonia XR

Clinical Presentation: Aspiration pneumonia/lung abscess is found in patients with large volume aspiration who are not adequately treated. Some commonly seen scenarios are aspiration secondary seizures, intoxication, CVA, and ET intubation/general anesthesia, and it presents with cough, foul smelling sputum, fever. Patients who are mostly upright may aspirate into the right lower lobe. Patients who are hospitalized or bed-ridden and lie mostly horizontally are more likely to aspirate into the right middle lobe.

PPx: Prompt treatment of aspiration pneumonia

MoD: Infected lung tissue becomes necrotic and forms cavitary lesions, and aspiration pneumonia/lung abscess is caused mainly by bacteria colonizing the oropharynx.

Dx: CXR will show a thick-walled cavity. May see air fluid levels.

Tx/Mgmt: Clindamycin for anaerobic coverage, ampicillin for gram-positive cocci. May need to add coverage if gram-negative organisms are suspected.

Fungal Infections

Allergic Bronchopulmonary Aspergillosis

Buzz Words: Asthma or CF + new or worsening cough + brown mucous plugs

Clinical Presentation: Allergic bronchopulmonary aspergillosis is found most commonly in patients with asthma or CF, and is characterized by chronic asthma, recurrent pulmonary infiltrates, and bronchiectasis. It presents with cough, dyspnea, increased sputum production, expectoration of brown-black mucous plug, and wheezing.

PPx: None

MoD: Hypersensitivity of the lungs to fungal antigens that colonize the bronchial tree

Dx:
1. CBC (peripheral blood eosinophilia)
2. Skin test reactivity to Aspergillus antigen
3. Elevated IgE
4. Antibodies against Aspergillus

Tx/Mgmt:
1. Oral steroids
2. Itraconazole for recurrent episodes

Histoplasmosis

Buzz Words: Ohio and Mississippi river valleys + exposure to bird and bat droppings + erythema nodosum (round rashes often on shins)

Clinical Presentation: Histoplasmosis is the most prevalent endemic mycosis in the United States, and it is found in the Ohio and Mississippi river valleys. Most infections are asymptomatic, and some individuals develop

99 AR
ABA radiographs

acute pulmonary infections. Histoplasmosis presents with fever, chills, anorexia, cough, and chest pain usually 2–4 weeks after exposure. An extensive exposure can lead to diffuse disease, which can progress to respiratory failure; and it is often accompanied by joint pain and erythema nodosum.

PPx: None

MoD: *Histoplasma capsulatum* proliferates best in soil contaminated with bird or bat droppings. Organisms are inhaled and cause localized or patchy bronchopneumonia, and macrophages are unable to ingest and kill the fungi. Infected macrophages then can spread the disease throughout the body.

Dx: Histoplasmosis is often confused with CAP on CXR, and CXR shows focal infiltrates with lymphadenopathy.

1. Clinical presentation
2. CXR/Chest CT
3. Lesion biopsy
4. Serologic
5. PCR
6. Blood culture

Tx/Mgmt:

1. Most patients recover without treatment.
2. Extensive exposure can be treated with antifungal therapy, such as Itraconazole/amphotericin B.

Coccidioidomycosis

Buzz Words: Pneumonia + meningitis

Clinical Presentation: Coccidioidomycosis is found in Southwestern United States, Northern Mexico, and South/Central America. The disease ranges from self-limited acute pneumonia (Valley fever) to disseminated disease, and more significant illness is correlated to more intensive exposure. Primary infection most frequently manifests as CAP about 21 days after exposure, and the most common symptoms are chest pain, cough, and fever. Coccidioidomycosis may also present with fatigue, arthralgias, and erythema nodosum.

PPx: None

MoD: Inhalation of spores, usually from stirred up dust

Dx:

1. Clinical presentation
2. CXR/Chest CT
3. Lesion biopsy
4. Serologic
5. PCR
6. Blood culture

Tx/Mgmt:
1. Most patients recover without therapy.
2. Antifungals in immunosuppressed patients or those with severe disease. Fluconazole, Amphotericin B, Itraconazole

Blastomycosis

Buzz Words: Pneumonia + skin/bone disease
Clinical Presentation: Shadows histoplasmosis in Midwestern and Southeastern United States (Fig. 7.3)
PPx: None
MoD:
Dx:
1. Clinical presentation
2. CXR/Chest CT
3. Lesion biopsy
4. Serologic
5. PCR
6. Blood culture
Tx/Mgmt: Itraconazole, Amphotericin B, Fluconazole

Pneumocystis Pneumonia

Buzz Words: Human immunodeficiency virus (HIV) + low CD4 count + dry cough
Clinical Presentation: Pneumocystis pneumonia occurs almost exclusively in AIDS patient with a CD4 count <200 and presents with dyspnea on exertion, dry cough, and fever.

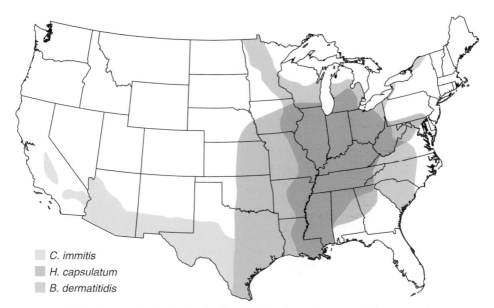

C. immitis
H. capsulatum
B. dermatitidis

FIG. 7.3 Geographic distribution for *Coccidioides*, *Histoplasma*, and *Blastomycosis*.

PPx: TMP/SMX in any patient with CD4 count under 200

MoD: Caused by *P. jirovecii*

Dx: CXR showing bilateral interstitial infiltrate, elevated LDH levels. The most accurate test is lavage.

Tx/Mgmt:

1. TMP/SMX (dapsone or atovaquone if sulfa allergic)
2. Add steroids is pO_2 is less than 70 or A-a gradient is greater than 35

Obstructive Airway Disease

Asthma

Buzz Words: Reversible + wheezing with prolonged expiratory phase + chest pain/tightness + tachypnea, dyspnea

Clinical Presentation: Asthma is the most common chronic disease of childhood and is exacerbated by viral infections, exposure to allergens and irritants, exercise, and changes in weather. Nighttime symptoms are also common. Symptoms reversible with bronchodilator therapy differentiate asthma from COPD, and acute exacerbation presents with wheezing, prolonged expiratory phase, chest tightness, tachypnea, and dyspnea. Asthma is also associated with eczema.

PPx: Avoid exposure to triggers, and carefully adhere to medications.

MoD: Inflammatory cells, chemical mediators, and chemotactic factors mediate the underlying inflammatory response; and inflammation contributes to airway hyperresponsiveness. Asthma results in edema, increased mucous production, and influx of inflammatory cells; and chronic inflammation leads to airway remodeling.

Dx: Most accurate are PFTs, and they are usually normal between exacerbations.

- PFTs: decreased FEV1/FVC, increase in FEV1 >12% with use of albuterol, decrease in FEV1 >20% with methacholine challenge, increased DLCO
- In acute exacerbation: Peak expiratory flow or ABG are more useful. Peak expiratory flow approximates FVC
- CXR can be obtained to exclude pneumonia and CHF

Tx/Mgmt: To determine treatment, you must first determine the classification of asthma and use the step-wise method. The patient can be moved up or down based on the severity and control of symptoms.

Acute Asthma Management

1. Best initial therapy: oxygen, nebulized short-acting beta agonist (SABA) (albuterol), bolus of IV steroids
2. Ipratropium given in combination with albuterol as a DuoNeb. Ipratropium does not work as quickly as albuterol.
3. Magnesium can be used to help relieve bronchospasm. It is only given in severe exacerbations that have been unresponsive to multiple rounds of nebulizers.
4. If patient is not responding to treatment and has an increasing PCO_2 on ABG, intubation needs to be considered.

Long-Term Asthma Management

1. **Intermittent**: symptoms ≤ 2 days/week
   - Nighttime awakenings ≤ 2×/month
   - SABA use ≤ 2 days/week
   - No interference with normal activity
   - Normal FEV1 between exacerbations, FEV1 > 80% predicted, FEV1/FVC normal
   - Step 1 Treatment: SABA

High-yield asthma video

2. **Mild Persistent**: symptoms ≥ 2 days/week but not daily
   - Nighttime awakenings 3–4×/month
   - SABA use > 2 days/week, but not daily. Not more than once per day
   - Minor limitation with activity
   - Step 2 Treatment: SABA + low dose inhaled glucocorticoid
3. **Moderate Persistent**: symptoms daily
   - Nighttime awakenings >1× per week, but not nightly
   - SABA use daily
   - Some limitation with activity
   - Step 3: SABA + low-dose inhaled glucocorticoid + long-acting beta agonist (LABA)
4. **Severe**: symptoms throughout the day
   - Nighttime awakenings: nightly
   - SABA use several times per day
   - Extreme limitation of activity
   - Step 4: SABA + medium-dose inhaled glucocorticoid + LABA
   - Step 5: SABA + high-dose inhaled glucocorticoid + LABA
   - In severe cases, can move up to step 6 and add oral systemic glucocorticoids

Chronic Obstructive Pulmonary Disease

Buzz Words (Fig. 7.4): Cough + sputum production + dyspnea

Clinical Presentation: Patients may have a combination of chronic bronchitis and emphysema or just one of the two.

- Chronic Bronchitis
  - Clinical diagnosis, cough + sputum 3 months per year for 2+ years
  - Blue Bloaters
  - Overweight and cyanotic, chronic cough, cor pulmonale (right heart failure) with no use of accessory muscles and not in respiratory distress
- Emphysema
  - Pathologic diagnosis with enlargement of air spaces
  - Pink Puffers
  - Thin, increased energy expenditure during breathing with a tendency to lean forward with a barrel chest, in obvious distress, and using accessory muscles

PPx: Smoking cessation. COPD patients must get pneumococcus vaccination.

MoD: Chronic bronchitis: mucus production narrows airways → inflammation/scarring → obstruction

Emphysema: Increased protease activity from tobacco smoking → breakdown of alveolar walls

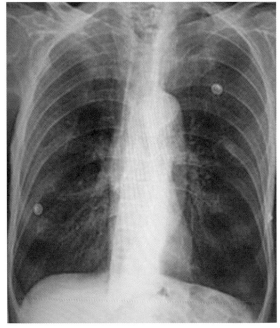

FIG. 7.4 Chronic obstructive pulmonary disease.

Dx:
1. PFT (obstruction FEV1 <70% of normal value, TLC, RV, FRC increased)
2. CXR (hyperinflammation, flattened diaphragm, diminished vasculature markings). Low sensitivity.
3. ABG

Tx/Mgmt:
1. B2 agonists (albuterol or salmeterol)
2. Inhaled anticholinergics (ipratropium bromide)
3. Corticosteroids (budesonide, fluticasone)
4. Acute exacerbation (persistent increase in sputum and cough → respiratory failure)
   - Bronchodilators + systemic corticosteroids + antibiotics + supplemental O_2
   - Intubation if patient is struggling or going downhill

GOLD 2017 Guidelines for COPD management

Pneumoconioses

These diseases are caused by occupational exposure. You will only be tested on the ability to recognize a pneumoconiosis from a clinical presentation. The organizing principle here is the **occupation**. Use the diagnostic modalities of CXR and biopsy to help refine your diagnosis (Table 7.2).

Hypersensitivity Pneumonitis

Buzz Words: Fever, chills, cough, dyspnea + pulmonary infiltrates after exposure to inhaled agent

Clinical Presentation: Hypersensitivity pneumonitis can lead to restrictive lung disease. Three big associations to make for the medicine shelf:
- Farmer's lung—moldy hay
- Bird breeder's lung—avian droppings
- Bagassosis—moldy sugar cane

PPx: Prevent exposure.

MoD: Inhalation of antigenic agent → immune-mediated pneumonitis

Dx: CXR (pulmonary infiltrates)

Tx/Mgmt: Glucocorticoids

Interstitial Lung Disease/Idiopathic Pulmonary Fibrosis

Buzz Words: Dyspnea + nonproductive cough + digital clubbing +/− cyanosis/pulmonary HTN

Clinical Presentation: Interstitial lung disease (ILD) is inflammation of alveolar wall leading to fibroblast proliferation and collagen deposition. This causes irreversible fibrosis that impairs gas exchange and can be caused

TABLE 7.2 Occupational Exposures and Their Pulmonary Sequelae

Exposure	Occupation	CXR/Biopsy Findings
Silica	Mining/tunnel perforation	Nodular pattern, mediastinal adenopathy, collagen in nodules
Coal	Coal miner	Coal laden macrophages, nodular patterns in middle lung fields
Asbestos	Asbestos mining, ship building, insulation material use	Interstitial pneumonia + pattern on CXR, increased risk of bronchogenic carcinoma
Beryllium "Berylliosis"	Aerospace industry, ceramics, fluorescent lighting	**Sarcoid granulomas** + reticular and nodular pattern, hilar and mediastinal adenopathy; always Tx with glucocorticoids
Iron/tin/ barium "Siderosis"	Mining, welding, polishing, Barium in glass and paper manufacturing	Hyperdense nodules
Aluminum "Aluminosis"	Explosives manufacturer	Interstitial fibrosis + irregular nodules + opacities in upper/lower fields
Mercury	Electrical industry + scientific equipment	Tracheobronchitis, pneumonia, pulmonary edema

CXR, Chest x-ray.

by several etiologies. Any of the pneumoconiosis or pneumonitis or COP can cause ILD, and other diseases to know include sarcoidosis, granulomatosis with polyangiitis, eosinophilic granulomatosis with polyangiitis (Churg-Strauss), and Goodpasture syndrome. High-yield drugs causing pulmonary fibrosis include amiodarone and bleomycin; an idiopathic cause is idiopathic pulmonary fibrosis. Know this well for the medicine shelf.

PPx: N/A

Dx:

1. CXR—diffuse reticulonodular pattern, honeycombing
2. Chest CT (Fig. 7.5)
3. PFTs FEV1/FVC is elevated
4. Tissue biopsy

Tx/Mgmt:

1. Supplemental O_2
2. Corticosteroids + cyclophosphamide
3. Transplant

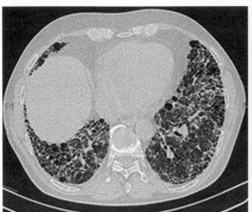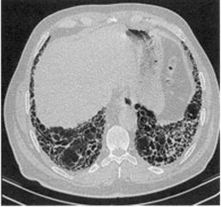

FIG. 7.5 Computed tomography for idiopathic pulmonary fibrosis. (From Wikimedia Commons. https://commons.wikimedia.org/wiki/File:HR_tomography_of_the_chest_of_an_IPF_patient.jpg. By IPFeditor. Used under the Creative Commons Attribution-Share Alike 3.0 Unported License.)

Benign Neoplasms of Upper Airways

Vocal Cord Polyps

Buzz Words: Hoarseness + scratchiness, lump in throat + unilateral + smoker

Clinical Presentation: Vocal cord polyps presents with hoarseness, scratchy throat, or "lump in throat" sensation in the setting of chronic irritation. Polyps tend to be unilateral and present in the anterior one-third of the vocal fold. It is more common in males and in smokers, in which it may be caused by HPV.

PPx: Smoking cessation

MoD: Chronic vocal cord irritation

Dx:

1. Physical examination focusing on quality of patient's voice, oral cavity, and cranial nerve function.
2. Laryngoscopy

Tx/Mgmt:

1. Voice rest
2. Smoking cessation
3. Surgery

Nasal Polyps

Buzz Words: Chronic rhinosinusitis + aspirin/NSAID-induced bronchospasm

Clinical Presentation: Nasal polyps present with recurrent nasal discharge/congestion with bilateral, shiny mucoid masses; and anosmia leads to a possible change in taste. Bilateral nasal polyps in a child on the shelf should raise suspicion of CF, and unilateral nasal polyps on the shelf suggests aspirin-induced asthma.

PPx: N/A
MoD: Unknown
Dx:
1. Physical exam including rhinoscopy
2. Nasal endoscopy
3. Head CT or magnetic resonance imaging (MRI)
4. Allergy tests
5. Test for CF
Tx/Mgmt:
1. Intranasal glucocorticoids
2. Oral glucocorticoids if severe or refractory to intranasal delivery
3. Surgery, although polyps tend to return

Benign Neoplasms of Lung and Pleura

Solitary Pulmonary Nodule

Buzz Words: Singular nodule/lesion + accidental finding
PPx: N/A
Clinical Presentation: Solitary pulmonary nodule presents as single, well defined, round opacity surrounded completely by pulmonary parenchyma that is less than 3 cm. If imaging also depicts atelectasis, lymph node enlargement, or pleural effusion the lesion is not a solitary pulmonary nodule (SPN). Solitary pulmonary nodule is usually found accidently on CXR. For SPN, it is more important to focus on the Dx and Mgmt rather than the cause of the nodule.
MoD:
• **Infectious**: tuberculosis, fungal infection, abscess, nocardia, nontuberculosis mycobacteria, round pneumonia, septic embolus
• **Benign neoplasm:** hamartoma, fibroma, or chondroma
• **Malignant neoplasm**: bronchogenic carcinoma, carcinoid/neuroendocrine, metastasis, lymphoma, teratoma, leiomyoma
• **Inflammatory:** granulomatosis with polyangiitis, rheumatoid nodule, sarcoidosis
• **Vascular:** arteriovenous malformation, hematoma, pulmonary artery aneurysm, pulmonary venous varix, pulmonary infarct
• **Bronchial**: bronchogenic cyst, mucocele, lung sequestration
Dx:
1. Compare with previous imaging
   a. If low risk for malignancy (see Table 7.1), or 2-year radiographic stability, no further testing is needed and follow yearly with serial chest CT scans

b. If intermediate risk of malignancy, either fine-needle aspiration (FNA) or positron emission tomography (PET) scan is acceptable

c. If the results suggest malignancy, surgical resection is the next step.

d. However, if the results are nondiagnostic, active surveillance is the correct course of action.

Tx/Mgmt:

1. Serial chest CT scans
2. CT-FNA
3. PET scan
4. Surgical excision

Bronchial Carcinoid Tumor

Buzz Words: Recurrent PNA in same pulmonary segment + indolent course

Clinical Presentation: Most of these tumors arise in the proximal airways and lead to symptoms due to obstruction from the mass or bleeding from its hypervascularity. Patients may have a cough or wheeze, chest pain, recurrent pneumonia in same pulmonary segment, or hemoptysis. Bronchial carcinoid tumors produce less serotonin than midgut carcinoid tumors. Therefore, they are less likely to present with cutaneous flushing, diarrhea, bronchospasms, and right-sided valvular heat disease.

PPx: N/A

MoD: Thought to arise from specialized Kulchitsky cell, a type of neuroendocrine cell

Dx:

1. Chest CT scan
2. Bronchoscopic biopsy for central lesions
3. Transthoracic needle biopsy for peripheral lesions
4. Abdominal CT scan looking for metastatic liver lesions

Tx/Mgmt: Surgical resection

Malignant Neoplasms of Upper Airways

Lip—Squamous Cell Carcinoma (SCC)

Buzz Words: Smoker + alcohol use + "persistent" papules + plaques + erosions/ulcers

PPx: Smoking cessation, alcohol cessation, adequate sun protection

Clinical Presentation: Lip SCC presents as an exophytic or ulcerative lesion often associated with pain. It is a slow growing, local tumor with a low potential to metastasize.

MoD: Malignant proliferation of squamous keratinocytes

99 AR

Management of SPN

QUICK TIPS

Despite being a rare tumor, bronchial carcinoid tumors are the most common primary lung neoplasm of children. The most common metastatic site for carcinoid tumors is the liver.

QUICK TIPS

Lip SCC is more commonly found on lower lip due to greater sun exposure.

Dx:
1. Physical exam
2. Biopsy

Tx/Mgmt:
1. Mohs surgery or excision
2. Topical imiquimod and 5-fluorouracil

Oral Cavity—Squamous Cell Carcinoma

Buzz Words: Smoker + alcohol use + "non-healing" ulcer + immunocompromised

PPx: Smoking cessation, alcohol cessation

Clinical Presentation: Oral cavity SCC presents with a persistent, nonhealing ulcer or mass associated with pain. It may also present as a bleeding sore, growth or lump, painful chewing or swallowing, sore throat, and poorly fitting dentures. More likely to occur in smokers, alcohol abusers, and the immunocompromised. The effect of smoking and alcohol is multiplicative with the increased risk of developing cancers of the oral cavity, and a subset of oropharyngeal SCC is associated with HPV infection (HPV-16). Also, remember that oral leukoplakia is a precancerous lesion presenting as white patches or plaques.

MoD: Malignant proliferation of squamous keratinocytes, progression from untreated leukoplakia

Dx:
1. Physical exam
2. Biopsy
3. Head and neck CT scan

Tx/Mgmt:
1. Surgical removal of tumor and any involved lymph nodes
2. Radiation
3. May require chemotherapy with cisplatin plus fluorouracil if more advanced

Pharynx—Squamous Cell Carcinoma

Buzz Words: Smoker + painful swallowing + cystic neck mass

PPx: Smoking cessation, alcohol cessation

Clinical Presentation: Pharynx SCC presents with dysphagia and odynophagia often in the setting of smoking and alcohol abuse. It may also present with snoring and obstructive sleep apnea (OSA), bleeding, or a neck mass. HPV associated oropharyngeal cancers (HPV-16) often present with cystic neck masses, and these may often be mistaken for branchial cleft cyst carcinomas, although these are remarkably rare. If the patient is presenting with a cystic neck mass, metastatic cystic SCC should be excluded.

MoD: Malignant proliferation of squamous keratinocytes
Dx:
1. Physical exam
2. Head and neck CT scan
3. Triple endoscopy if smoking and/or alcohol abuse history
4. Direct laryngoscopy if lack of smoking and/or alcohol abuse history
5. Biopsy
6. Chest CT scan to rule out metastatic disease
Tx/Mgmt: Same as SCC of oral cavity

Larynx—Squamous Cell Carcinoma

Buzz Words: Smoker + alcohol use + hoarseness
PPx: Smoking cessation, alcohol cessation
Clinical Presentation: Larynx SCC presentation depends on location of tumor. Persistent hoarseness is the initial complaint in glottic lesions; and symptoms may progress to dysphagia, referred otalgia, persistent cough, hemoptysis, and stridor. Supraglottic lesions are more indolent and are often discovered later from airway obstruction or from palpable lymph nodes.
MoD: Malignant proliferation of squamous keratinocytes
Dx:
1. Physical exam
2. Head and neck CT scan
3. Triple endoscopy if smoking and/or alcohol abuse history
   a. Direct laryngoscopy if lack of smoking and/or alcohol abuse history
4. Biopsy
5. Chest CT scan to rule out metastatic disease
Tx/Mgmt: Same as SCC of oral cavity

Malignant Neoplasms of Lower Airway

Squamous Cell Carcinoma

Buzz Words: Smoker + persistent cough + hemoptysis + hypercalcemia + superior vena cava (SVC) syndrome (swelling of face, neck, chest) + Horner syndrome (ptosis, meiosis, anhidrosis)
Clinical Presentation: Intrathoracic symptoms of SCC include a persistent cough, hemoptysis, chest pain, dyspnea, hoarseness, and wheezing. Constitutional symptoms, especially in a smoker, such as weight loss, decreased appetite, and weakness should raise your suspicion for lung cancer. Be on the lookout for recurrent pneumonia in the same lobe, as this could be a sign of postobstructive pneumonia.

99 AR
Lung Cancer Review

99 AR
Paraneoplastic Syndromes

Local invasion may lead to SVC syndrome, Horner syndrome, Pancoast syndrome, phrenic nerve palsy, recurrent laryngeal nerve palsy, and malignant pleural effusion. SVC syndrome presents with facial and upper extremity edema, dilated neck and chest veins, and a feeling of facial fullness.

Horner syndrome presents with unilateral facial anhidrosis, ptosis, and miosis (PAM: Ptosis, Anhidrosis, Miosis).

Pancoast syndrome presents with shoulder pain that may radiate down the arm, atrophy of hand muscles, and upper extremity weakness. Phrenic nerve palsy presents with dyspnea from hemidiaphragmatic paralysis.

Recurrent laryngeal nerve presents with persistent hoarseness.

Malignant pleural effusion shows up on imaging and has a poor prognosis, as it is considered incurable. Paraneoplastic syndromes seen in SCC include hypertrophic pulmonary osteoarthropathy and PTHrP secretion. Hypertrophic osteoarthropathy presents with clubbing and a symmetrical, painful arthropathy in the ankles, knees, wrists, and elbows. PTHrP secretion will lead to symptoms of hypercalcemia such as decreased appetite, nausea, vomiting, constipation, lethargy, polyuria, polydipsia, and dehydration. Labs in such instances will depict decreased PTH and increased PTHrP. Do not forget that hypercalcemia in cancer patients may also be due to other causes such as bony metastasis.

Frequent site of metastasis of lung cancer includes liver, adrenal glands, bones, and brain.

PPx: Smoking cessation, avoiding asbestos, and avoiding radon. Low-dose CT screening for patients aged 55–77 without symptoms but a 30 pack-year smoking history.

MoD:
- SCC-malignant proliferation of squamous keratinocytes.
- SVC syndrome-obstruction of the SVC.
- Horner syndrome-infiltration of cervical sympathetic chain by an apical tumor.
- Pancoast syndrome-apical tumor infiltration of C8 and T1–T2.
- Phrenic nerve palsy-tumor infiltration of phrenic nerve.
- Recurrent laryngeal nerve palsy-infiltration of recurrent laryngeal nerve.
- Malignant pleural effusion-extension of tumor into the visceral and/or parietal pleura.

- Hypertrophic pulmonary osteoarthropathy-periosteal proliferation of tubular bones.
- Hypercalcemia-tumor secretes PTH analog (PTHrP) is secreted directly from tumor cells.

Dx:

1. Physical exam
2. CXR (compare to previous images)
3. Chest CT scan
4. Cytology of sputum-may diagnose central tumors (SCC tends to be central)
5. Whole body PET scan
6. Biopsy: Bronchoscopy with endobronchial ultrasound (EBUS)-directed biopsy for central primary tumors and mediastinal lymph nodes; transthoracic needle biopsy for peripheral lesions
7. Mediastinoscopy for staging the mediastinum
8. Pulmonary function tests. (Patients must meet minimal requirements to be able to tolerate surgery.)

Tx/Mgmt:

Stage I and II: primarily surgical management
Stage III: chemotherapy, radiation
Stage IV: chemotherapy

Lung Cancer Staging

Adenocarcinoma

Buzz Words: Persistent cough + hemoptysis + peripheral location in lung + osteoarthropathy + normal calcium level

Clinical Presentation: Similar to SCC of the lung, see above. However, adenocarcinoma tends to be found in a more peripheral location, has higher incidence of hypertrophic pulmonary osteoarthropathy, and does not produce PTHrP. It is the most common primary lung malignancy in smokers and nonsmokers. Suspect adenocarcinoma when presenting symptoms are found in a nonsmoker.

PPx: Smoking cessation (although adenocarcinoma has the lowest association with smoking), avoiding asbestos, and avoiding radon. Low-dose CT screening for those age 55–77 who have no symptoms and have a 30 pack-year smoking history.

MoD: Malignant neoplastic gland formation possibly containing intracytoplasmic mucin

Dx: Same as lung SCC

Tx/Mgmt: Same as lung SCC

Large Cell Carcinoma

Buzz Words: Smoker, persistent cough, hemoptysis, no paraneoplastic syndrome

Clinical Presentation: Similar to SCC of the lung, see above. However, large cell carcinoma (LCC) tends to be found both centrally and peripherally. It is rare to encounter paraneoplastic syndromes in LCC except hypereosinophilia.

PPx: Smoking cessation. Low-dose CT screening for patients aged 55–77 who have no symptoms and have a 30 pack-year smoking history.

MoD: Undifferentiated epithelial neoplasm lacking both glandular and squamous cells. Highly aggressive with a poor prognosis.

Dx: Same as lung SCC

Tx/Mgmt: Same as lung SCC

Small Cell Carcinoma

Buzz Words: Smoker, persistent cough, hemoptysis, hyponatremia, Cushing's

Clinical Presentation: Similar to SCC of the lung, see above. However, small cell carcinoma tends to be found more centrally and has different paraneoplastic syndromes. Paraneoplastic syndromes associated with small cell carcinoma include syndrome of inappropriate antidiuretic hormone secretion (SIADH), Cushing syndrome, and Eaton-Lambert syndrome. SIADH presents with symptoms of hyponatremia including anorexia, nausea, and vomiting. If the onset of hyponatremia is rapid, symptoms of cerebral edema such as irritability, restlessness, confusion, and seizures may occur.

Cushing syndrome presents with muscle weakness, weight loss, hypertension, hirsutism, osteoporosis, hypokalemic, alkalosis, and hyperglycemia. Eaton-Lambert presents with symmetrical, proximal muscle weakness (that improves with use) and autonomic dysfunction such as dry mouth and erectile dysfunction.

MoD: Malignant, poorly differentiated small cells arising from neuroendocrine (Kulchitsky) cells. SIADH-ectopic secretion of ADH. Cushing syndrome-ectopic secretion of ACTH. Eaton-Lambert syndrome antibodies against presynaptic voltage-gated calcium channel leads to decreased release of acetylcholine.

PPx: Smoking cessation. Low-dose CT screening for patients aged 55–77 who have no symptoms and have a 30 pack-year smoking history.

Dx: Same as lung SCC

Tx/Mgmt: Surgery and chemoradiation

Malignant Neoplasms of Pleura

Mesothelioma

Buzz Words: Asbestos, plumber, construction worker, unilateral pleural effusion

Clinical Presentation: Mesothelioma presents with gradual onset of symptoms such as chest pain, dyspnea, hoarseness, night sweats, or dysphagia. Majority of cases occur in older patients, and mesothelioma tends to present decades after exposure to asbestos. Constitutional symptoms may also be present such as fatigue and weight loss. It can also present with a large, unilateral pleural effusion, which leads to unilateral dullness to percussion and decreased aeration at the lung base during a physical exam. It has a very poor prognosis.

PPx: Avoiding asbestos, avoiding radiation

MoD: Malignant proliferation of mesothelial surfaces of the pleura

Pleural thickening in mesothelioma

Dx:

1. CXR (Fig. 7.6)
2. Chest CT scan
3. Thoracentesis of pleural effusion
4. Closed pleural biopsy
5. If still not adequate tissue for diagnosis, VATS biopsy and/or EBUS-guided biopsies of mediastinal pleural lesions
6. PET scan for staging

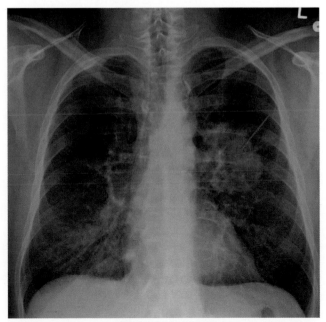

FIG. 7.6 Lung tumor

Tx/Mgmt: Surgical resection, chemoradiation

Metastasis to Lung

Buzz Words: Multiple dense pulmonary nodules

Clinical Presentation: Symptoms of metastasis to lung include persistent cough, hemoptysis, chest pain, dyspnea, hoarseness, and wheezing. Constitutional symptoms such as weight loss, decreased appetite, and weakness may also be present. Imaging depicts multiple pulmonary nodules that are ≥1 cm in diameter and in different stages of growth. Metastatic lesions tend to be round with sharply demarcated borders and have a predilection for the bases.

PPx: N/A

MoD: Tumors that tend to metastasize to the lungs include breast cancer, colon cancer, prostate cancer, bladder cancer, and sarcoma.

Dx:

1. Spiral CT scan
2. PET scan
3. Biopsy (see Dx section of lung SCC)

Tx/Mgmt: Treatment based on primary tumor.

Respiratory Failure/Respiratory Arrest and Pulmonary Vascular Disorders

Acute Respiratory Distress Syndrome

Buzz Words: Dyspnea + hypoxemia refractory to oxygen + bilateral diffuse pulmonary infiltrates + "White-out" on CXR

Clinical Presentation: Acute respiratory distress syndrome (ARDS) presents with respiratory distress with dyspnea, tachypnea, hypoxemia, and diaphoresis. CXR clearly depicts bilateral alveolar infiltrates. In addition, ARDS presents with $PaO_2/FiO_2 \leq 200$ mm Hg, brain natriuretic peptide (BNP) <100 pg/mL, and pulmonary capillary wedge pressure (PCWP) ≤ 18 mm Hg. It is important to remember cardiogenic pulmonary edema presents in a similar manner and must be distinguished from ARDS (look for signs of volume overload, CHF, jugular venous distension (JVD), edema, and hepatomegaly. Complications include permanent lung injury or barotrauma from high-pressure mechanical ventilation.

PPx: N/A

MoD: ARDS is a consequence of alveolar injury producing massive alveolar damage. This injury leads to the release of pro-inflammatory cytokines, which recruit

gg AR

ARDS chest x-ray

neutrophils to the lungs. These neutrophils release toxic mediators that lead to damage to the capillaries and alveoli. Ultimately, the airspaces will fill with edema fluid and debris from damaged cells causing: ventilation-perfusion mismatching from physiologic shunting (A-a gradient), decreased lung compliance from lung stiffness, increased dead space from obstruction and destruction of pulmonary capillary bed, and pulmonary hypertension (PH) from hypoxic vasoconstriction.

Dx:
1. CXR ("White-out")
2. Arterial blood gas
3. Calculate PaO_2/FiO_2
4. BNP
5. Swan-Ganz catheter-PCWP

Tx/Mgmt:
1. Mechanical ventilation: high FiO_2 for appropriate oxygenation, low tidal volume (will lead to permissive hypercapnia) to protect from barotrauma, and positive end-expiratory pressure (PEEP) to open collapse alveoli and decrease shunting
2. Manage fluids to prevent volume overload
3. Treat underlying condition

Pulmonary Hypertension

Buzz Words: Loud pulmonic heart sound + exertional fatigue + right heart failure + mean pulmonary arterial pressure (mPAP) $\geq$ 25 mm Hg at rest or 30 mm Hg during exercise

Clinical Presentation: PH is defined by an mPAP $\geq$ 25 mm Hg at rest or 30 mm Hg during exercise. Patients often present with dyspnea on exertion, fatigue, atypical chest pain, and syncope. On physical exam, the patient may have a loud pulmonic component of the second heart sound. As the disease progresses and right ventricular failure occurs, signs will include JVD, hepatomegaly, ascites, and peripheral edema/anasarca.

PPx: None

MoD: PH occurs ultimately due to vascular remodeling and increased pulmonary vascular resistance. PH is classified as one of five groups.

- **Group 1, Pulmonary arterial hypertension (PAH):** causes such as sporadic idiopathic PAH, heritable PAH, drugs and toxins, systemic sclerosis, HIV, and congenital heart disease
- **Group 2, PH from left heart disease:** causes such as mitral and aortic valve disease, left ventricular systolic or diastolic dysfunction, or restrictive cardiomyopathy

QUICK TIPS

Causes of ARDS: sepsis, aspiration of gastric contents, severe trauma, fractures, acute pancreatitis, massive transfusions, near drowning, and drug overdose

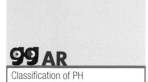

- **Group 3: PH from lung disease:** causes such as COPD and interstitial lung disease
- **Group 4, PH from thromboembolic disease:** causes such as chronic thromboembolic occlusion of pulmonary vessels
- **Group 5: PH from multifactorial causes**

Dx:
1. EKG
2. CXR
3. Echocardiogram
4. Right heart catheterization

Tx/Mgmt:
1. Fluid management with diuretics
2. Oxygen
3. Anticoagulant therapy (Group 4)
4. Calcium channel blocker such as dihydropyridine or diltiazem (Group 1)
5. Prostacyclin analogs such as epoprostenol (Group 1)
6. Endothelin agonists such as ambrisentan, bosentan, or macitentan (Group 1)
7. Oral phosphodiesterase inhibitors such as sildenafil (Group 1)
8. Lung transplant

Pulmonary Arteriovenous Malformations (PAVMs)

Buzz Words: Hereditary hemorrhagic telangiectasia, hemoptysis

Clinical Presentation: PAVMs are most commonly asymptomatic and are found incidentally on imaging. If a patient has symptoms, they may include dyspnea and hemoptysis. Complications from PAVM also include stroke, brain abscesses, and PH.

PPx: N/A

MoD: Abnormal communications between pulmonary arteries and veins, which may lead to right-to-left shunt.

Dx:
1. Echocardiography scan
2. Chest CT

Tx/Mgmt:
1. Many patients just require yearly clinical observation and a CT every 3–5 years
2. If symptomatic, use embolotherapy via angiographic occlusion of the feeding artery
3. Surgery for patients who fail multiple embolization
4. Lifelong antibiotics prophylaxis prior to dental procedures

QUICK TIPS

The most common cause of PAVMs is hereditary hemorrhagic telangiectasia.

Noncardiogenic Pulmonary Edema

Buzz Words: Respiratory distress, crackles

Clinical Presentation: Noncardiogenic pulmonary edema presents with dyspnea, hypoxemia, and crackles on lung auscultation. It is important to rule out cardiogenic causes.

PPx: N/A

MoD: Movement of excess fluid into the alveoli. In noncardiogenic pulmonary edema (PCWP ≤18 mm Hg), this accumulation of fluid and protein in the alveolar leads hinders diffusion capacity. Major causes include ARDS, high altitude, neurogenic pulmonary edema, opioid overdose, massive pulmonary embolism, and eclampsia.

Dx:

1. CXR
2. BNP
3. ABG
4. ECG
5. Echo

Tx/Mgmt:

1. Oxygen
2. Manage fluids to prevent volume overload
3. Treat underlying condition

Cardiogenic Pulmonary Edema

Buzz Words: Respiratory distress + crackles + history of orthopnea and/or paroxysmal nocturnal dyspnea (PND) + S3 or S4 + JVD

Clinical Presentation: Cardiogenic pulmonary edema presents with dyspnea, hypoxemia, and crackles on lung auscultation. Patients may have tachycardia and hypertension. S3 or S4, JVD, and peripheral edema may also be present.

PPx: Adherence to medications and low sodium dietary restrictions

MoD: Most often, cardiogenic pulmonary edema is the result of acute decompensated heart failure (ADHF) due to ventricular systolic or diastolic dysfunction leading to a rapid and acute increase in left ventricular filling pressures and left atrial pressure. Ultimately, this causes increased transudation of protein-poor fluid into the alveolar spaces. Causes of left ventricular systolic dysfunction include coronary heart disease, hypertension, valvular disease, and dilated cardiomyopathy. Causes of left ventricular diastolic dysfunction include hypertrophic and restrictive cardiomyopathies.

99 AR
Great Breath Sounds Review

QUICK TIPS
The most common mechanism of noncardiogenic pulmonary edema is an increase in capillary permeability.

Dx:

1. CXR
2. BNP
3. ABG
4. ECG
5. Echo

Tx/Mgmt:

1. Place patient sitting up with legs dangling from bed
2. Diuresis with daily assessment of weight
3. Supplemental oxygen and assisted ventilation
4. Nitrates
5. Morphine

Pulmonary Embolism

Buzz Words: Dyspnea, tachycardia + chest pain + post-op, long travel + OCPs + normal CXR

Clinical Presentation: The most common presenting symptoms of pulmonary embolism are tachycardia and dyspnea followed by pleuritic chest pain, cough, and signs of a deep vein thrombosis (DVT). Rarely, as in the case of a massive PE, do patients present with hemoptysis, shock, syncope, and/or right bundle branch block. Many patents are asymptomatic or have mild symptoms. What is important to remember are the risk factors for PE. Inherited risk factors include factor V Leiden mutation, prothrombin gene mutation, protein S or C deficiency, and antithrombin deficiency. Acquired risk factors include malignancy, surgery (especially orthopedic procedures), trauma, prior DVT/PE, pregnancy, oral contraceptives, immobilization, congestive heart failure, obesity, and nephrotic syndrome.

PPx: Early mobility after surgery. Anticoagulants for high-risk patients.

MoD: Virchow triad leads to a thrombus.

This thrombus, originating in another location of the body, embolizes to the pulmonary vasculature, leading to three possible pathophysiologic responses: pulmonary infarction, abnormal gas exchange, and cardiovascular compromise. Pulmonary infarction is due to small thrombi traveling distally to the segmental and subsegmental vessels. Abnormal gas exchange is due to mechanical obstruction altering the ventilation to perfusion ratio, which creates dead space. Cardiovascular compromise is caused by increased pulmonary vascular resistance, which ultimately leads to an impeded right ventricular outflow and causes right heart strain.

QUICK TIPS

Virchow triad: venous stasis, endothelial injury, and hypercoagulable state

QUICK TIPS

Common sources of emboli include deep veins of the lower extremity (iliac, femoral, and popliteal) and deep veins of the pelvis.

Dx:
1. Use Modified Wells Criteria determined to determine likelihood of PE
2. D-dimer for unlikely probability of PE
3. Spiral CT for likely probability of PE
4. Leg ultrasound if spiral CT is inconclusive or cannot be performed
5. Ventilation–perfusion (V/Q) scan is reserved for those with suspected PE in whom spiral CT is contraindicated (renal insufficiency), inconclusive, or negative in the face of high clinical suspicion.

Tx/Mgmt:
1. Oxygen and fluids
2. Low-molecular-weight heparin or unfractionated heparin
3. Inferior vena cava filter placement for those with contraindications to anticoagulation
4. Thrombolytic therapy, catheter-directed therapy, and/or thrombectomy for hemodynamically unstable patients
5. Long-term anticoagulation with factor Xa inhibitors (apixaban, edoxaban, rivaroxaban), direct thrombin inhibitors (dabigatran), or warfarin

99 AR
Criteria for pulmonary embolism

99 AR
Algorithm for diagnosing PE

Air Embolism

Buzz Words: Dyspnea + trauma, surgery + audible air suction during a procedure

Clinical Presentation: In cases of venous embolism, dyspnea is accompanied by substernal chest pain, lightheadedness, or dizziness. Massive air embolism can present with acute onset right-sided heart failure, syncope, shock, or cardiac arrest. Signs may include tachypnea, tachycardia, hypotension, wheezing, crackles, and elevated jugular venous pressure. Arterial embolism presents differently based on what organ is affected. The most commonly affected organ is the brain, and these patients present with an abrupt change in mental status and/or focal neurologic deficits.

PPx: N/A

MoD: Most common causes include surgery, trauma, vascular interventions, and barotrauma from mechanical ventilation.

Dx:
1. ABG
2. CXR
3. ECG
4. Echocardiogram
5. Chest or head CT scan

Tx/Mgmt:
1. Position patient in left lateral decubitus or Trendelenburg for venous air embolism
2. Position patient in supine position for arterial embolism
3. Oxygen
4. Mechanical ventilation
5. Fluids
6. Vasopressors
7. Hyperbaric oxygen, manual removal of air, and closed chest cardiac massage for severe cases

Fat Embolism

Buzz Words: Dyspnea + **petechial rash** + post op or trauma + **long bone fracture (e.g., femur)**

Clinical Presentation: Fat embolism presents 24–72 hours after the original insult (e.g., femur fracture) with the classical triad of hypoxemia, neurologic abnormalities, and a petechial rash, often on the chest.

PPx: Early immobilization of fractures, prophylactic corticosteroids

MoD: Result of fat globules entering the bloodstream usually from bone marrow or adipose tissue

Dx: Clinical presentation

Tx/Mgmt:
1. Supportive care
2. Oxygen
3. Fluid management

QUICK TIPS
Fat globules are usually disturbed by surgery or trauma.

Respiratory Failure Due to Enteral Feeding

Buzz Words: Dyspnea + enteral nutrition

Clinical Presentation: Respiratory distress after enteral feeding (e.g., TPN). Patient will present with dyspnea and hypoxia and may also have a delayed presentation that includes cough, fever, tachypnea, or frothy sputum.

PPx: Backrest elevation, post-pyloric feeding, enteral feeding via percutaneous gastrostomy, and use of motility agents to promote gastric emptying

MoD: Enteral nutrition is associated with an increased incidence of aspiration. Patients who are very ill or post op are unable to protect their airways during tube feedings. Large volumes of aspiration may lead to hypoxia or pneumonitis.

Dx: CXR

Tx/Mgmt:
1. Supportive care
2. Oxygen
3. Antibiotics if aspiration pneumonia is suspected (clindamycin)

QUICK TIPS
Enteral feeding may lead to aspiration pneumonia.

Disorders of the Pleura, Mediastinum, and Chest Wall

Pleural Effusion

Buzz Words: Orthopnea + PND + blunted costophrenic angles

Clinical Presentation: Most cases of pleural effusions are indolent; therefore, the patient is asymptomatic. If symptomatic, signs and symptoms include dyspnea on exertion, peripheral edema, orthopnea, PND, dullness to percussion, decreased breath sounds, and decreased tactile fremitus (Table 7.3).

PPx: N/A

MoD: Pleural effusions are caused by an increased drainage of fluid into the pleural space, increased fluid production in the pleural space, or decreased drainage from the pleural space. The causes of pleural effusions are broken down into two categories, transudative or exudative, based on the Light's Criteria (Box 7.1) (Transudative effusions are caused by increased hydrostatic pressure or decreased plasma or intrapleural oncotic pressures. On the other hand, exudative effusions are due to increased capillary or pleural membrane permeability.)

Dx:
1. CXR (lateral decubitus films more reliable for detecting small effusions)
2. Thoracentesis and analysis of pleural effusion

Tx/Mgmt:
1. Treat underlying condition
2. Therapeutic thoracentesis if symptomatic

QUICK TIPS

The most common causes of transudative pleural effusions include CHF, constrictive pericarditis, cirrhosis, PE, nephrotic syndrome, hypoalbuminemia, and atelectasis.

QUICK TIPS

The most common causes of exudative pleural effusions include bacteria pneumonia, tuberculosis, malignancy, PE, and collagen vascular disorder.

TABLE 7.3 Analyses of Pleural Effusion Fluid

Description	Likely Diagnoses
Elevated pleural fluid amylase	Esophageal rupture, pancreatitis, or malignancy
Milky fluid	Chylothorax
Frank pus	Empyema
Bloody effusion	Malignancy
Exudative and primarily lymphocytic	Tuberculosis (TB)
pH < 7.2	Parapneumonic effusion or empyema
Glucose < 60	Rheumatoid arthritis, TB, esophageal rupture, malignancy, or lupus

> **BOX 7.1** Light's Criteria
>
> Pleural fluid protein/serum protein ration > 0.5
> Pleural fluid LDH/serum LDH ration > 0.6
> Pleural fluid LDH > two-thirds the upper limits of the normal serum LDH

Chylothorax

Buzz Words: Milky white fluid + pleural effusion + dyspnea

Clinical Presentation: Patients present with gradual signs and symptoms that are due to the mechanical effects of a pleural effusion such as decreased exercise tolerance, dyspnea, fatigue, and a heavy feeling in the chest. Remember that chyle in the pleural space does not create an inflammatory response; therefore, patients may not present with fever and chest pain.

PPx: N/A

MoD: Chylothorax is due to the disruption or obstruction of the thoracic duct that leads to the leakage of lymphatic fluid known as chyle into the pleural space. The etiology of chylothorax is broken down into nontraumatic and traumatic causes. Nontraumatic causes are often caused by malignancy such as lymphoma, chronic lymphocytic leukemia, and metastatic cancer. Surgical procedures near the thoracic duct account for most cases of traumatic chylothorax. Esophagectomy, pulmonary resection, and heart surgery appear to carry the greatest risk of resulting in chylothorax.

Dx:
1. CXR
2. Thoracentesis
3. Analysis of pleural fluid, which can be milky, sanguineous, or serous
4. Chest CT scan

Tx/Mgmt:
1. Treat underlying disease
2. Therapeutic pleural drainage accompanied by therapeutic thoracentesis, tube thoracostomy, or indwelling pleural catheter
3. Dietary control with high protein-low fat
4. Talc via thoracoscope for pleural sclerosing
5. Surgical thoracic duct ligation
6. Surgical pleurodesis

Empyema

Buzz Words: Prolonged duration of pneumonia + effusion

Clinical Presentation: Signs and symptoms of bacterial pneumonia such as cough, fever, pleuritic chest pain, dyspnea, and increased sputum production. Patients with increased duration of such signs and symptoms of pneumonia are more likely to develop empyema. On auscultation, patients may have decreased breath sounds and decreased fremitus (unlike the crackles, egophony, and increased fremitus typical of consolidation).

PPx: Early treatment of pneumonia

MoD: Bacterial infection of the pleural fluid that leads to either pus or the presence of bacterial organisms on Gram stain

Dx:
1. CXR
2. Chest ultrasound
3. Chest CT scan
4. Thoracentesis + analysis of pleural fluid

Tx/Mgmt:
1. Antibiotics specific to cultured organism
2. Pleural drainage: tube thoracostomy, open decortication

Mediastinitis

Buzz Words: Sternal purulent discharge + bacteremia

Clinical Presentation: Mediastinitis presents with fever, tachycardia, chest pain, and/or signs of sternal wound infection. This is a life-threatening condition that must be recognized immediately. Postoperative mediastinitis can be either fulminant or subacute. Risk factors include diabetes, obesity, peripheral artery disease, tobacco use, and prolonged surgical procedures.

PPx: Smoking cessation. Preoperative antibiotic prophylaxis with first- or second-generation cephalosporins in high-risk patients.

MoD: Before the modern area of cardiothoracic surgery, most cases of mediastinitis were due to esophageal perforation or from spread of odontogenic or retropharyngeal infections. However, currently, the majority of cases of mediastinitis occur as a postoperative complication of cardiothoracic procedures due to wound contamination during surgery. The most common organisms isolated from cases of mediastinitis are *S. aureus* (MSSA and MRSA), gram-negative bacilli, coagulase-negative staphylococci, and streptococci.

QUICK TIPS

Start with antibiotic that includes anaerobic coverage such as clindamycin, amoxicillin-clavulanate, piperacillin-tazobactam, or imipenem

Dx:
1. Physical exam (Hamman sign—crunching sound heard with stethoscope)
2. Blood cultures
3. Chest CT scan
4. Subxiphoid aspiration

Tx/Mgmt:
1. Antibiotics: vancomycin plus third-generation cephalosporin (ceftazidime), a quinolone, or an aminoglycoside
2. Surgical debridement
3. Vacuum-assisted closure before delayed closure

Pleuritis

Buzz Words: Sharp pain, worse with breathing
PPx: Early treatment of pneumonia
Clinical Presentation: Pleuritis presents with sharp, stabbing pain that worsens with deep breathing.
MoD: Inflammation of the lung pleura most often due to autoimmune diseases

Dx:
1. CXR
2. EKG

Tx/Mgmt:
1. Pain management
2. Treat underlying cause
3. Screen for SLE: ANA, anti-ds DNA Ab, anti-Sm Ab, antihistone Ab
4. Screen for RA: RF, anticitrullinated peptide/protein Ab

Spontaneous Pneumothorax

Buzz Words: Tall, lean, young men, acute respiratory distress
PPx: Smoking cessation
Clinical Presentation: Spontaneous pneumothorax presents with tachypnea, pleuritic chest pain, hypoxia, unilateral diminished or absent breath sounds, and unilateral hyperresonance to percussion. Primary spontaneous pneumothorax is more common in tall, lean, and young men and in smokers.
MoD: Pneumothorax is an abnormal collection of air in the pleural spaces the leads to an uncoupling of the lung from the chest wall. This leads to decreased lung volume and therefore hypoxia. Spontaneous pneumothorax may be classified as primary or secondary. Primary spontaneous pneumothorax occurs due to rupture of subpleural blebs without a precipitating event in a person who does not have lung disease. Secondary pneumothorax occurs in patients with underlying lung disease.

QUICK TIPS
Autoimmune diseases that may causes pleuritis: systemic lupus erythematosus (SLE) or rheumatoid arthritis (RA), complicated pneumonia, and drugs

QUICK TIPS
Drugs that may cause pleuritis: procainamide, hydralazine, and isoniazid

QUICK TIPS
Causes of secondary spontaneous pneumothorax: COPD, asthma, interstitial lung disease, neoplasm, cystic fibrosis, and tuberculosis

Dx:
1. CXR
2. Chest CT scan

Tx/Mgmt:
1. Supplemental oxygen if patient stable and small pneumothorax
2. Pleural aspiration if patient stable and large pneumothorax
3. Chest tube if clinically unstable
4. Pleurodesis via VATS for recurrent cases

Costochondritis

Buzz Words: Chest pain reproduced with palpation

Clinical Presentation: Musculoskeletal chest pain often presents as an insidious and persistent pain. It can also be sharp and localized to a specific area. Pain is often reproducible upon palpation, which is key to differentiating costochondritis from other more serious causes of chest pain. Most chest wall pain associated with costochondritis is positional and will be exacerbated by deep breathing and movement. Patients often do not have the typical risk factors for cardiac causes of chest pain.

PPx: N/A

MoD: Inflammation of cartilage that connects ribs to sternum. This can be caused by physical strain, a blow to the chest, arthritis, or joint infection.

Dx:
1. Physical exam
2. ECG
3. CXR

Tx/Mgmt:
1. Avoid strenuous activity
2. Stretching
3. Heat/Cold packs
4. NSAIDs

Traumatic and Mechanical Disorders of Upper Airways

Epistaxis

Buzz Words: Nosebleed, fall/winter season

PPx: No nose picking

Clinical Presentation: Patient presents with a nosebleed, a common occurrence that most patients do not seek care for.

MoD: Epistaxis can be broken down into two categories: anterior bleeds and posterior bleeds.

Anterior nosebleeds are often a result of mucosal trauma such as nose picking, but they can also be due to low moisture. Posterior nosebleeds arise from the postero-lateral branches of the sphenopalatine artery. Anterior and posterior nosebleeds may be associated with the following conditions: anticoagulation, hereditary hemorrhagic telangiectasia, platelet disorders, and aneurysm of the carotid artery.

Dx: Coagulation study if frequent or severe occurrence
Tx/Mgmt:
1. Self-resolve
2. Nasal packing
3. Balloon catheter for continuous posterior bleeding

Barotrauma

Buzz Words: Respiratory distress, mechanical ventilation

Clinical Presentation: Barotrauma presents with symptoms that may range from asymptomatic to tachypnea, tachycardia, acute respiratory distress, hypoxemia, and hemodynamic collapse.

PPx: Protective ventilator practices such as limiting plateau pressure, using low tidal volume, and cautious use of PEEP

MoD: Most often due to alveolar rupture from mechanical ventilation, leading to release of air into extra-alveolar areas

Dx:
1. CXR
2. Chest CT
3. Chest ultrasound

Tx/Mgmt:
1. Manage ventilatory settings: lower tidal volume and/or PEEP
2. Increase sedation
3. Tube thoracostomy for pneumothorax
4. Supportive measures for pneumoperitoneum, pneumomediastinum, and subcutaneous emphysema as they tend to be self-limiting in such cases

Laryngeal/Pharyngeal Obstruction

Buzz Words: Sudden respiratory distress

Clinical Presentation: Laryngeal/pharyngeal obstruction presents with acute onset respiratory distress with dyspnea, tachypnea, wheezing, tachycardia, and hypoxemia. It also presents with decreased breath sounds.

PPx: N/A

MoD: Narrowing or blocking of upper airways due to many causes including allergic reactions, foreign bodies, chemical burns, epiglottitis, peritonsillar abscess, retropharyngeal abscess, and neoplasm

Dx:
1. Chest/neck x-ray
2. Laryngoscopy/pharyngoscopy

Tx/Mgmt:
1. Manage airway
2. Removal of foreign body via laryngoscopy/ pharyngoscopy if cause of obstruction
3. Treat underlying condition

Tracheal Stenosis

Buzz Words: Dyspnea + multiple intubations

Clinical Presentation: Tracheal stenosis presents with a gradual onset of symptoms, which can usually be mistaken for other disorders such as difficult-to-treat adult asthma. Patient presents with cough, dyspnea, hypoxia, wheezing, stridor, and fatigue.

PPx: N/A

MoD: Narrowing or constriction of trachea. Most cases develop due to tracheal injury after prolonged intubation or from a tracheostomy. Rarely, it may be congenital.

Dx:
1. CXR
2. Chest CT
3. Fluoroscopy
4. Bronchoscopy

Tx/Mgmt:
1. Surgical correction: tracheal resection and reconstruction, tracheal laser surgery (breaks up scar tissue)
2. Tracheal dilation with either balloon or tracheal dilators
3. Tracheobronchial airway stent

Tracheomalacia

Buzz Words: Dyspnea, positional wheezing

Clinical Presentation: Tracheomalacia may be asymptomatic. However, as the severity of airway narrowing increases, patients may have dyspnea, cough, sputum retention, wheezing, and stridor. Certain maneuvers can elicit signs of tracheomalacia: forced expiration, cough, Valsalva maneuver, and laying down.

PPx: N/A

MoD: Caused by diffuse of segmental tracheal weakness. The acquired causes of tracheomalacia include

QUICK TIPS

Other less common causes of tracheal stenosis include trauma, radiotherapy, neoplasm, and autoimmune conditions such as sarcoidosis or Wegener granulomatosis.

damage via tracheostomy or endotracheal intubation, external chest trauma, thoracic surgery, chronic compression of trachea (commonly due to a benign goiter), chronic inflammation from smoking and severe emphysema, and recurrent infections such as those seen in chronic bronchitis and CF patient. It may also be congenital.

Dx:
1. Bronchoscopy
2. Chest CT scan
3. Pulmonary functional tests

Tx/Mgmt:
1. No treatment for asymptomatic patients
2. Treat underlying condition
3. Continuous positive airway pressure (CPAP) if in respiratory distress
4. Insert silicone stents (long-term stenting for non-surgical candidates)
5. Surgery: tracheobronchoplasty with polypropylene mesh for patients who improve with stenting and are surgical candidates

Blunt Tracheal Injury

Buzz Words: Motor vehicle collision (MVC) + respiratory distress + subcutaneous emphysema

Clinical Presentation: Blunt trauma more commonly affects the intrathoracic trachea. Diagnosis is often delayed, as intrathoracic injury may be subtle and indolent, presenting with retained secretions, recurrent pneumothoraces, and obstruction. The telltale sign of blunt tracheal injury is a pneumothorax or pneumomediastinum that reoccurs despite tube thoracostomy. Radiographic signs include subcutaneous emphysema, rising of the larynx above the third cervical vertebra, and abnormal location of endotracheal tube.

PPx: None

MoD: Blunt tracheal injury post MVC is a rare occurrence, occurring in less than 1% of patients with blunt thoracic trauma. This is the case because the trachea is protected from injury by its position relative to the mandible, sternum, and its relative elasticity. Most of the patients who do have blunt trauma to the trachea die at the scene.

Dx:
1. CXR
2. Chest CT
3. Bronchoscopy
4. Visualization during surgery

Tx/Mgmt:
1. Manage airway
2. Primary surgical repair with possible lung resection

Penetrating Neck/Tracheal Injury

Buzz Words: Gunshot or stab wound in the neck, respiratory distress

Clinical Presentation: Tracheal injury due to penetrating wounds is predominantly confined to the cervical trachea. Patients present with respiratory distress, stridor, subcutaneous air, hemoptysis, odynophagia, dysphonia, or anterior neck tenderness. Patients may appear stable initially but may quickly decompensate.

PPx: N/A

MoD: Gunshot wounds, stab wounds, or penetrating debris such as glass or shrapnel. Penetrating neck injuries are defined as any injury that penetrates the platysma.

Dx:
1. Primary assessment: Airway, Breathing, and Circulation (ABCs)
2. Secondary evaluation: head-to-toe exam with a focus on determining if the platysma has been penetrated, what zones of the neck are involved, and hard vs. soft signs of penetrating neck injury
3. Head/neck x-ray
4. Multidetector helical computed tomography with angiography (MDCT-A)
5. Nasopharyngoscopy, laryngoscopy, bronchoscopy

Tx/Mgmt:
1. Manage ABCs: Secure airway, ensure adequate ventilation, control bleeding, two large-bore IV catheters
2. No-Zone approach: surgical exploration/intervention for unstable patients regardless of which zone was injured (patients with hard signs), MDCT-A for stable patients (patients with soft signs), treat underlying injuries accordingly

Penetrating Neck Trauma Anatomy

3. Zone approach: surgical exploration/intervention for injuries located in Zone II, MDCT-A for patients with injuries located in Zone I or III

Penetrating Neck Trauma Management

Foreign Body Aspiration (Pharynx, Larynx, and Trachea)

Buzz Words: Acute asphyxiation + cyanosis

Clinical Presentation: Unlike foreign bodies in the lower airways, obstruction of the upper airway is more likely to present as choking with acute asphyxiation leading to respiratory distress. Monophasic wheeze and/or stridor may be present due to tracheal foreign body aspiration. This is more common in children, psychiatric patients, and the elderly.

PPx: Chew food thoroughly. Do not leave small children unattended.

MoD: Aspiration of foreign body. In adults, commonly inhaled objects include incompletely chewed foods, nails, pins, and dental debris/prostheses. In children, nuts, seeds, and other food account for most cases of foreign body aspiration. Most foreign bodies are radiolucent. One third of aspiration presenting with acute asphyxiation is in the supraglottic position.

Dx:
1. Assess ABCs
2. Neck x-ray
3. Chest CT
4. Laryngoscopy or Bronchoscopy

Tx/Mgmt:
1. Secure airway in acute asphyxiation: Heimlich maneuver, proper oxygenation, cricothyrotomy or tracheotomy
2. Retrieve foreign body via laryngoscopy or bronchoscopy

Septal Perforation

Buzz Words: Young adult + nasal erythema and discharge + cocaine + nasal surgery

Clinical Presentation: Septal perforation may be asymptomatic with only minor erythema. Small perforations may present with whistling noise. Larger perforations may lead to more severe symptoms such as crusting, bloody discharge, pressure, and nasal discomfort.

PPx: Cessation of nasal cocaine usage

MoD: Septal perforation is a condition often seen with intranasal cocaine use. Other causes include septal surgery, atrophic rhinitis, rheumatologic disorders, and granulomatosis with polyangiitis.

Dx: Physical exam

Tx/Mgmt:
1. Humidification
2. Observation for asymptomatic patients
3. Tox screen
4. Surgical closure for symptomatic patients

Traumatic Disorders of Lower Airways and Pleura

Atelectasis

Buzz Words: Fever, hypoxemia, postoperative day two

Review of postop fever

Clinical Presentation: Atelectasis presents with increased work of breathing, hypoxemia, and fever usually occurring on postoperative day two. Atelectasis is one of the most common postoperative pulmonary complications, especially following abdominal and thoracoabdominal procedures.

PPx: Smoking cessation at least 8 weeks before surgery

Deep breathing, incentive spirometry, early mobilization, adequate pain control (epidural analgesia or intercostal nerve blocks)

CPAP

MoD: Collapse of lung tissue leading to loss of lung volume. Caused by decreased compliance of lung tissue, impaired regional ventilation, retained secretions, and pain interfering with deep breathing and coughing.

Dx: CXR

Tx/Mgmt:

1. Chest physiotherapy and suctioning
2. CPAP

Blunt Chest Wall and Diaphragm Injury

Buzz Words: MVCs, respiratory distress, seatbelt sign

Clinical Presentation: The common presentation of blunt chest wall and diaphragm injury consists of respiratory distress, signs of shock, and possibly hypoxia. The remainder of the clinical presentation depends on the specific injury sustained. Patients with clavicular fracture will often present with a complaint of pain exacerbated by shoulder movement and have a palpable deformity of the clavicle. Patients with sternal fracture will often present with severe pain localized to the sternum (may have a pleuritic component) and have a palpable deformity of the sternum. Patients with rib fractures will have focal tenderness and palpable deformities. On the other hand, patients with flail chest will depict a paradoxical motion with breathing (opposite motion of the uninjured chest wall). Lastly, patients with diaphragmatic rupture will often present with abdominal pain along with referred shoulder pain.

PPx: N/A

MoD: The most common mechanism of this injury are MVCs. Blunt trauma to the thoracic region has the potential to cause various injuries to the chest wall and diaphragm including clavicle fracture, sternum fracture, rib fracture, flail chest, diaphragmatic rupture, pneumothorax, and pulmonary contusion. Of note, flail chest occurs due to three or more adjacent ribs being fractured in two different locations, creating a "floating" segment of ribs.

Dx:

1. Primary assessment with a focus on ABCs
2. Secondary evaluation via a head-to-toe exam
3. Extended Focused Assessment with Sonography (E-FAST)
4. Chest and abdominal XR
5. Chest & abdominal CT scan

Tx/Mgmt:

1. Manage ABCs: secure airway, ensure adequate ventilation, control bleeding, two large-bore IV catheters
2. Clavicular fracture: surgical open reduction and internal fixation if displaced; otherwise, immobilization via sling
3. Sternal and rib: adequate pain control and follow-up as the majority are nondisplaced and heal on their own
   a. Flail chest: conservative management via ventilatory support or surgical open reduction and internal fixation
   b. Diaphragmatic rupture: surgical repair usually done via trauma laparotomy

Penetrating Chest Wound

Buzz Words: Respiratory distress + knife wound, gunshot wound

Clinical Presentation: We will focus on the general presentation and approach to penetrating chest wound, as individual injury to the respiratory system will be discussed separately. Presentation is variable from stable to hemodynamically unstable patients. Clinical picture depends on what structures were injured and its resulting pathophysiology. Serious injury to respiratory system presents with respiratory distress, decreased breath sounds, and/or hemodynamically instability. Although less common than blunt trauma, penetrating chest trauma tends to be deadlier.

PPx: N/A

MoD:

Penetrating trauma to thorax. Possible injuries include pneumothorax, pulmonary contusion, hemothorax, tracheobronchial injury, pericardial tamponade, diaphragmatic rupture, and esophageal injury.

Dx:

1. Primary assessment with a focus on ABCs
2. Secondary evaluation via a head-to-toe exam
3. E-FAST

4. Chest and abdominal x-ray
5. Chest & abdominal CT scan
6. Esophagoscopy
7. Bronchoscopy

Tx/Mgmt:
1. Manage ABCs: secure airway, ensure adequate ventilation, control bleeding, two large-bore IV catheters
2. Urgent thoracotomy for cardiac tamponade and significant hemorrhage or a persistent air leak from a chest tube
3. Management of pneumothorax, pulmonary contusion, and hemothorax will be discussed separately

Traumatic Pneumothorax/Tension Pneumothorax

Buzz Words: Respiratory distress + trauma + tracheal deviation + decreased breath sounds unilaterally

Clinical Presentation: Traumatic pneumothorax presents with tachypnea, chest pain, hypoxia, unilateral diminished or absent breath sounds, and unilateral hyperresonance to percussion. Tension pneumothorax is more serious; it presents with severe respiratory distress, hypotension, distended neck veins, and tracheal deviation away from pneumothorax. This is an emergency.

PPx: CXR after procedures or trauma with potential to disrupt pleura

MoD: Pneumothorax is an abnormal collection of air in the pleural spaces the leads to an uncoupling of the lung from the chest wall. This leads to decreased lung volume and therefore hypoxia. Pneumothorax is a common serious injury associated with penetrating or blunt chest trauma.

A tension pneumothorax occurs when a pneumothorax leads to tissues surround the opening into the pleural cavity to act as a one-way valve allowing air to enter but not leave.

Dx:
1. CXR
2. Chest CT scan

Tx/Mgmt:
1. Manage ABCs
2. Needle decompression in second intercostal space, midclavicular line for tension pneumothorax for tension pneumothorax
3. Sterile occlusive dressing taped on three sides for open pneumothorax
4. Chest tube
5. Serial CXR for small/asymptomatic pneumothorax

QUICK TIPS

Pneumothorax can also be iatrogenic due to chest tube placement, thoracentesis, transthoracic needle aspiration, and central line placement.

99 AR

Great review and images of tension pneumothorax

Hemothorax

Buzz Words: Respiratory distress + trauma + pleural effusion

Clinical Presentation: Hemothorax presents with tachypnea, chest pain, hypoxia, unilateral diminished or absent breath sounds, and unilateral dullness to percussion.

PPx: N/A

MoD: Blood in the pleural space is most commonly a result of blunt chest trauma. Injuries leading to hemothorax include aortic rupture, myocardial rupture, injuries to hilar structures, injuries to lung parenchyma, and injuries to intercostal or mammary blood vessels.

Dx:
1. Ultrasound
2. CXR
3. Chest CT scan

Tx/Mgmt:
1. Manage ABCs
2. Chest tube
3. Surgical thoracotomy for immediate bloody drainage of 1500 mL or shock with persistent, substantial bleeding (>3 mL/kg per hour)

Pulmonary Contusion

Buzz Words: Respiratory distress + bilateral patchy, alveolar infiltrates + blunt trauma

Clinical Presentation: Pulmonary contusion presents with tachypnea, chest pain, and hypoxia usually within 24 hours of trauma. Initial CXR may not depict contusion, and symptoms worsen with IV fluids.

PPx: N/A

MoD: Bruising after lung trauma (blunt or penetrating) resulting in hemorrhage/edema within the lung parenchyma.

Dx:
1. CXR
2. Chest CT scan

Tx/Mgmt:
1. Manage ABCs
2. Pain control
3. Pulmonary toilet
4. Restrict fluids to euvolemia
5. Self resolves within seven days

Pneumomediastinum

Buzz Words: Chest crepitus + trauma

Clinical Presentation: Pneumomediastinum presents with dyspnea, chest pain, neck pain, tachycardia, tachypnea, or hypertension. Crepitus may be heard during physical exam.

PPx: N/A

MoD: Air in the mediastinum. May be due to blunt/penetrating trauma, esophageal rupture, alveolar rupture, bowel rupture, or iatrogenic (esophagoscopy, barotrauma)

Dx:

1. CXR
2. Chest CT scan

Tx/Mgmt:

1. Manage ABCs
2. Treat underlying cause (air usually resorbs)

Foreign Body Aspiration (Bronchi and Lungs)

Buzz Words: Recurrent pneumonia, unilateral wheeze

Clinical Presentation: Foreign body aspiration depends on the degree of obstruction as well as the location and length of time the foreign body has been in the airway. In adults, the clinical presentation is often subtle. Therefore, a chronic cough due to distal obstruction is the most common symptom followed by symptoms that may mimic pneumonia such as fever, chest pain, and hemoptysis. Patient may not remember inhalation of foreign body. Dyspnea is an uncommon presentation for adults. Patient may have a unilateral wheeze from main stem or lobar obstruction. The most common site of aspiration is the right bronchus.

PPx: Chew food thoroughly.

MoD: Aspiration of foreign body. In adults, commonly inhaled objects include incompletely chewed foods, nails, pins, and dental debris/prostheses. In children nuts, seeds, and other foods account for most cases of foreign body aspiration.

Dx:

1. Assess ABCs
2. CXR
3. Chest CT-scan
4. Laryngoscopy or Bronchoscopy

Tx/Mgmt:

1. Manage ABCs
2. Retrieve foreign body via bronchoscopy
3. Treat pneumonia if present

Upper and Lower Respiratory Tract

Obstructive Sleep Apnea

Buzz Words: Snoring + daytime somnolence + overweight

Clinical Presentation: Obstructive sleep apnea presents with obstructive apneas, snoring, and resuscitative snorts at night. Daytime symptoms may include sleepiness,

> **QUICK TIPS**
> Foreign body aspiration is more common in children, psychiatric patients, and the elderly.

> **QUICK TIPS**
> Majority of foreign bodies are radiolucent.

> **QUICK TIPS**
> One third of aspiration presenting with acute asphyxiation is located in the supraglottic position.

fatigue, or poor concentration, and it may cause secondary hypertension. Risk factors include advanced age, male gender, obesity, and craniofacial or upper airway soft tissue abnormalities.

PPx: Weight loss

MoD: Recurrent, functional collapse during sleep of the velopharyngeal and/or oropharyngeal airway leading to reduced or complete cessation of airflow despite breathing efforts. It ultimately leads to hypercapnia and hypoxemia and fragmented sleep.

Dx:

1. In-laboratory polysomnography
2. Home sleep apnea testing

Tx/Mgmt:

1. Weight loss
2. CPAP
3. Oral appliances
4. Upper airway surgery to remove floppy tissue
5. Hypoglossal nerve stimulation

Central Sleep Apnea

Buzz Words: Cheyne-Stokes breathing + daytime somnolence + heart failure + stroke

Clinical Presentation: Central sleep apnea presents with symptoms of disrupted sleep, such as excessive daytime sleepiness, poor sleep quality, and poor concentration. It may also present with PND, morning headaches, and nocturnal angina. Patients with heart failure or previous stroke are more likely to exhibit central sleep apnea with Cheyne-Stokes breathing.

Risk factors include advanced age, male sex, heart failure, stroke, and chronic opioid use.

PPx: N/A

MoD: Central nerves system fails to transmit proper signals to respiratory muscles. The most common type of central sleep apnea is due to hyperventilation: Hypoxia (possibly due to secretions) triggers hyperpnea during sleep. This causes a ventilator overshoot leading to hypocapnia, which induces central apnea.

Dx: In-laboratory polysomnography

Tx/Mgmt:

1. CPAP
2. Adaptive servo-ventilation for patients without heart failure
3. Nocturnal oxygen
4. Medical management of heart failure

99 AR

Cheyne-Stokes breathing

99 AR

ACV

Obesity-Hypoventilation Syndrome

Buzz Words: Symptoms of OSA + right-sided heart failure

Clinical Presentation: Most patients presenting with obesity-hypoventilation syndrome have coexisting OSA; therefore, the presentation is almost identical: obstructive apneas, hypopneas, snoring, and resuscitative snorts. Daytime symptoms may include sleepiness, fatigue, or poor concentration. Patients often have severe obesity (BMI >50 kg/m^2) and may have signs of right-sided heart failure.

Untreated, it can progress to acute, life-threatening cardiopulmonary compromise and is associated with high mortality syndrome.

PPx: Weight loss

MoD: The result of the complex interaction of several physiologic abnormalities such as sleep-disordered breathing (OSA), altered pulmonary function, and altered ventilatory control

Dx:

1. ABG
2. Pulmonary function tests
3. Serum bicarbonate In-laboratory polysomnography
4. CXR

Tx/Mgmt:

1. Weight loss
2. Abstain from alcohol and drugs that diminish respiratory drive such as benzodiazepines, opioids, and barbiturates
3. CPAP

Congenital Disorders

Bronchogenic Cysts

Buzz Words: Recurrent cough, pneumonia, second decade of life

Clinical Presentation: Bronchogenic cysts present with recurrent cough, wheezing, and pneumonia usually during the second decade of life. It may also be detected as neck masses or incidental findings on imaging.

PPx: N/A

MoD: They arise from anomalous budding of the foregut during development and can occur at any point throughout the tracheobronchial tree.

Dx:

1. CXR
2. Chest CT scan

Tx/Mgmt: Surgical excision

Congenital diaphragmatic hernia x-ray

Congenital Diaphragmatic Hernia

Buzz Words: Acute respiratory distress in neonates + PH + bowel in chest on XR

Clinical Presentation: Congenital diaphragmatic hernia is usually diagnosed prenatally. Neonates present in the first few hours of life with acute respiratory distress that may be mild or severe to the point of incompatibility with life. It may also present with persistent pulmonary hypertension of the newborn (PPHN) and adrenal insufficiency, and it may be isolated or associated with additional abnormalities including trisomy 18, 13, and 21.

PPx: N/A

MoD: Congenital defect of the diaphragm that allows the abdominal viscera to herniate into the chest. In most cases, the herniation occurs on the left, and the herniation compresses the lungs during its development. This compression decreases bronchial and pulmonary artery branching, leading to increasing degrees of pulmonary hypoplasia. This hypoplasia is most severe on the ipsilateral side, but it may also occur on the contralateral side due to shift of the mediastinum, and hypoplasia may also lead to PPHN.

Dx:
1. Prenatal ultrasound
2. Ultrafast fetal MRI
3. Fetal echocardiography
4. Umbilical artery line for monitoring of blood gas and blood pressure
5. Fetal genetic studies

Tx/Mgmt:
1. Fetal monitoring via nonstress testing or biophysical profile testing at 33–34 weeks
2. Antenatal glucocorticoids
3. Intubation and ventilation
4. Nasogastric tube
5. Isotonic fluids, dopamine and/or dobutamine, and hydrocortisone for BP support
6. Surfactant
7. Inhaled nitric oxide
8. Extracorporeal membrane oxygenation
9. Surgical correction consisting of reduction of the abdominal viscera and primary closure of the defect

QUICK TIPS

Nitric oxide decrease in pulmonary hypertension

Pulmonary Sequestration

Buzz Words: Respiratory distress + nonfunctioning lung mass

Clinical Presentation: Pulmonary sequestration is usually diagnosed prenatally. Most affected neonates are asymptomatic; however, the minority that are symptomatic at birth present with respiratory distress. The patients that have intralobar sequestration tend to present later in life with symptoms of recurrent infections such as fever, cough, hemoptysis, and chest pain. It may also be found as an accidental finding on imaging. In addition, cases can be isolated or associated with congenital diaphragmatic hernia, vertebral anomalies, congenital heart disease, and colonic duplication.

PPx: N/A

MoD: A rare abnormality of the lower airways consisting of a nonfunctioning mass of lung tissue. This abnormal lung receives its arterial blood supply from the systemic circulation tissue as it lacks normal communication with the tracheobronchial tree.

Dx:

1. Prenatal ultrasound
2. CXR
3. Chest CT scan

Tx/Mgmt:

1. Manage airway and ventilation
2. Surgical resection for symptomatic patients and asymptomatic patients with large lesions (occupies ≥20% of the lobe)
3. Observation or surgical resection for asymptomatic patients with small lesions

Immotile Cilia Syndrome/Primary Ciliary Dyskinesia

Buzz Words: Chronic rhinitis since childhood + infertility + bronchiectasis + **Dextrocardia** (think Kartagener syndrome)

Clinical Presentation: Immotile cilia syndrome/primary ciliary dyskinesia symptoms are variable depending on the extent of ciliary defect. The most common presenting features are recurrent infections of the upper and lower respiratory tract with most patients presenting in childhood. Patients may also present with bronchiectasis manifesting as auscultatory crackles. Of note, men with this condition are infertile, and women have decreased fertility and increased risk of ectopic pregnancy. This condition is associated with cardiac abnormalities, pyloric stenosis, and epispadias.

PPx: N/A

MoD: Inherited autosomal recessive disease that leads to a congenital impairment of mucociliary clearance.

QUICK TIPS

Pulmonary sequestration is characterized by its location, either intralobar (most common) or extralobar.

QUICK TIPS

If a patient presents with situs inversus, chronic sinusitis, and bronchiectasis, they have Kartagener syndrome (a subset of immotile cilia syndrome).

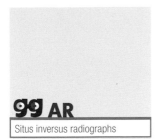

99 AR

Situs inversus radiographs

It is a highly heterogeneous that can be caused by a defect in any of the many polypeptide species within the axoneme of cilia or of sperm flagella. The cilia may be unable to beat, unable to beat normally, or absent altogether.

Dx:
1. CXR
2. Measuring nasal nitric oxide (low or absent in immotile cilia syndrome)
3. Inhalation of tagged colloid albumin to measure mucociliary transport
4. Biopsy with electron microscopy to assess ciliary motion and structure
5. Genetic testing

Tx/Mgmt:
1. Daily chest physiotherapy
2. Humidified air
3. Smoking cessation
4. Amoxicillin-clavulanate for serious infections. Vaccination against influenza and pneumococcus
5. Intranasal glucocorticoids
6. Surgery for debulking nasal polyposis

Tracheoesophageal Fistula

Buzz Words: Excessive drooling in newborn + polyhydramnios + inability to feed at birth

Clinical Presentation: Tracheoesophageal fistula symptoms depend on the presence or absence of esophageal atresia (EA). In patients with EA (95%), polyhydramnios occurs during the gestational period. Infants with EA are symptomatic with excessive secretions causing drooling, choking, respiratory distress, and inability to feed. If a fistula between the trachea and distal esophagus is present, infant can present with gastric distension and aspiration pneumonia.

PPx: N/A

MoD: A common congenital anomaly of the respiratory tract and typically occurs with EA, and this malformation is characterized according to their anatomic configuration

Dx:
1. Attempt to pass a catheter into the stomach
2. CXR
3. Upper gastrointestinal series with water-soluble contrast

Tx/Mgmt:
1. Manage airway
2. Surgical ligation of fistula with primary anastomosis of the esophageal segment if necessary

3. Staged procedures for long distance between esophagus and stomach that include elongation of the esophagus, interposition of the jejunum or colon, and gastric transposition

GUNNER PRACTICE

1. A 63-year-old male is brought to the hospital by his wife due to fever, shortness of breath, and chest pain. She says that he returned from a business trip to Arizona a few days ago with fevers, headache, muscle aches, a sore throat, and a cough. He had been feeling much better yesterday, but this morning, his fever had returned and become quite high, with shaking chills and chest pain when breathing. His medical history includes hypertension and sciatica, and he smokes cigars occasionally. His vital signs are T 102.4 HR 115 BP 98/62 RR 24 SpO_2 87% on room air. On exam, he is ill-appearing and in moderate respiratory distress. Crackles are auscultated at the upper lung lobes bilaterally, and egophony is noted at the left lower lobe. Blood and sputum cultures are acquired, and a chest x-ray is obtained (Fig. 7.7). Of the following, which is the most likely infectious agent?
   A. *Mycobacterium tuberculosis*
   B. *Staphylococcus aureus*
   C. *Coccidioides immitis*
   D. *Chlamydophila pneumoniae*
   E. *Pneumocystis jirovecii*

2. A 72-year-old woman refers herself to your Pulmonology practice for "difficulty breathing." She tells you that she had not seen a doctor in over 20 years until last month, when she was admitted to a hospital in another state for shortness of breath. She was kept there for two days and discharged with antibiotics and a set of pills that made her "feel superhuman." The patient does not know of any medical history aside from low back pain, but she has noticed that she has gotten "winded" more and more easily over the past few years and has had a nagging cough with some white sputum in the morning for around a decade. She has smoked a pack of cigarettes a day since she was in her 30s. Her vital signs are T 98.8 HR 87 BP 149/96 RR 16 SpO_2 93% on room air. On exam, you note a disproportionately long expiratory phase with faint apical wheezing. She is also distinctly barrel-chested. After counseling her on her smoking habits, you refer her for pulmonary function testing and a chest x-ray, which can be seen below (Fig. 7.8).

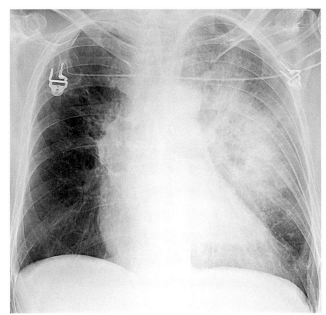

FIG. 7.7 Pneumonia (*Staphylococcus aureus*). (From: Nestor L. Müller, MD, PhD, C. Isabela, S. Silva, MD, PhD: *High-Yield Imaging: Chest*, 132–133.)

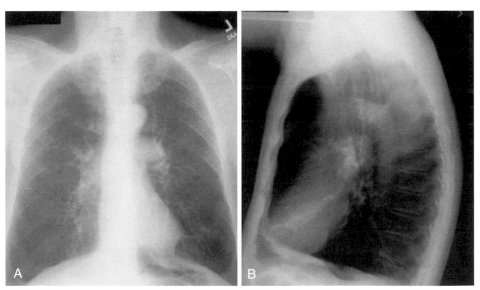

FIG. 7.8 Chronic obstructive pulmonary disease. (From Niewoehner DE: Chronic obstructive pulmonary disease. In Goldman L, Schafer AS, editors: *Goldman-Cecil Medicine*, ed 25. Philadelphia, 2016, Elsevier.)

You find out that, pre- and post-bronchodilator challenge, her FEV_1 = 35% and her FEV_1/FVC = 46%. What is your diagnosis?

A. GOLD 4 Chronic Obstructive Pulmonary Disease
B. Asthma
C. Cystic Fibrosis
D. GOLD 1 Chronic Obstructive Pulmonary Disease
E. GOLD 3 Chronic Obstructive Pulmonary Disease

3. A 69-year-old male is brought to the Emergency Department by his wife. She explains that he has been progressively short of breath with a dry cough for the last month. He has also become more confused and less talkative during the past two days. He has a medical history that includes hypertension, osteoarthritis, and appendicitis. He smoked a pack of cigarettes a day for 45 years, but quit last year when his granddaughter was born. His vital signs are T 98.1 HR 87 BP 128/85 RR 20 SpO_2 93% on room air. On exam, he appears somnolent and in mild respiratory distress. Initial labs show serum Na 127 and Cr 1.3, but CBC, basic metabolic panel, and liver function tests are otherwise unremarkable. Chest x-ray reveals a large, right-sided hilar mass. CT chest confirms the presence of the mass and reveals bulky mediastinal lymphadenopathy. A head CT is performed and shows two masses at the gray-white matter junction, with corresponding edema. Biopsy is performed and reveals nests of small, round, blue cells, some of which are obscured by crush artifact. The cells are chromogranin(+) and TTF-1(+). What is the diagnosis and appropriate first step in treatment?

A. Squamous cell lung cancer, surgical resection with adjuvant chemotherapy
B. Small cell lung cancer, surgical resection with adjuvant chemotherapy, and radiation
C. Squamous cell lung cancer, chemotherapy
D. Small cell lung cancer, chemotherapy
E. Large cell lung cancer, surgical resection with adjuvant chemotherapy and radiation

ANSWERS: What Would Gunner Jess/Jim Do?

1. WWGJD? A 63-year-old male is brought to the hospital by his wife due to fever, shortness of breath, and chest pain. She says that he returned from a business trip to Arizona a few days ago with fevers, headache, muscle aches, a sore throat, and a cough. He had been feeling much better yesterday, but this morning his fever had returned and become quite high, with shaking chills and chest pain when breathing. His medical history includes hypertension and sciatica, and he smokes cigars occasionally. His vital signs are T 102.4 HR 115 BP 98/62 RR 24 SpO$_2$ 87% on room air. On exam, he is ill-appearing and in moderate respiratory distress. Crackles are auscultated at the upper lung lobes bilaterally, and egophony is noted at the left lower lobe. Blood and sputum cultures are acquired, and a chest x-ray is obtained (see below). Of the following, which is the most likely infectious agent?

Answer: B, *Staphylococcus aureus*

Explanation: This man presents with acute pneumonia and possible sepsis (he meets SIRS criteria and his qSOFA score is at least 2 as well) after nearly recovering from what is described as a likely viral syndrome. The exam and x-ray suggest a patchy, bilateral pneumonia with consolidation of the left lower lobe (see Fig. 7.7). This is a classic presentation of *S. aureus* pneumonia, which frequently superimposes a viral infection.

A. *Mycobacterium tuberculosis* → Incorrect. This would be expected to present as an indolent reactivation of infection, with subacute cough, fevers, and night sweats, or as miliary tuberculosis, which would yield a chest x-ray with innumerable, small areas of infection in the lungs and/or other organs. Additionally, he does not have classic risk factors (including homelessness, incarceration, or immunocompromising condition).

C. *Coccidioides immitis* → Incorrect. While he has just returned from an endemic area, this is another infection that would be expected to progress in a less acute manner and is less likely to show the large consolidated area on this chest x-ray. Also, this agent would not fit with the patient's story of having a recent infection that became superinfected.

D. *Chlamydophila pneumonia* → Incorrect. Though this is a common cause of "atypical" bacterial pneumonia and can look quite similar to this radiograph, it classically occurs in teenagers and young adults (e.g., college students and military recruits) and presents with a more subacute course. This severe, abrupt presentation in an older patient with a story suggesting superinfection argues against this.

E. *Pneumocystis jirovecii* → Incorrect. This is yet another infection that typically presents with a more indolent course. It also classically occurs in immunocompromised patients, especially those on corticosteroids or certain chemotherapeutic agents, or who have AIDS.

2. WWGJD? A 72-year-old woman refers herself to your Pulmonology practice for "difficulty breathing." She tells you that she had not seen a doctor in over 20 years until last month, when she was admitted to a hospital in another state for shortness of breath. She was kept there for two days and discharged with antibiotics and a set of pills that made her "feel superhuman." The patient does not know of any medical history aside from low back pain, but she has noticed that she has gotten "winded" more and more easily over the past few years, and has had a nagging cough with some white sputum in the morning for around a decade. She has smoked a pack of cigarettes a day since she was in her 30s. Her vital signs are T 98.8 HR 87 BP 149/96 RR 16 SpO_2 93% on room air. On exam, you note a disproportionately long expiratory phase with faint apical wheezing. She is also distinctly barrel-chested. After counseling her on her smoking habits, you refer her for pulmonary function testing and a chest x-ray, which can be seen below.

You find out that, pre- and post-bronchodilator challenge, her FEV_1 = 35% and her FEV_1/FVC = 46%. What is the most likely diagnosis?

Answer: E, GOLD 3 Chronic Obstructive Pulmonary Disease

Explanation: This is an elderly woman with a 30–40 pack-year smoking history who complains of chronic, progressive dyspnea and cough with morning sputum. She recently had an acute exacerbation of dyspnea that was likely due to the same disease and that was treated with antibiotics and what might have been steroids. Her physical exam (barrel chest, prolonged expiratory phase, and apical wheeze) and chest x-ray (hyperinflation without obvious infiltrates) (see Fig. 7.8) are consistent with COPD, and her PFTs reveal an obstructive pattern that is not alleviated by bronchodilator treatment. Therefore, this is most likely COPD. The staging of COPD is complex and has evolved significantly, but a major component has rested upon stratification by FEV_1 into GOLD categories 1–4 (mild, moderate, severe, and very severe). $30\% </= FEV_1 < 50\%$ classifies this patient as having severe (GOLD 3) COPD.

A. GOLD 4 Chronic Obstructive Pulmonary Disease → Incorrect. This requires $FEV_1 < 30\%$.

B. Asthma → Incorrect. While it is not uncommon to have obstructive lung disease due to concurrent asthma and COPD, we are given a clear story of progressive disease in older age with a long history of smoking and cough with sputum production. The failure to improve post-bronchodilator on PFTs and the chronic air-trapping apparent on exam and by CXR are further indicative of COPD as the likely diagnosis.

C. Cystic Fibrosis → Incorrect. A congenital disease such as cystic fibrosis would have likely presented far earlier in life and would not present in such a progressive manner this late in life. We are given no information regarding failure to thrive, a family history of pulmonary disease, or repeated infections, and the patient's CXR is indicative of COPD and lacks infiltrates or bronchiectasis that might accompany CF.

D. GOLD 1 Chronic Obstructive Pulmonary Disease → Incorrect. This requires $FEV_1 >= 80\%$.

3. **WWGJD?** A 69-year-old male is brought to the Emergency Department by his wife. She explains that he has been progressively short of breath with a dry cough for the last month. He has also become more confused and less talkative during the past 2 days. He has a medical history that includes hypertension, osteoarthritis, and appendicitis. He smoked a pack of cigarettes a day for 45 years, but quit last year when his granddaughter was born. His vital signs are T 98.1 HR 87 BP 128/85 RR 20 SpO$_2$ 93% on room air. On exam, he appears somnolent and in mild respiratory distress. Initial labs show serum Na 127 and Cr 1.3, but CBC, basic metabolic panel, and liver function tests are otherwise unremarkable. Chest x-ray reveals a large, right-sided hilar mass. CT chest confirms the presence of the mass and reveals bulky mediastinal lymphadenopathy. A head CT is performed and shows two masses at the gray-white matter junction, with corresponding edema. Biopsy is performed and reveals nests of small, round, blue cells, some of which are obscured by crush artifact. The cells are chromogranin(+) and TTF-1(+). What is the diagnosis and appropriate first step in treatment?

Answer: D, Small cell lung cancer, chemotherapy

Explanation: This patient is an elderly ex-smoker with 45 pack-years who presents with subacute, progressive dyspnea and cough, found to have a large hilar mass and likely metastases to the brain. The features of the pathologic specimen are classic for small cell lung cancer (SCLC). Because this is extensive disease (as opposed to limited disease, which exists only within the hemi-thorax), the treatment would be chemotherapy. Of note, the patient's low serum sodium is likely due to SIADH, a paraneoplastic syndrome associated with SCLC.

A. Squamous cell lung cancer, surgical resection with adjuvant chemotherapy → Incorrect. This might present similarly (or with hemoptysis or postobstructive pneumonia), but the pathologic specimen would reveal intercellular bridges and, perhaps, keratin pearls.

B. Small cell lung cancer, surgical resection with adjuvant chemotherapy and radiation → Incorrect. Extensive SCLC is not treated with surgical resection.

C. Squamous cell lung cancer, chemotherapy → Incorrect. See answer for A.

E. Large cell lung cancer, surgical resection with adjuvant chemotherapy and radiation → Incorrect. While the pathologic diagnosis of this cancer is a complicated subject, it inherently does not display features of squamous cell or small cell lung cancer. Not only is the sample in the question classic for SCLC, but the cells are noted to be "small" in the stem and therefore would not classify as "large."

Nutritional and Digestive Disorders

Alejandro Suarez-Pierre, William Plum, Leo Wang, Hao-Hua Wu, Daniel Gromer, Rebecca Gao, and Nadia Bennett

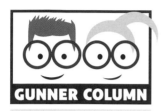

GUNNER COLUMN

Introduction

This chapter on Nutritional and Digestive Disorders encompasses the disease processes and conditions that affect the alimentary and para-alimentary tracts. The alimentary tract begins at the mouth and ends at the anus, and the para-alimentary organs include the pancreas, liver, and gallbladder.

At first glance, this chapter may seem expansive and difficult to structure. Disorders listed here vary from infectious to malignant, drug-related to traumatic, congenital to immunologic. Presentations can be limited and nonspecific, as symptoms like nausea or jaundice can signal the reader to suspect several etiologies, some of which are severe and require intensive medical therapy, while others are relatively benign and can resolve with minimal or no intervention.

However, DO NOT be discouraged by the breadth of the material. Understanding a limited set of simple principles will allow you to easily parse diseases apart.

First, recall the basic organization of the gut. By the end of this chapter, you will be able to generate differential diagnoses for vague signs, like rectal bleeding, by understanding that all processes causing bleeding will likely affect a mucosal (or epithelial) layer.

Second, keep in your mind the general goal of the gastrointestinal (GI) tract organs: to ingest, digest, and absorb nutrients. Many disorders will present with weight loss, diarrhea, and the like. *The underlying issue here will almost always relate to a broad problem with ingestion, digestion, or absorption of digested material.*

Third, maintain confidence in your interpretation of the HPI. While gastroenterologists often make use of images and laboratory data, there are few data points (aside from endoscopy) that provide conclusive evidence. Therefore, trust in your knowledge of the spectrum of disease and your ability to differentiate causes sometimes on history alone. We will provide you with the key terms and tools to do so.

This chapter is organized into (1) Infectious disorders (bacterial, viral, fungal, parasitic); (2) Immunologic and inflammatory disorders; (3) Neoplasms; (4) Signs, symptoms and ill-defined disorders; (5) Disorders of the salivary gland and esophagus; (6) Disorders of the stomach, small intestine, colon, rectum, anus; (7) Disorders of the liver and biliary system, noninfectious; (8) Disorders of the pancreas; (9) Traumatic and mechanical disorders; (10) Congenital disorders; (11) Adverse drug effects; and (12) Gunner practice.

General Signs and Symptoms

Dysphagia

Clinical Presentation: Difficulty swallowing
PPx: N/A
MoD: Dysphagia may be classified into oropharyngeal versus esophageal, primary/secondary to obstruction versus motility disorder.
Dx: Oropharyngeal dysphagia is usually described as difficulty initiating a swallow and is accompanied by coughing, nasopharyngeal regurgitation, choking, or aspiration. Esophageal dysphagia occurs a couple of seconds after successfully initiating the swallow and is accompanied by the sensation of food getting stuck lower down in the throat and chest.
Tx/Mgmt: Depends on the etiology

QUICK TIPS

Dysphagia = difficulty swallowing.
Odynophagia = painful swallowing.

Paralytic Ileus

Clinical Presentation: Obstipation and oral intolerance usually lasting more than 3–5 days. Symptoms of prolonged ileus include distention, bloating, nausea and vomiting, the inability to pass flatus and stool, and abdominal pain. Important risk factors for postoperative ileus are: prolonged abdominal or pelvis surgery, open procedures, delayed initiation of enteral nutrition, and intra-abdominal inflammation.
PPx: Avoid medications known to impede peristalsis, such as opioids.
MoD: Inflammatory process involving the intestinal smooth muscle cells, which disrupts normal peristaltic activity. Common causes are postoperative ileus, the use of opiates or anticholinergics, severe illness, and hypothyroidism.
Dx: Exclude other causes of ileus (i.e., bowel obstruction, intraabdominal infections, bowel perforation, etc.) Abdominal films show retained air in colon and rectum without a visible transition zone.

Tx/Mgmt:
1. Nasogastric tube for decompression
2. Fluid and electrolyte replacement
3. Pain management
4. Serial abdominal examinations

Impaction

Buzz Words: Fecal loading in abdominal films

Clinical Presentation: Elderly patient who chronically suffers from constipation with abdominal distention and prolonged failure to pass stool

PPx: Eliminate potential causes of constipation + dietary fiber intake of 20–25 g/day

MoD: Inability to sense and respond to the presence of stool in the bowel plays a role in the development of intestinal impaction.

Dx:
1. Digital rectal exam would show copious amount of stool in the rectum
2. Abdominal x-ray may aid in the diagnosis when proximal loops of bowel are involved in the absence of rectal impaction

Tx/Mgmt:
1. Digital disimpaction. Once disimpaction has been successfully performed, oral administration of polyethylene glycol can serve to prevent re-impaction
2. Osmotic enemas may aid in the softening of the fecal matter
3. Refractory cases can be managed with the injection of local anesthetics to relax the pelvic floor; an abdominal massage can be performed; or a colonoscope can be used to fragment distal fecal matter

Intestinal Obstruction/Stricture

Clinical Presentation: Intermittent abdominal pain, cramping, nausea, vomiting, and distention. Exam will be noteworthy for signs of hypovolemia, increased peristalsis, and high-pitched bowel sounds (which can disappear as the bowel distends).

PPx: N/A

MoD: Normal flow of bowel contents is interrupted leading to dilation, edema of the bowel wall, and proximal increase in intraluminal pressure. An excessive increase in pressure will obstruct blood flow and lead to bowel perforation. Postoperative adhesions are the most common cause of obstruction, followed by hernias, volvulus, intestinal inflammation, neoplasms, and prior irradiation.

Dx:
1. Clinical diagnosis. Digital rectal examination should be performed to rule out impaction
2. Abdominal computed tomography (CT) scan may help identify location and severity of obstruction

Tx/Mgmt:
1. Decompression with nasogastric tube, volume replacement, and adequate management of pain
2. Patients with partial obstruction may be observed with frequent reassessments in expectation of spontaneous resolution
3. Prompt surgical exploration in complicated obstructions by ischemia, necrosis, or perforation

Fecal Incontinence

Clinical Presentation: Involuntary loss of feces or flatus. Urge incontinence is characterized by an intense desire to defecate, with incontinence occurring despite efforts to retain stool. Passive incontinence consists in a lack of awareness of the need to defecate.

PPx: Avoid foods known to worsen symptoms.

MoD: Incontinence can occur by alteration in any of the physiologic components of defecation: sphincter function, stool volume/consistency, rectal compliance, cognitive function, anorectal awareness, and reflexes.

Dx:
1. Flexible sigmoidoscopy to rule out malignancy or mucosal inflammation
2. Patients with sphincter defects should be evaluated with endoscopic ultrasound, and those with intact sphincters should have a rectal manometry performed

Tx/Mgmt: Reduce frequency and increase consistency of stool with bulking agents (i.e., methylcellulose) or antidiarrheal agents (i.e., loperamide).

Proctitis

Clinical Presentation: Rectal urgency, tenesmus, pain worsened by bowel movements, and mucus discharge. Risk factors for developing proctitis include previous radiation therapy and unprotected anal intercourse.

PPx: Use of condom during anal intercourse

MoD: *Clamydia trachomatis* and *herpes simplex virus* (HSV) *type 2* are common causes of proctitis on patients who engage in anal intercourse.

Dx:

1. Clinical diagnosis
2. Sigmoidoscopy might show erythematous, friable, and ulcerated rectal mucosa

Tx/Mgmt:

1. Pain relief: Sitz baths, topical anesthetics, and oral analgesics
2. Tetracycline or doxycycline for chlamydia proctitis

Ascites

Buzz Words: Abdominal fullness + fluid wave + flank dullness on percussion + shifting dullness

Clinical Presentation: Accumulation of fluid in the peritoneal cavity. The most common cause is chronic liver failure, but other processes may induce it as well (e.g., nephrotic syndrome, malnutrition, protein-losing enteropathy, heart failure, carcinomatosis, etc.). Patients with abdominal hernias may suffer an exacerbation due to the high pressure with thinning of the overlying skin. Approximately 10% of patients will develop spontaneous bacterial peritonitis (SBP), which carries a mortality of 50% at 1 year.

PPx: Fluid and sodium restriction

MoD: Transudation of fluid usually occurs from the intravascular space to the hepatic parenchyma, then leaks into the peritoneal cavity, which is due to increased hydrostatic pressure (in the setting of portal hypertension) and decreased colloid oncotic pressure.

Dx:

1. Abdominal exam reveals dullness to percussion and fluid wave on palpation. These signs become evident when accumulation is greater than 1.5 L.
2. Ultrasound/CT can detect lower volumes of fluid in the peritoneal cavity
3. Diagnostic paracentesis aids in differential diagnosis (cell count, amylase level, triglyceride level, pH, and albumin)
4. Anyone with ascites + fever must undergo paracentesis; SBP is diagnosed with more than 250 cells/mm^3

99 AR

Radiograph findings in ascites

Tx/Mgmt:

1. Fluid and Na^+ restriction (<2 g/day) and diuresis with spironolactone (to promote Na^+ excretion) ± furosemide
2. When respiration or mobility become severely limited, therapeutic paracentesis (8–10 L) is performed while administering intravenous (IV) albumin (8 g/L of fluid removed)

Ischemic Hepatitis

Buzz Words: Liver shock + hypoxic hepatitis

Clinical Presentation: Right upper quadrant (RUQ) pain, nausea, vomiting, anorexia, and malaise. This is a rare phenomenon since the liver receives a dual blood supply (proper hepatic artery and portal vein).

PPx: N/A

MoD: Diffuse hepatic infarction from acute hypoperfusion, severe hypoxemia, severe respiratory failure, or it can be associated with acute lower limb ischemia. There is an imbalance between oxygen demand and supply. Zone 3 of the hepatic acinus is the most susceptible to injury; this is the furthest away from oxygenated blood supply.

Dx: Alanine aminotransferase (ALT) and aspartate aminotransferase (AST) may surpass the normal range by 50×.

Tx/Mgmt: Restoration of cardiac output

Jaundice

Clinical Presentation: Yellow pigmentation in skin and eyes. Unconjugated bilirubin (UGB) is lipophilic and can cross the blood-brain barrier (BBB), leading to kernicterus (accumulation in basal ganglia). Leakage of bile salts, bile acids, and cholesterol into the blood would manifest pruritus and xanthomas.

PPx: Depends on mechanism

MoD: Accumulation of bilirubin, the end product of heme degradation. Table 8.14 briefly depicts the distinct mechanisms in which jaundice may be produced.

Dx: Adequate identification of the risk factors for disease and the interpretation of liver function tests (LFTs) (see Table 8.11) are key to narrowing down the mechanism for the presentation.

Tx/Mgmt: Phototherapy is a safe method to treat severe unconjugated hyperbilirubinemia in newborns by increasing the solubility of UGB and allowing it to be excreted in urine. Administration of calcium carbonate modestly enhances the effect of phototherapy.

Infectious Disorders

Bacterial

Pseudomembranous Colitis (Clostridium difficile)

Buzz Words: Watery diarrhea + broad-spectrum antibiotics + obligate anaerobe Gram-positive rods

Clinical Presentation: Classic presentation is secretory diarrhea. *C. difficile* is part of the normal gut flora. Patients who are exposed to long-term antibiotics (most commonly clindamycin, quinolones, ampicillin) lose a significant portion of their normal flora. It is the most common cause of nosocomial and healthcare-associated diarrhea.

PPx: Avoid overuse of broad-spectrum antibiotics.

MoD: Exotoxin A and B alter the structural integrity of actin filaments, leading to increased permeability of tight junctions, which promote watery diarrhea; these cells end up undergoing apoptosis due to caspase activation and Rho protein inactivation. Exotoxin damage leads to the formation of a shaggy layer of fibrin and dead epithelial cells (pseudomembrane), which cover the mucosal lining.

Dx:

1. Cytotoxins in diarrhea
2. Glutamate dehydrogenase antigen test

Tx/Mgmt:

1. Oral metronidazole
2. Oral vancomycin
3. IV metronidazole for high severity and/or toxic megacolon

Enteric Infections

Staphylococcus aureus

Buzz Words: N/V + abdominal pain + recent ingestion of dairy product (e.g., old mayonnaise)

Clinical Presentation: Fast onset (1–6 hours) food poisoning; nausea, vomiting, abdominal cramps

PPx: Adequate refrigeration of food products; hand hygiene

MoD: Heat-stable enterotoxin B acts as a superantigen by forming a bridge between MHC-II on antigen-presenting cells and T-cell receptors on T-cells. It grows in dairy products, meats, and salads that are kept at room temperature.

Dx:

1. Clinical diagnosis
2. Vomitus and/or food can be tested for the enterotoxin

Tx/Mgmt: Self-limited; supportive therapy

Escherichia coli

Buzz Words: Hemolytic uremic syndrome (HUS) + schistocytes + hemorrhagic diarrhea + recently ate undercooked meat (e.g., hamburgers)

Clinical Presentation: There are four types of *E. coli* that can be tested by the NBME (Table 8.1). Of the four, EHEC is the most high-yield. If pressed for time, skip EPEC, ETEC, and EIEC.

- **Enterohemorrhagic *E. coli* (EHEC)**—Shiga-like toxin from undercooked meat leading to HUS

TABLE 8.1 Most Common Diarrheal Illnesses Caused by *Escherichia coli*

	ETEC (i.e., Traveler's Diarrhea)	EHEC (*O157:H7 Serotype*)	EIEC
Presentation	Watery diarrhea	Hemorrhagic colitis and HUS in 8% of cases	Dysentery 12–72 h after ingestion
MoD	Heat-labile (LT) and heat-stable (ST) toxins activate adenylate and guanylate cyclase respectively → secretory diarrhea	Shiga toxin (verotoxin) → inactivates ribosomal 60S component → endothelial damage (gut, kidney, lung) → hemorrhage	Mucosal cell invasion causing membrane disruption
Clinical cues	Traveler's and children <5 year old	Children and elderly; transmitted through undercooked ground beef	Developing countries; invasion rarely goes beyond submucosa
Management	Fluid replacement Ciprofloxacin	Fluid replacement Avoid antibiotics! These may precipitate HUS	Fluid replacement

EHEC, Enterohemorrhagic *E. coli*; *EIEC*, enteroinvasive *E. coli*; *ETEC*, enterohemorrhagic *E. coli*; *HUS*, hemolytic uremic syndrome; *MoD*, mechanism of disease.

Most commonly tested. Make sure to learn how to identify this one only.

- Enteropathogenic *E. coli* (EPEC)—Mostly children, nonbloody diarrhea
- Enterotoxigenic *E. coli* (ETEC)—Travelers' diarrhea, nonbloody
- Enteroinvasive *E. coli* (EIEC)—Inflammatory bowel, bloody diarrhea

PPx: Hand washing, adequate sanitization of water, and avoiding food contamination.

Patients traveling to endemic areas can take antibiotics (fluoroquinolones first-line, azithromycin if going to Asia) and use them in case of developing diarrhea during their trip; these decrease symptom duration.

MoD:

For EHEC: Shiga toxin (verotoxin) → inactivates ribosomal 60S component → endothelial damage (gut, kidney, lung) → hemorrhage

- No need to know MoD of ETEC, EIEC, or EPEC for shelf
- Know that EHEC and EIEC → bloody diarrhea = bacteria invades mucosa
  - ETEC and EPEC do not invade and inflame gut mucosa

Dx:

1. Blood culture and Gram stain (motile, encapsulated Gram-negative rod, catalase [+], and oxidase [–])
2. MacConkey agar (pink; lactose fermenter)
3. DNA assays, enzyme immunoassays for toxin
4. For EHEC: complete blood count (CBC), basic metabolic panel (BMP)

Tx/Mgmt:

1. Supportive therapy (i.e., fluids)
2. Avoid antiperistaltic agents (loperamide) as these might prolong the duration of infection
3. For EHEC: Fluid replacement; Avoid antibiotics, which may precipitate HUS

Listeria monocytogenes

Buzz Words: Pasteurized milk + dark/cloudy amniotic fluid + newborn meningitis

Clinical Presentation: Febrile gastroenteritis, which might progress to systemic disease in pregnant patients, during steroid therapy, or in the immunosuppressed. Listeria is also the third most common cause of meningitis in newborns and is the reason why **ampicillin** is added to the treatment regimen at times with ≤6-month-olds with sepsis.

PPx: N/A

MoD: Motile by actin filament polymerization. Transmitted through contaminated dairy products and deli meat. The organism can survive refrigerator temperatures and a wide range of pH.

Dx: Stool culture and Gram stain (shows tumbling motility; catalase (+), Gram-positive; facultative anaerobe)

Tx/Mgmt:
1. Ampicillin
2. TMP/SMX (antibiotic resistance is rare)

Yersinia enterocolitica

Buzz Words: Gram-negative coccobacillus with bipolar staining ("*safety-pin*" appearance) + resistant to cold temperatures + pseudo appendicitis in children

Clinical Presentation: Enterocolitis in children may be accompanied by pharyngitis (no other cause of bacterial diarrhea). Mesenteric lymphadenitis that simulates acute appendicitis. It is associated with human leukocyte antigen (HLA)-B27 tissue type (seronegative spondyloarthropathies); it may have erythema nodosum and reactive arthritis as sequelae.

PPx: Avoid contact with canine feces, and ensure hand washing after exposure to swine products.

MoD: Organism courses through the stomach, attaches and invades the gut wall to end up localizing in regional lymphoid tissue.

Dx: Culture isolation from stool, pharynx, or mesenteric nodes

Tx/Mgmt: Ciprofloxacin (adults) or TMP-SMX (children) only in patients with severe disease only

> **MNEMONIC**
> Diseases associated with HLA-B27 subtype (**PAIR**): **P**soriasis, **A**nkylosing spondylitis, **I**nflammatory bowel disease, and **R**eactive arthritis

Campylobacter spp.

Buzz Words: Bloody diarrhea, fever + cramping periumbilical abdominal pain

Clinical Presentation: Bloody diarrhea, fever, and cramping periumbilical abdominal pain. Children may manifest abdominal pain that mimics appendicitis or colitis. Guillain-Barré syndrome (ascending paralysis), HUS, and reactive arthritis are late onset complications.

PPx: Avoid eating raw/undercooked meat.

MoD: Invasive with a low infective dose (~500 bacteria). Poultry reservoir. Puppies are the most common source of infection for children. Produces crypt abscesses resembling ulcerative colitis. The disease is self-limited with a mean duration of 7 days.

Dx:
1. Stool culture
2. Serologic test may be used to detect recent infection once the organism is no longer in the stool

Tx/Mgmt:
1. Sortive therapy
2. Fluoroquinolones, azithromycin, or erythromycin in the setting of severe diarrhea

Vibrio cholera

Buzz Words: Rice-water stools + comma-shaped Gram-negative rod, acid-labile, oxidase (+)

Clinical Presentation: High-volume secretory diarrhea (10 L stool/day) ± vomitus, significant hypovolemia, and electrolyte abnormalities, which may occur hours after onset of disease.

PPx: Adequate hygiene and keeping a clean water supply.

MoD: Fimbriae allow attachment to gut wall. Toxin attaches to GM1 ganglioside → activates G_s pathway → increases cAMP → opens CFTR Cl^- channels → secretory diarrhea

Dx: Clinical diagnosis

Tx/Mgmt:
1. Aggressive oral rehydration therapy is the best initial therapy
2. IV fluids for patients in hypovolemic shock
3. Supplement zinc and vitamin A in children

Salmonella spp.

Buzz Words:
- Fever + abdominal cramps + diarrhea + chicken + fever + 60% lymphocytes
- Sickle cell patient + osteomyelitis

Clinical Presentation: Inflammatory diarrhea, nausea, vomiting, fever, and abdominal cramps. It is an important cause of osteomyelitis in patients with sickle cell disease.

PPx: Adequate hygiene; live-attenuated (Ty21a) or Vi capsular vaccines exist

MoD: Transmitted through the ingestion of poultry, eggs, and milk products. The organism invades the intestinal wall and submucosal lymphoid system and into the circulation, and finally finds shelter within macrophages of the reticuloendothelial system. Type III secretion system and lipid A are the two main virulence factors. Chronic carriage state (>1 year) most usually occurs in elderly patients with biliary tract abnormalities (gallstones most commonly).

Dx: Stool culture (H2S (+), motile, acid-labile, capsulated, Gram-negative bacilli, black colonies on Hektoen agar, "pea-soup" diarrhea
Tx/Mgmt:
1. Supportive therapy
2. Antibiotics (fluoroquinolones) only for severe infection or patients with risk factors

Shigella spp.
Buzz Words: Bloody diarrhea + day-care center, mental institution + beef ingestion
Clinical Presentation: Patient with frequent, small volume, bloody stools with fever, abdominal cramps, and tenesmus. Intestinal complications involve toxic megacolon, colonic perforation, intestinal obstruction, proctitis, and rectal prolapse. Thrombocytopenia and HUS are common in young children (similar to EHEC); other systemic complications include protein-loss enteropathy, leukemoid reaction, neurologic manifestation, and reactive arthritis.
PPx: Adequate hygiene
MoD: Invasion of M cells. Toxin inactivates ribosomal 60S subunit (similar to verotoxin in EHEC). Glomerular damage. Spreads fecal-oral, hand-hand.
Dx: Stool culture to isolate bacteria (acid-stable, immotile, Gram-negative bacilli; green colonies on Hektoen agar).
Tx/Mgmt:
1. Supportive therapy; self-limited infection
2. Antibiotics (ceftriaxone or azithromycin) are appropriate for children and immunosuppressed patients

Hepatic Abscess
Pyogenic
Buzz Words: History of appendicitis or diverticulitis
Clinical Presentation: A patient with a history of peritonitis and developed leakage of bowel contents is now presenting with RUQ pain, fever, leukocytosis, and elevated alkaline phosphatase.
PPx: Adequate antibiotic therapy in GI/biliary tract infections
MoD: Bacteria usually find their way to the liver from a GI or biliary tract source of infection. Nonetheless, hematogenous seeding may also be the etiology in the setting of bacteremia.
Dx:
1. Ultrasound (hypoechoic mass with a hyperechoic wall)
2. CT (well-demarcated, encapsulated, fluid-filled lesion)

Tx/Mgmt:

1. Percutaneous catheter drainage (when >5 cm). The catheter should remain in place until drainage ceases (~7 days)
2. Bacterial cultures on collected fluid to narrow down the antimicrobial therapy
3. Surgical drainage should be considered in the setting of multiple abscesses, loculated abscesses, viscous contents, and inadequate clearing with drainage

Amebic Abscess

Buzz Words: Immigrant/recent travel to Central or South America + abscess with *"anchovy-paste"* fluid

Clinical Presentation: Adult male with 1–2 weeks of RUQ and fever ± diarrhea, hepatosplenomegaly, and point-tenderness over the liver on abdominal exam.

PPx: N/A

MoD: *Entamoeba histolytica* trophozoites invade the colon wall and migrate to the liver through the portal circulation. Liver abscesses occur in 10% of patients with amebiasis. Although most occur in the right lobe, lesions in the left hepatic lobe are at a higher risk of spontaneous rupture.

Dx:

1. Ultrasound-guided percutaneous aspiration (sterile fluid with anchovy-paste appearance)
2. Antiamebic antibodies are useful in patients who are not from endemic areas (individuals from endemic areas will test positive even in the absence of infection)

Tx/Mgmt:

1. Metronidazole or tinidazol
2. Subsequent treatment with paromomycin is warranted to eliminate intraluminal cysts
3. Surgical drainage is required in the setting of the rupture of secondary bacterial infection

Echinococcus

Buzz Words: Sheep + dogs + cystic mass in liver + abdominal pain + fever + eosinophilia

Clinical Presentation: Echinococcus is a parasitic infection that causes hydatid cysts in the liver and can lead to anaphylaxis if the cystic contents leak out through biopsy. Thus, biopsy or rupture of cysts is avoided. It is associated with sheep and dogs.

PPx: Do NOT **biopsy** (leakage of fluid in cysts → anaphylaxis)

MoD: Echinococcus granulosus infection carried by sheep and dog feces.

Dx:

1. CBC (eosinophilia)
2. Casoni skin test (positive)

Tx/Mgmt:

1. Albendazol
2. Surgical removal of entire cyst (do NOT rupture)

Peritonitis

Definition:

Peritonitis is an acute inflammatory process involving the peritoneum, which is most commonly (but not exclusively) due to infection. Inflammation causes increased regional blood flow, permeability, and the formation of fibrinous exudates, making the surrounding loops of bowel to slow down, which causes ileus and allows the omentum to adhere. Intra-abdominal infections represent a major cause of morbidity and mortality.

Buzz Words: *Washboard* abdomen + Blumberg sign (rebound tenderness) + involuntary guarding + tenderness to percussion

Clinical Presentation: Diffuse poorly-defined pain should make you think of inflammation of the visceral peritoneal layer; divided by embryologic derivatives: epigastrium—foregut, periumbilical—midgut, hypogastrium—hindgut. Pin-point and well-localized pain should make you think of inflammation of the parietal peritoneal layer. Progression from the first to the second is a valuable clue to identify progression of peritonitis (e.g., appendicitis).

Primary Peritonitis

Buzz Words: SBP + fever in liver disease patient with ascites

Clinical Presentation: Most commonly in the setting of chronic liver disease and ascites (10% of patients with ascites); nonetheless, it may also occur in nephrotic syndrome, acute viral hepatitis, malignancy, and SLE. Clinical cues are fever, altered mental status, and diffuse abdominal pain in a patient with liver disease.

PPx: Antibiotics (i.e., TMP-SMX, ciprofloxacin, or norfloxacin) in patients at high risk for developing SBP (grade 1A evidence to support this). High-risk patients:

- Patients who had SBP (recurrence rate is 70% at 1 year)
- Cirrhosis + GI bleed
- Ascitic fluid protein less than 1.5 g/dL + impaired renal function OR liver failure

MoD: Occurs in the absence of an evident intra-abdominal source of infection. The route of infection is usually hematogenous. Most common pathogens: *E. coli*, *Klebsiella*, and *Streptococcus* spp. The fluid separates the visceral and parietal surfaces, preventing the development of a rigid abdomen; therefore, some patients are asymptomatic at the time of diagnosis.

Dx: Paracentesis prior to initiating antibiotics (ascitic fluid absolute PMN count $\geq$ 250 cells/mm^3 and positive fluid culture)

Tx/Mgmt:
1. Empiric cefotaxime and bacterial culture
2. Start albumin infusion on patients with borderline renal function (decreased risk of developing renal failure)
3. Discontinue nonselective β-blockers (associated with worst transplant-free survival, greater incidence of hepatorenal syndrome, and prolonged hospitalization)

Secondary Peritonitis

Buzz Words: Free air in the belly + anastomotic dehiscence

Clinical Presentation: Very rare compared to SBP but with high (>50%) mortality. Manifestations may also be subtle, such as nonspecific abdominal pain. The identification of symptoms requires a high clinical suspicion.

PPx: N/A

MoD: Ascitic fluid infection in the setting of a surgically treatable source of infection. Secondary bacterial peritonitis is lethal when treatment only consists of antibiotics and no surgery. The mortality for an unnecessary laparotomy in the setting of SBP ~80%.

Dx:
1. Paracentesis
2. Polymicrobial infection. On analysis of ascitic fluid, Ruyon criteria (⅔ findings) are indicative of secondary bacterial peritonitis:
   - Total protein greater than 1 g/dL
   - Glucose less than 50 mg/dL
   - LDH > upper limit of normal for serum

Tx/Mgmt:
1. Empiric antibiotics (e.g., cefotaxime)
2. Exploratory laparotomy should be done emergently in the setting of "*free air*" or if a surgically treatable source of infection is found
3. Repeat paracentesis at 48 hours to assess the response to treatment

Whipple Disease

Buzz Words: Steatorrhea + confusion + foamy macrophages on pathology

Clinical Presentation: Middle-aged patient (male > female) with intermittent steatorrhea, colicky abdominal pain, fever, recurrent polyarthritis, generalized lymphadenopathy, and increased skin pigmentation. Central nervous system (CNS) involvement may present as cognitive dysfunction and confusion. Can ultimately lead to severe wasting syndrome.

PPx: N/A

MoD: *Tropheryma whippelii* enters macrophage → macrophage unable to digest *T. whippelii* → decreased lymphatic drainage and chylomicron transportation into the blood (similar MoD to apoB48 deficiency).

Dx:

1. Polymerase chain reaction (PCR) or stool test for *T. whippelii* (shows PAS-positive, non-acid-fast, Gram-positive rod)
2. EGD with small intestine biopsy showing PAS-positive foamy macrophages

Tx/Mgmt:

1. Long-term antibiotics (6–12 months) ceftriaxone
2. Maintenance with TMP/SMX or doxycycline plus hydroxychloroquine

Viral Infections of the Gastrointestinal Tract

Infectious Esophagitis

Buzz Words: Esophageal erosions on EGD

Clinical Presentation: Often an immunosuppressed patient with odynophagia and dysphagia. Keep a high clinical suspicion in all immunosuppressed patients.

PPx: N/A

MoD: Most common viral agents are HSV and cytomegalovirus (CMV). CMV usually damages the colon as well.

Dx: EGD to take biopsies or brushing from the edge of the ulcer.

Tx/Mgmt:

1. HSV-esophagitis should receive acyclovir PO 2–3 weeks for immunosuppressed patients
2. CMV-esophagitis should receive ganciclovir

Hepatitis A

Buzz Words: Travel to rural area or developing country + jaundice + elevated LFTs + no history of hepatitis A virus (HAV) vaccine + ingestion of uncooked shellfish

Clinical Presentation: Patients who travel to endemic areas are at higher risk. It presents as jaundice in adults; anicteric hepatitis might present in children. There is a 1-month duration of symptoms.

99 AR

Whipple disease overview

PPx:
1. Inactivated vaccine
2. Hygienic practices, such as handwashing, heating food appropriately, and avoiding drinking tap water in areas of poor sanitization

MoD: Fecal-oral transmission. Uncooked shellfish is a common source of infection in developed countries.

Dx: Serum immunoglobulin (Ig)M anti-HAV antibodies. HAV RNA can be detected in stool prior to onset of symptoms.

Tx/Mgmt: Self-limiting infection, supportive therapy and fluids

Hepatitis B

Buzz Words: History of blood transfusion/IV drug use/ unprotected sex + painful hepatomegaly + polyarteritis nodosa/membranous GN/membranoproliferative GN + no history of vaccination

Clinical Presentation: Variable fever, purpuric macules, painful hepatomegaly, profound malaise, and urticaria. Polyarteritis nodosa and secondary kidney disease. Associated with membranous and membranoproliferative glomerulonephritis. Second most common cause of fulminant hepatitis (7% of cases). 10% of adult infections progress to chronic infections and 90% of neonatal infections progress to chronic infections. Associated with hepatocellular carcinoma (10%–15% of cases).

PPx: Immunization with recombinant vaccine

MoD: Uses a reverse transcriptase to infect hepatocytes. Spread by maternal-fetal, blood, or sexual activity.

Dx: ALT rises during adult symptomatic infection (ALT > AST) but does not vary significantly in children (Table 8.2).

Tx/Mgmt: Interferon-α, lamivudine, NRTIs, and liver transplantation.

Hepatitis C

Buzz Words:
- **Acute HCV:** Elderly adult w/ blood transfusion OR young adult w/ IV drug use + elevated LFTs
- **Chronic HCV:** Elderly adult w/ blood transfusion OR young adult w/ IV drug use + cirrhosis/HCC + decreased LFTs

Clinical Presentation: 60% 80% will progress to a chronic infection. May lead to cirrhosis and hepatocellular carcinoma. Most common cause of fulminant hepatitis,

TABLE 8.2 Hepatitis B Virus Serologic Studies

Interpretation	HBsAg	HBV DNA	Anti-HBc IgM	Anti-HBc IgG	Anti-HBs
Early infection	+	−	−	−	−
Acute infection	+	+	+	−	−
Window phase	−	−	+	−	−
Recovery	−	−	−	+	+
Immunized	−	−	−	−	+
Healthy carrier	+	−	−	+	−
Infective carrier	+	+	−	+	−

Anti-HBc, Antibody to hepatitis B core antigen; *anti-HBs;* antibody to hepatitis B surface antigen; *HBV,* hepatitis B virus; *IgG,* immunoglobulin G; *IgM,* immunoglobulin M.

hepatitis in healthcare workers, and main indication for liver transplantation in the United States.

PPx: Avoid needle sharing. Once infected, avoid habits known to accelerate progression of liver disease such as alcohol, marijuana, and obesity. Those who develop cirrhosis require abdominal US q2 years for early detection of HCC.

MoD: Lacks proofreading enzymes (3′–5′ exonuclease), which allows for significant antigenic variability of envelope. The virus has 6 different genotypes which modify preferred therapy.

Dx:
1. Anti-HCV antibodies or HCV RNA in serum
2. ALT rises during symptomatic infection (ALT > AST)
3. Chronic HCV infection is diagnosed by detectable HCV viral level more than 6 months. Also, LFTs are decreased with chronic HCV 2/2 cirrhosis

Tx/Mgmt: Different treatment regimens exist depending on the genotype of the virus, but combination therapy is the cornerstone of treatment with ribavirin and/or interferon-α. Liver transplant for advanced cirrhosis.

Hepatitis D

Buzz Words: Concomitant hepatitis B virus (HBV) infection

Clinical Presentation:
- Coinfection = HBV + hepatitis D virus (HDV) at the same time (usually transient and self-limited).
- Superinfection = chronic HBsAg carrier + HDV infection.
- Severity of infection is dependent on viral genotype. Genotype 1, which is most common in the Western

world, has a fulminant course with rapid progression towards cirrhosis. Infection tends to occur in children and young adults. It is endemic in the Mediterranean region.

PPx: Mode of transmission is unclear.

MoD: Although HDV can replicate autonomously, it requires HBsAg for virion assembly and secretion.

Dx: Serum HDAg, HDV RNA, or anti-HDV antibodies (both IgM and IgG)

Tx/Mgmt: Pegylated interferon-α

Hepatitis E

Buzz Words: Elevated LFTs + self-limited + pregnancy/pre-existing disease

Clinical Presentation: Self-limited acute viral hepatitis. Fulminant hepatitis may occur in pregnant patients or those with preexisting liver disease.

PPx: Hand-washing and avoiding consumption of untreated water

MoD: Fecal-oral transmission with outbreaks associated with the contamination of water sources

Dx: Detection of hepatitis E virus (HEV) in serum or stool by PCR, anti-HEV IgM antibodies in serum

Tx/Mgmt: Supportive therapy

Rotavirus Enteritis

Buzz Words: Double-stranded RNA virus + telescoping of the bowel

Clinical Presentation: Secretory diarrhea, nausea, low-grade fever, and vomiting in small children. Occurs most frequently in the winter months.

PPx: Oral live-attenuated vaccine exists; it has been associated with intussusception

MoD: Most common cause of severe diarrhea in children. NSP4 toxin causes chloride permeability through the intestinal cell membranes.

Dx: Rotazyme test on stool

Tx/Mgmt: Oral rehydration

Mumps

Buzz Words: Chipmunk facies (b/l parotitis) + orchitis + fever/headache + no vaccination history

Clinical Presentation: Vague viral prodrome, which consists low-grade fever, malaise, headache, myalgias, and anorexia. Bilateral parotitis occurs in 70% of cases. Unilateral orchitis occurs most commonly in an older child or adult.

PPx: Measles, mumps, and rubella vaccine, and isolation of any infected individual

MoD: Neuraminidase and hemagglutinin are the main virulence factors. Caused by RNA paramyxovirus.

Dx:
1. CBC (leukopenia with a relative lymphocytosis)
2. Increased serum amylase (released from salivary glands)

Tx/Mgmt: Supportive therapy with analgesics and antipyretics

Gingivostomatitis, Herpetic

Buzz Words: Cowdry bodies + dew drops on a rose petal + multinucleated giant cells in Tzanck smear/prep + dsDNA virus

Clinical Presentation: Viral prodrome (fever + constitutional symptoms) followed by oral lesions (initially vesicles on erythematous base → painful ulcers cover by greyish membrane), halitosis, refusal to drink, anorexia, and regional lymphadenitis. Affected age group 6 months to 5 years of age.

PPx: Contact precautions with affected children

MoD: HSV type 1 (HSV-1). Affect resolution of symptoms the virus migrates to the trigeminal ganglion to establish latent infection. Reactivation can be induced by exposure to sunlight, trauma, cold, stress, or immunosuppression.

Dx: Clinical diagnosis

Tx/Mgmt:
1. Supportive therapy
2. Acyclovir if disease is prolonged (>72 hours)

Fungal

Thrush

Buzz Words: White plaques that are easy to scrape from oral mucosa

Clinical Presentation: Fuzzy white plaques on oral mucous membranes that come off by scraping with a tongue depressor, revealing inflamed and friable mucosa. Differentiate from hairy leukoplakia (Epstein-Barr virus), which does not come off by scraping and is usually associated with human immunodeficiency virus (HIV).

PPx: N/A

MoD: Oropharyngeal colonization of *Candia albicans.* It may happen in the immunocompetent neonate or the immunocompromised adult. Infection may be transmitted by the passage through the birth canal, the mother's nipple, or the environment.

Dx:
1. Clinical diagnosis
2. May also confirm by KOH smear or fungal culture

Tx/Mgmt: Topical nystatin or fluconazole. If the mother's breasts are also infected treat them at the same time.

Parasitic

Most of the parasitic organisms that produce enterocolitis are opportunistic (AIDS < 50 cells/mm^3) and tend to present as patients who have traveled or migrated from endemic regions and have had diarrhea for more than 7 days.

Cryptosporidium

Buzz Words: AIDS patient with CD_4 < 100 cells + intracellular protozoan + banana-shaped motile sporozoites

Clinical Presentation: Most common cause of diarrhea in AIDS, and diarrhea from swimming in municipal pools. Also associated with children who attend daycare.

PPx: Strict hand-washing; avoidance of untreated water and undercooked food when traveling to endemic regions

MoD: Organisms can be present in stool, duodenal aspirates, and bile or respiratory secretions.

Dx:
1. Stool antigen test (high sensitivity and specificity)
2. Modified acid-fast stain
3. Alkaline phosphatase (ALP) may be elevated in patients with biliary tract involvement

Tx/Mgmt:
1. Nitazoxanide in immunocompetent patients (less effective in immunodeficient) who have symptoms greater than 2 weeks
2. For AIDS patients, antiretroviral therapy should be initiated

Cyclospora

Buzz Words: AIDS patient or international traveler to endemic area + pink acid-fast oocysts

Clinical Presentation: Low-grade fever, diarrhea, abdominal cramping, flatulence, anorexia, and nausea in an AIDS patient

PPx: Strict hand-washing and avoiding the consumption of untreated water and undercooked food when traveling to endemic regions

MoD: Oocysts passed in the stool are shed in a non-infective form and require several days before they become infectious. Low infectious does (10–100 organisms). Causes food-borne and water-borne infection.

Dx: Stool microscopy with acid-fast staining (oocysts are larger than cryptosporidium oocysts, which are also acid-fast)

Tx/Mgmt: TMP-SMX

Entamoeba histolytica

Buzz Words: Flask-shaped ulcers in a patient who recently visited or migrated from a developing country + bloody diarrhea + spherical cysts

Clinical Presentation: Symptoms range from mild diarrhea to dysentery with severe abdominal pain and bloody stools. Fulminant colitis or toxic megacolon with bowel perforation can also occur.

PPx: Strict hand-washing. Avoid untreated water and undercooked food when traveling to endemic regions.

MoD: Transmission by ingestion of cysts in contaminated food/water; cysts become trophozoites in the cecum and secrete histolytic agents, which produce flask-shaped ulcers. Trophozoites can invade into hepatic veins and produce a liver abscess (discussed before) or systemic disease.

Dx: Stool antigen test

Tx/Mgmt:
1. Metronidazole for symptomatic patients
2. Paromomycin (eliminated intraluminal cysts) for asymptomatic carriers

Giardia

Buzz Words: Camper or hiker with nonbloody diarrhea + oval cysts in liver

Clinical Presentation: Steatorrhea with frequent burping, bloating, distention, and flatus (i.e., malabsorption). Malaise and weight loss can occur when with chronic infection.

PPx: Strict hand-washing. Avoid untreated water and undercooked food when traveling to endemic regions.

MoD: *Giardia lamblia* is a flagellated protozoan that produces a water-borne infection. Conditions with absent IgA production (IgA deficiency, Bruton agammaglobulinemia) make the perfect setting for giardiasis in a test question.

Dx: Ova and parasite test (O&P), ELISA stool antigen test, and nucleic acid detection assays

QUICK TIPS

Be able to differentiate Giardia lamblia cysts, which are oval-shaped and cause **nonbloody** diarrhea

QUICK TIPS

Be able to differentiate Echinococcus vs. Entamoeba; the former presents 3 months post-infection; the latter presents 1–2 weeks post-infection w/ abdominal pain.

Tx/Mgmt: Metronidazole, tinidazole, or nitazoxanide for symptomatic patients. Treatment is warranted for (1) asymptomatic patients who are food-handlers, (2) those in contact with pregnant women, (3) those who are immunocompromised, or (4) children in day-care.

Cystoisospora (isospora) belli

Buzz Words: Partially acid-fast, opportunistic protozoan + watery diarrhea

Clinical Presentation: In the immunocompetent, self-limited watery diarrhea. In AIDS patients (<50 cells/mm^3), a severe debilitating chronic diarrhea with wasting.

PPx: Adequate sanitization of food and water sources. Prophylactic antibiotics in AIDS < 200 cells/mm^3 with TMPX-SMX.

MoD: Acquired by ingestion of sporulated oocysts (fecal-oral). Common pathogen in AIDS diarrhea along with Cyclospora and microsporidia.

Dx:
1. Detection of oocysts in feces through acid-fast staining
2. Severe diarrhea may progress to hypokalemia, hypomagnesemia, and bicarbonate wasting

Tx/Mgmt:
1. Aggressive fluid and electrolyte replacement
2. For the immunosuppressed, TMP-SMX is the preferred treatment and prophylactic

Strongyloides stercoralis

Buzz Words: Abdominal pain + Worm infection after walking barefoot ± AIDS patient

Clinical Presentation: Immunosuppressed patient with waxing and waning GI (abdominal pain and diarrhea), cutaneous, and respiratory symptoms (cough and wheezing) that persist for years

PPx: Strict hand-washing. Avoid untreated water and undercooked food when traveling to endemic regions.

MoD: Intestinal nematode. Peculiar mode of transmission: larvae penetrate feet → larva migrate to the lungs and ascend the airway to get swallowed → molt into adult form and penetrate in intestinal mucosa and lay eggs → eggs hatch and rhabditiform larvae that go back into the stool → develop into the filarial form, which is infective. Autoinfection may occur, which significantly increases the burden of adult worms

Dx: Eosinophilia, stool sampling for rhabditiform larvae, or serologic testing

Tx/Mgmt: Ivermectin

Immunologic and Inflammatory Disorders

Autoimmune Hepatitis

Buzz Words: Abnormal LFTs + ANAs + anti-smooth muscle Abs

Clinical Presentation: Broad range of presentations from abnormal LFTs to fulminant hepatitis and cirrhosis. Most common in young women. May be associated with other autoimmune disorders such as Graves disease or Hashimoto thyroiditis.

PPx: N/A

MoD: Two types exist. Type 1 is the most common in the United States. Association with HLA DR3 and DR4.

Dx:
1. Anti-smooth muscle antibodies in serum (>85% of cases) and antinuclear antibodies (>60% of cases)
2. Liver biopsy is the most accurate test. (3) Decreased serum albumin and prolonged PT in severe disease
3. Decreased serum albumin and prolonged PT in severe disease

Tx/Mgmt:
1. Steroids and azathioprine
2. Liver transplantation if disease progresses to fulminant hepatitis

99 AR

Autoimmune hepatitis—definition and pathology

Celiac Disease

Buzz Words: Malabsorption in diabetic with skin lesions + flattened/atrophic intestinal villi

Clinical Presentation: Steatorrhea, weight loss, failure-to-thrive, microcytic (Fe^{2+} deficiency) anemia. Prevalence of 1% in the United States.

PPx: Gluten-free diet (avoid wheat, barley, and rye products).

MoD: Inappropriate T-cell and IgA-mediated response against gluten; more specifically, gliadin, a breakdown product of gluten. Duodenum is the most commonly injured site. Significant clinical associations are dermatitis herpetiformis, T1DM, IgA deficiency, small bowel lymphoma, Turner syndrome, Down syndrome, and other autoimmune diseases (Hashimoto and PBC). Associated to HLA DQ2 (95% of cases) and HLA DQ8 (5% of cases).

Dx:
1. Anti-tissue transglutaminase and anti-endomysial antibodies have specificities >95%
2. Anti-gliadin antibodies is usually also elevated

Celiac disease—symptoms and pathophysiology

3. Mucosal biopsy will show villous atrophy, crypt hyperplasia, and intraepithelial lymphocytic infiltration

Tx/Mgmt: Prevention is key. Gluten-free diet and steroids in refractory cases.

Eosinophilic Esophagitis

Buzz Words: H/o food impaction + persistent dysphagia or gastroesophageal reflux disease (GERD) refractory to medical therapy

Clinical Presentation: Young men with h/o of atopy who present with vomiting, abdominal pain, dysphagia, and food impaction. Esophageal perforation after dilation of a stricture is also a presentation, which should trigger the thought of this disease.

PPx: Some patients might find success in preventing their disease by pursuing elimination diets (testing-directed, empiric, or elemental).

MoD: Chronic immune-mediated disease characterized by esophageal dysfunction with an eosinophil-predominant inflammatory process. Genetic defects of calpain-14 may predispose to disease.

Dx:
1. EGD with mucosal biopsies (>15 Eos/HPF) after 2 months of PPI therapy
2. Common visual findings in EGD are stacked circular rings (*feline* esophagus), strictures, linear furrowing, and white papules (eosinophilic micro-abscesses)

Tx/Mgmt:
1. Topical steroids (i.e., fluticasone or budesonide) and elimination diet
2. Refractory cases may benefit from oral prednisone or esophageal dilation

Inflammatory Bowel Disease

Definition:

Inflammatory bowel disease (IBD) is the collective term to for Crohn disease (CD) and ulcerative colitis (UC). The etiology of both is poorly understood and their management is quite similar. See Table 8.3 for differences between CD and UC. In general, CD and UC share elements of presentation and treatment, such as:

Clinical Presentation: Abdominal pain, diarrhea, blood, and mucus in stool. Other relevant findings are joint involvement, uveitis, erythema nodosum, and pyoderma

TABLE 8.3 Differences Between Crohn Disease and Ulcerative Colitis

	Crohn Disease	Ulcerative Colitis
Epidemiology	Children > adults, Jews > non-Jews, smoking is a risk factor	Smoking is protective, lower incidence if appendectomy <20 years old
Location	May occur anywhere along the GI tract, most commonly affects ileum	Rectum with continuous extension into L colon
Depth	Transmural	Mucosa and submucosa
Macroscopic findings	Thick wall, narrow lumen, aphthous ulcers, skip lesions, strictures, fistulas, "*cobble-stone*" pattern	Pseudopolyps, ulceration, hemorrhage
Microscopic findings	Noncaseating granulomas and lymphoid aggregates	Ulcers and crypt abscesses; dysplasia/cancer may be present. Mononuclear infiltration isolated to mucosa
Clinical cues	RLQ colicky pain, diarrhea, and weight loss. Ulcers in oral mucosa. Perianal fistulae	Left-sided cramping, diarrhea with blood and mucus, fever, and tenesmus. Non-GI: primary sclerosing cholangitis, HLA B27 positive arthritis. p-ANCA antibodies present (>45% of cases)
Complications	Anal fistulas, calcium oxalate renal stones (increased absorption of oxalate through inflamed mucosa), malabsorption, megaloblastic (B_{12}) anemia	Mortality rate 50% Toxic megacolon and adenocarcinoma
Treatment	TNF inhibitors for fistulas and surgery for bowel obstruction	Total colectomy with ileostomy can be curative

GI, Gastrointestinal; *HLA*, human leukocyte antigen; *p-ANCA*, perinuclear anti-neutrophil cytoplasmic antibodies; *RLQ*, right lower quadrant; *TNF*, tumor necrosis factor.

gangrenosum. Erythema nodosum is a panniculitis characterized by tender, erythematous nodules symmetrically involving the lower extremities. Pyoderma gangrenosum begins as a pustule that evolves into an ulcer with rolled, undermined borders.

Tx/Mgmt:
1. Steroids for acute episodes
2. Other immunosuppressants (azathioprine/6-MU) are used to wean off steroids
3. Sulfasalazine and mesalamine for maintenance and long-term therapy
4. Any form of IBD is associated with an increased risk of developing colon cancer. A colonoscopy is required after 10 years with IBD

Crohn Disease

Buzz Words: Skip lesions on colonoscopy + noncaseating granulomas + *string*-sign in terminal ileum from narrowing

Clinical Presentation: Postprandial diarrhea, weight loss, low-grade fever, abdominal pain, and palpable abdominal masses. Viscus perforation, perianal fistula, fissures, and abscesses are characteristic (help differentiate from ulcerative colitis).

PPx: Avoid smoking.

MoD: Segmental, transmural inflammation that can occur anywhere along the GI tract. The terminal ileum is the most commonly affected segment. Fistulae develop from transmural granulomas; these can form between intestines, into the bladder, or through the skin. Immune-mediated free radical damage to the cells of the GI tract. May be triggered by pathogens such as *Mycobacterium paratuberculosis*, *Pseudomonas*, and *Listeria*. A frameshift mutation of the NOD2/CAR15 gene predisposes to CD.

99 AR

Crohn disease (Crohn disease)— symptoms and pathophysiology

99 QUICK TIPS

If the patient has sclerosing cholangitis in the question stem, she/he also has UC.

Dx:
1. FOBT
2. Colonocopy + biopsy

Tx/Mgmt: Anti-tumor necrosis factor (TNF)-alpha drugs (adalimumab, infliximab, etanercept) are used for when fistulae occur. Antibiotics, such as ciprofloxacin or metronidazole, are used for perianal disease; these are preferred due to their additional anti-inflammatory effect.

Ulcerative Colitis

Buzz Words: IBD symptomatology with tenesmus and rectal urgency, *lead-pipe* radiographical appearance, **sclerosing cholangitis**

Clinical Presentation: Young woman with diarrhea, bright red blood per rectum, vague abdominal cramping, and tenesmus

PPx: N/A

MoD: Continuous and circumferential mucosal inflammation that begins in the rectum and ascends the GI tract; usually confined to the colon

Dx:

1. FOBT
2. Colonoscopy + biopsy

Tx/Mgmt:

1. Initial management of mild presentation is with 5-ASA enema, steroid (hydrocortisone) foams, or suppositories
2. Resistant cases should be managed with systemic steroids (oral prednisone)
3. Colectomy and ileostomy can be curative

Ulcerative colitis—definition, symptoms, and causes

Microscopic Colitis

Buzz Words: Chronic diarrhea + negative stool cultures + normal appearing colonic mucosa

Clinical Presentation: Inflammatory disease characterized by chronic watery diarrhea. Other symptoms are fecal urgency, fecal incontinence, and abdominal pain. Most commonly occurs in middle-aged women.

PPx: Discontinue medications associated with microscopic colitis (nonsteroidal antiinflammatory drugs [NSAIDs], aspirin, PPIs, ranitidine, sertraline, clozapine, to name a few).

MoD: Multifactorial disease with poorly understood pathogenesis

Dx: Mucosa appears normal on colonoscopy. Diagnosis established by biopsy.

Tx/Mgmt:

1. Budesonide ± cholestyramine (depending on initial response)
2. Anti-TNF agents may be used for patients with disease refractory to treatment

Toxic Megacolon

Buzz Words: Toxic-appearing patient with altered sensorium and abdominal distention

Clinical Presentation: Severe bloody diarrhea, abdominal distention, tenderness, fever, tachycardia, and shock

PPx: Earlier management of etiologic condition

MoD: May occur as a complication of IBD (UC > CD), ischemia, volvulus, diverticulitis, infectious colitis, or obstructive colon cancer.

Dx: Megacolon can be identified by abdominal film shows dilation of the R colon >6 cm in diameter, loss of haustral markings, and mucosal ulcerations. Toxic megacolon = colonic dilation + systemic involvement.

Tx/Mgmt:
1. Fluid replacement, management of electrolytes abnormalities, initiation of broad-spectrum antibiotics (vancomycin if *C difficile* is the culprit), IV steroids, bowel rest, and decompression (nasogastric/orogastric tube)
2. Failure with medical therapy requires a subtotal colectomy with end-ileostomy

Neoplasms

Benign Neoplasms

Polyps

Gastric Polyps

Buzz Words: Mucosal outgrowth

Clinical Presentation: Asymptomatic presentation, found incidentally in the majority of cases. Important association with *Helicobacter pylori* chronic infection. Hyperplastic polyps are the most common, have a hamartomatous architecture, and have no malignant potential. Adenomatous polyps are neoplastic and have potential for malignant transformation.

PPx: N/A

MoD: Mucosal protuberance. Complication of chronic gastritis and achlorhydria.

Dx: EGD/biopsy

Tx/Mgmt:
1. All gastric polyps should be biopsied and complete resection should be attempted
2. Triple therapy for *H. pylori*

Small and Large Bowel Polyps

Buzz Words: Mucosal outgrowth

Clinical Presentation: Usually asymptomatic, but may twist around their own stalk and bleed, cause tenesmus if they are in the rectum, or produce intestinal obstruction of they are large

PPx: N/A

MoD: Mucosal protuberance from the normally flat mucosa. Nonneoplastic polyps are usually classified as hyperplastic, mucosal, inflammatory, hamartomatous, or submucosal.

Dx: Colonoscopy with biopsy of all the lesions.

Tx/Mgmt:
1. Endoscopic resection should be attempted
2. Surveillance should be repeated every 5–10 years in patients with nonneoplastic polyps

Oral Leukoplakia

Buzz Words: White plaques in the oral cavity that do not scrape off with a tongue depressor

Clinical Presentation: White lesions that arise in trauma-prone regions of the oral cavity. The risk of progression to squamous cell carcinoma is 20% within 10 years.

PPx: Avoid consumption of tobacco products.

MoD: Precancerous lesion of the oral mucosa that has a strong association with the human papillomavirus (HPV).

Dx:
1. Clinical diagnosis
2. Lesions should be biopsied to document the degree of dysplasia

Tx/Mgmt: Topical retinoids might aid in regression of the lesion.

Oral Cancer

Squamous Cell Carcinoma

Buzz Words: Nonhealing ulcer or nodule in oral cavity

Clinical Presentation: Squamous cell carcinoma (SCC) manifests as papules, plaques, or nodules, which may be associated with hyperkeratosis, ulceration, or hyperpigmentation. It is most commonly located on the lower lip, the floor of the mouth, and the lateral border of the tongue. It metastasizes to the super jugular node.

PPx: Known risk factors are light-colored skin, HPV (most common, vaccination is protective), use of tobacco products, alcohol abuse (synergistic with tobacco), irritation from dentures, and lichen planus.

MoD: Erythroplakia and oral leukoplakia are precursor lesions. It usually develops in sites of chronic inflammation or scarring.

Dx: Biopsy

Tx/Mgmt: Surgery ± chemoradiation depending on stage

Salivary Gland Neoplasm

Buzz Words: Mucoepidermoid carcinoma + Bells palsy

Clinical Presentation: Painless mass or swelling arising from a salivary gland. May manifest signs of peripheral facial nerve involvement (Bell palsy). Tumors of the submandibular and sublingual are more likely than parotid to be malignant.

PPx: Avoid exposure to radiation.

MoD: Mucoepidermoid carcinoma is the most common malignant tumor of the salivary glands. Composed of mucinous and squamous cells. It usually arises from parotid and involves CN-VII (facial nerve).

Dx:
1. Fine-needle aspiration (FNA) or US-guided core needle biopsy
2. As with any other tumor, imaging studies (i.e., CT, magnetic resonance imaging [MRI], positron emission tomography [PET]/CT) aid in staging and assessment of surgical candidacy

Tx/Mgmt: Surgical resection for region-confined lesions ± radiation. Patients who are not considered adequate surgical candidates should receive definitive radiation therapy.

Barrett Esophagus

gg AR
NEJM Barrett esophagus review

Buzz Words: Gland with different types of epithelium, goblet cells in esophageal epithelium

Clinical Presentation: Similar to GERD, no difference in symptoms. Found when performing EGD and mucosal biopsies. Complications include stricture formation and glandular dysplasia with increased risk for adenocarcinoma.

PPx: Adequate treatment GERD and dietary modifications (less coffee, wine, mints, etc.).

MoD: Premalignant lesion of the distal esophagus caused by long-standing GERD (years). Constant exposure to gastric acid induces metaplasia. Nonkeratinized, stratified, squamous epithelium (normal) to columnar, secretory epithelium (intestinal).

Dx: EGD with mucosal biopsy in the setting of long-standing GERD.

Tx/Mgmt: PPI and repeat scoping q2–3 years for early detection of adenocarcinoma.

Esophageal Cancer

Presentation of esophageal cancer is similar for both SCC and adenocarcinoma. Surgery alone is recommended for superficial esophageal adenocarcinoma or SCC. The 5-year survival rate for stage I is only 50%–70%. The tri-modality approach (chemoradiation followed by surgery) has proven to be superior to surgery alone. Definitive chemoradiation is a reasonable approach for patients who are not surgical candidates. The 5-year survival rate for stage IV is generally <5%.

Squamous Cell Carcinoma

Buzz Words: Nodular mass with central area of ulceration

Clinical Presentation: Dysphagia to solids, weight loss, anemia, nontender supraclavicular nodes. May also manifest hemoptysis (tracheal invasion), hoarseness (RLN compression), odynophagia, hypercalcemia (PTHrP secretion similar to small-cell carcinoma in the lung). Lesions in the proximal ⅔ of esophagus (but may also occur in distal third).

PPx: Avoid known risk factors; smoking, alcohol, achalasia, caustic injuries, HPV infection, and nitrosamine exposure.

MoD: Poor prognosis, overall 5-year survival rate is 13%.

Dx:

1. EGD with biopsy
2. CT scan and endoscopic ultrasonography are useful for initial staging of the tumor. Integrated PET/CT scans are warranted for patient with metastasis

Tx/Mgmt: *Stated before*

Adenocarcinoma

Buzz Words: Raised lesion at the junction of the distal esophagus and proximal stomach

Clinical Presentation: White middle-aged male with dysphagia, weight loss, and anemia. Lesions in the distal ⅓ of the esophagus.

PPx: Adequate management of GERD

MoD: Barrett esophagus is a significant risk factor; other risk factors are smoking and high body mass index. Involvement of celiac and perihepatic nodes is more common than in SCC. *H. pylori* does not increase the risk of developing adenocarcinoma.

Dx: Tumors >5 cm away from EGD are considered gastric adenocarcinoma.

Tx/Mgmt: *Stated before*

Gastrinoma and Zollinger-Ellison Syndrome

Buzz Words: Multiple peptic ulcers or ulcer in unusual locations + recurrent epigastric pain refractory to PPI

Clinical Presentation: Patient having recurrent epigastric pain and diarrhea refractory to treatment with PPI

PPx: N/A

MoD: Tumor arising from enteroendocrine gastrin-producing cells in the pancreas and/or small intestine. Hypergastrinemia results in an excessive amount of gastric acid production, which accounts for ulcers and diarrhea.

Dx:

1. Serum gastrin level after the patient has been off PPIs for at least a week

2. Secretin stimulation test to differentiate gastrinoma and other causes of hypergastrinemia
3. Somatostatin receptor scintigraphy localizes and helps stage the tumor

Most common endoscopic finding is a solitary ulcer in the first portion of the duodenum, although multiple ulcers in unusual locations are also common.

Tx/Mgmt:
1. PPIs, octreotide, and surgical excision
2. Screen for multiple endocrine neoplasia type 1 (MEN1) syndrome

Carcinoid Tumors

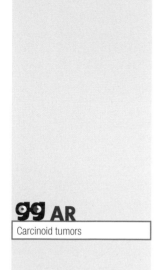

99 AR
Carcinoid tumors

Buzz Words: Flushing + diarrhea + wheezing + R-sided valvular disease

Clinical Presentation: Carcinoid syndrome is the most common manifestation; described as flushing, cramps, diarrhea (from hypermotility), intermittent wheezing, dyspnea, telangiectasia, and R-sided valvular disease (i.e., tricuspid regurgitation or pulmonary stenosis). Foregut and hindgut carcinoid tumors invade but rarely metastasize, while midgut carcinoid tumors invade and metastasize. The most common sites are the vermiform appendix (40% of cases) and terminal ileum.

PPx: N/A

MoD: The small bowel is the most common site of carcinoid tumors; however, these do not cause carcinoid syndrome because serotonin is metabolized by first-pass metabolism in the liver. Metastasis of the primary intestinal carcinoid to the liver or primary lung or ovarian carcinoid tumor results in carcinoid syndrome.

Dx:
1. Urine levels of 5-hydroxyindoleacetic acid
2. Abdominal CT scan to find metastasis
3. Neurosecretory granules visible on electron microscopy
4. Bright yellow tumor

Tx/Mgmt:
1. Octreotide to manage diarrhea and flushing
2. Surgical resection of primary tumor ± chemotherapy for metastatic disease

Gastrointestinal Stromal Tumors

Buzz Words: >40 year old + skin hyperpigmentation + dysphagia. Path reveals mesenchymal spindle-cell neoplasm + CD117-positive

Clinical Presentation: Varies with the site of lesion, the depth of penetration, and the stage of tumor progression. Most common age group is >40 years old, and the most common site is the stomach. Some of these might involve dysphagia or skin hyperpigmentation, or be accompanied by paragangliomas.

PPx: N/A

MoD: Mutation of *c-kit* proto-oncogene which activates KIT, a receptor tyrosine kinase. Gastrointestinal stromal tumors have a broad array of behaviors from benign to malignant aggressive tumors.

Dx:
1. Contrast-enhanced CT for screening and staging
2. Biopsy (endoscopic US-guided FNA) only recommended when metastatic disease is suspected or if preoperative imatinib is considered
3. Fluorodeoxyglucose (FDG)-PET is the best method to assess for metastatic disease

Tx/Mgmt:
1. Surgical resection of any tumor ≥2 cm in size through visceral resection; regional lymphadenectomy is not warranted
2. Imatinib (TK inhibitor) may be used as initial therapy for locally advanced or borderline resectable tumors

Stomach

Adenocarcinoma

Buzz Words: *Signet ring* cells + Sister Mary Joseph nodule

Clinical Presentation: Epigastric pain, weight loss, vomit ± melena. Increased incidence in Japanese and blood group A individuals. Most commonly located in lesser curvature (~50% of tumors), followed by cardia, body and fundus. Paraneoplastic skin findings: seborrheic keratosis (*Leser-Trélat* sign) and acanthosis nigricans.

PPx: Modifiable risk factors are dietary (high-sodium and low vegetable, smoked foods, nitrosamines) and substance abuse (i.e., alcohol and smoking). Adequate management of *H. pylori* infection is protective.

MoD: Gastric ulcer, adenomatous polyps, type A chronic atrophic gastritis, and intestinal metaplasia are associated with a higher risk of gastric cancer.

Dx: Endoscopic ultrasound-guided FNA to biopsy lesion, CT scan for staging. Serum tumor markers (i.e., CEA and CA-125) provide little to the management. Most common sites of metastasis are liver, lung, and ovaries. Hematogenous spread of signet ring cells to ovaries produce Krukenberg tumors.

Tx/Mgmt: Surgery, radiation, and chemotherapy. Open total gastrectomy is preferred for tumors involving the proximal ⅓ of the stomach, while a distal gastrectomy can be performed for tumors in the distal ⅔ of the stomach. The prognosis is poor prognosis. The 5-year survival is 10%–15%.

Gastric Lymphoma

Buzz Words: Sheets of neoplastic small lymphoid cells in gastric wall, lymphoepithelial lesions

Clinical Presentation: Epigastric pain, anorexia, weight loss, nausea, vomit, occult GI bleed, and early satiety. The majority are non-Hodgkin lymphomas with the stomach as the most common site (70% of cases), followed by small bowel, colon, rectum, and esophagus.

PPx: N/A

MoD: Gastric lymphomas are divided into extranodal marginal zone B cell lymphoma of mucosa-associated lymphoid tissue (i.e., MALToma) and diffuse large B cell lymphoma (DLBL).

Dx:

1. EGD findings
2. Characteristic translocation t(11;18) and fusion protein IAP2(API2)/MALT1
3. Neoplastic cells will be positive for B-cell markers (i.e., CD19, CD20, CD22)

Tx/Mgmt:

1. For patients with *H. pylori*-positive MALToma eradication therapy (Table 8.4) could induce regression in 50% of cases
2. *H. pylori*-negative MALToma require local radiotherapy. (3) DLBL requires chemotherapy + immunotherapy (i.e., rituximab) ± radiotherapy

TABLE 8.4 Simplified *Helicobacter pylori* Eradication Regimens

Consideration	Duration: 10–14 days
First-line	PPI + clarithromycin 500 mg bid + amoxicillin 1000 mg bid
Penicillin allergy	PPI + clarithromycin 500 mg bid + metronidazole 500 mg bid
Failed any of the regimens above	PPI + bismuth subsalicylate 525 mg qid + metronidazole 250 mg qid + tetracycline 500 mg qld

bid, Twice per day; *PPI,* proton pump inhibitor; *qid,* four times per day.

Colon, Rectum, Anus

Hereditary Colon Cancer Syndromes

Familial Adenomatous Polyposis

Buzz Words: Hundreds of colorectal polyps

Clinical Presentation: Colorectal cancer from malignant transformation of polyps usually develops by 45 years of age. Polyps begin to develop in the second decade with malignant transformation in the fourth decade. Also, there is an increased incidence of duodenal adenomas, duodenal cancer, papillary thyroid cancer, medulloblastomas, desmoid tumors, and congenital hypertrophy of retinal pigment epithelium.

PPx: Pre-implantation genetic diagnosis during preconception counseling

MoD: Inactivation of the adenomatous polyposis coli (APC) tumor suppressor gene on chromosome 5q. Autosomal dominant.

Dx: Genetic testing and counseling for patient and family members

Tx/Mgmt: Aggressive screening for colon (Table 8.5), duodenal, and other extraintestinal cancer is warranted. Eventually all patients will require a total colectomy; indications to perform the procedure include:
- Adenoma with high-grade dysplasia
- Concerning symptoms (i.e., GI bleed, weight loss, etc.)
- Marked increase in polyp number from one exam to the next

Hereditary Nonpolyposis Colon Cancer (Lynch Syndrome)

Buzz Words: Colorectal cancer and/or female reproductive tract cancer + family history + mutated mismatch repair genes

TABLE 8.5 Colonoscopy Screening Recommendations

Group	Recommendation
No risk factors	Age > 50 years old: screen every 10 years
First-degree relative w/ colon cancer	Age > 40 years old or 10 years earlier than family member: screen every 10 years
Hereditary nonpolyposis colon cancer	Age > 25 year old: screen every 1–2 years
Familial adenomatous polyposis	Age > 10: screen every year

Clinical Presentation: Lynch syndrome is the most commonly inherited genetic syndrome that predisposes one to early colorectal cancer. It is a syndrome characterized by mutations to the mismatch repair family (e.g., MLH1, MSH2, MSH6, and PMS2) that is autosomal dominant. There are two types to be aware of: Lynch syndrome I specific for only colorectal cancer (CRC) and Lynch syndrome II, which has all features of Lynch syndrome I with an increased occurrence of other cancers of the female reproductive tract, the GI tract, and the breast, brain, and skin.

PPx: Aspirin has a protective effect against the incidence of cancer in these patients.

MoD: Germline mutation that inactivates DNA mismatch repair genes (MLH1, MSH2, MSH6, PMS2), which causes a microsatellite repeat replication error (i.e., microsatellite instability). This leads to frameshift mutations affecting tumor suppressor genes.

Dx:
1. Family history
2. Loss of staining of mismatch repair proteins on immunohistochemistry

Tx/Mgmt:
1. Early screening for CRC
2. Surgery to remove precancerous lesions
3. Total colectomy with ileorectal anastomosis + yearly endoscopic surveillance for colorectal cancer

Peutz-Jeghers Syndrome (PJS)

Buzz Words: Perioral pigmentation + intestinal polyps

99 AR

Peutz-Jeghers syndrome overview

Clinical Presentation: Hamartomatous polyps predominate in the small intestine. Pigmentation macules on buccal mucosa and lips (95% of cases). Increased risk for colorectal, pancreas, breast, and gynecologic (ovarian sex cord tumors) cancer. Mean age at the time of cancer diagnosis is 42 years old.

PPx: Pre-implantation genetic diagnosis during preconception counseling for individuals with PJS.

MoD: Inactivation of the serine/threonine kinase 11 (STK11) tumor suppressor gene in chromosome 19p. Autosomal dominant inheritance

Dx: Genetic testing for STK11 mutations.

Tx/Mgmt: Aggressive cancer screening.
- GI tract: EGD, video capsule endoscopy, and colonoscopy at 8 years of age; to repeat q3 years if polyps are found.

- Gonads: Annual testicle exam (from birth for men) or pelvic exam + Pap smear (from 21 years of age for women).
- Breast: Monthly breast exams and annual mammograms starting at 18 and 25 years of age, respectively.
- Pancreas: Endoscopic retrograde cholangiopancreatography (ERCP)/magnetic resonance cholangiopancreatography (MRCP) q1–2 years starting at 30 years of age.

Gardner Syndrome

Buzz Words: Supernumerary teeth + bone osteomas + increased retinal pigmentation

Clinical Presentation: Constellation of colonic polyposis + extracolonic lesions. Benign osteomas, desmoid tumors, dental abnormalities, cutaneous lesions, adrenal adenomas, and nasal angiofibromas. Patients are at risk for neoplasms of pancreas, liver, thyroid, gallbladder, and biliary tract.

PPx: Pre-implantation genetic diagnosis during preconception counseling

MoD: Also associated with loss-of-function mutations to the APC gene. Autosomal dominant.

Dx: Genetic testing + clinical association

Tx/Mgmt:
1. Aggressive cancer screening
2. Total colectomy upon any of the indications for FAP

MUTYH-Associated Polyposis

Buzz Words: 10–100 colonic polyps and ruled out APC mutation

Clinical Presentation: Colonic polyposis in individual with >10 adenomatous polyps, which might be accompanied by dental cysts, desmoids, osteomas, or sebaceous hyperplasia. The lifetime risk of colorectal carcinoma is 75%. Also an increased risk for duodenal, ovarian, bladder, thyroid, and skin cancer.

PPx: N/A

MoD: The MUYTH gene codes for a glycosylase involved in DNA (base excision) repair. Autosomal recessive.

Dx: Genetic testing for biallelic germline mutations of MUTYH gene

Tx/Mgmt: Colonoscopy q1–2 years starting at 25 years of age. Same indications for colectomy + ileorectal anastomosis as in FAP (see above).

Biliary Tract

Gallbladder Adenocarcinoma

Buzz Words: Porcelain gallbladder

Clinical Presentation: Patients are usually asymptomatic. Usually affects elderly, Japanese women. A very uncommon but highly fatal malignancy.

PPx: N/A

MoD: Chronic cholecystitis, porcelain gallbladder, and development of gallstones at any point in life increases the risk significantly. Some hereditary neoplastic syndromes, like Gardner and neurofibromatosis, have also been associated.

Dx: CT, endoscopic ultrasound, and MRCP

Tx/Mgmt: Cholecystectomy ± radiation therapy

99 AR

Gallbladder cancer (adenocarcinoma)—signs, symptoms, and causes

Cholangiocarcinoma

Buzz Words: H/o PSC + elevated CEA, AFP or CA-19-9 + palpable gallbladder + elevated bili

Clinical Presentation: Extrahepatic cholestasis, Courvoisier sign (palpable gallbladder), and hepatomegaly. The tumor may be present anywhere along the extrahepatic biliary tract. Most common malignancy of the biliary tree.

PPx: N/A

MoD: Primary sclerosing cholangitis, *Clonorchis sinensis*, exposure to thorium dioxide, choledochal cysts, and Caroli disease are the most common causes of cholangiocarcinoma.

Dx:
1. Liver panel
2. MRI, MRCP, or CT
3. Tumor markers: Carcinoembryonic antigen (CEA), alpha-fetoprotein (AFP) or cancer antigen (CA) 19-9 may be elevated (Table 8.6)

Tx/Mgmt: Surgical resection ± chemoradiation depending on stage

Adenocarcinoma of the Ampulla of Vater

Buzz Words: FAP + acute pancreatitis + jaundice + palpable gallbladder

Clinical Presentation: Similar presentation to cholangiocarcinoma with obstruction of the biliary tree + possible complications from obstruction of the pancreatic ducts (i.e., acute pancreatitis). Males > females. Almost half of the patients have developed lymph node metastasis at the time of diagnosis.

PPx: N/A

TABLE 8.6 Tumor Cancer Markers Versus Type of Cancer

Tumor Cancer Markers	Type of Cancer
CEA	Colon cancer
AFP	HCC
Ferritin	HCC
CA 19-9	Pancreatic cancer
CA-50	Pancreatic cancer
Beta-hCG	Testicular cancer + choriocarcinoma (fast growing cancer of uterus)
CA-125	Ovarian cancer
Neuron-specific enolase	Small cell lung cancer
CA 15-3	Breast cancer

AFP, Alpha-fetoprotein; *CA*, cancer antigen; *CEA*, carcinoembryonic antigen; *HCC*, hepatocellular carcinoma; *hCG*, human chorionic gonadotropin.

MoD: *K-ras* mutations may play a role in pathogenesis. Associated with FAP.

Dx:

1. Liver panel
2. MRI, MRCP, or CT

Tx/Mgmt: Whipple procedure (pancreaticoduodenectomy)

Liver

Cavernous Hemangioma

Buzz Words: Contrast enhancement + mass in liver + asymptomatic

Clinical Presentation: Benign neoplasms of small blood vessel endothelial cells. Most common benign lesion of the liver. Focal, well-circumscribed, encapsulated, hypervascular lesion in liver parenchyma w/ spongy consistency. Can rarely rupture and produce intraperitoneal hemorrhage. No malignant potential.

PPx: Avoid biopsy to PPx against hemorrhage

MoD: Etiology not completely understood. Formed through ectasia of vasculature.

Dx:

1. CT scan w/ contrast
2. MRI or tagged red blood cell (RBC) scan
3. Angiography

Tx/Mgmt:

1. Observation
2. Surgical resection if painful or symptoms suggesting mass effect

Focal Nodular Hyperplasia

Buzz Words: Central scar on CT + asymptomatic + discovered incidentally

Clinical Presentation: Focal nodular hyperplasia is a common nonmalignant hyperplastic response to anomalous arteries. Females > males. Associated to hereditary hemorrhagic telangiectasia (Osler-Weber-Rendu disease). NOT associated with OCP use. No malignant potential. Second most benign liver tumor.

PPx: N/A

MoD: Nonmalignant localized aggregates of rapidly reproducing liver cells.

Dx:
1. CT (central scar, hypervascular mass with AV connections)
2. Angiography
3. Biopsy shows Kupffer cells and sinusoids (vs. hepatic adenoma, which shows glycogen and lipids)

Tx/Mgmt: Treatment is unnecessary in asymptomatic patients, unless the lesion is painful.

Hepatic Adenoma

Buzz Words: Young woman + OCP use + normal AFP + glycogen/lipids on biopsy

Clinical Presentation: Females > males. Most common cause is oral contraceptive use, followed by anabolic steroids and Von Gierke disease.

PPx: Avoid oral contraceptive pills (OCPs).

MoD: Benign epithelial tumor, frequently located in the R hepatic lobe. Highly vascular with a tendency to rupture during pregnancy (growth secondary to hyperestrogenemia) producing intraperitoneal hemorrhage.

Dx: CT scan

Tx/Mgmt:
1. Emergent surgery if ruptured/bleeding
2. Resection if greater than 4 cm or patient desires pregnancy. If less than 4 cm, d/c OCPs and monitor with serial CTs

Hepatocellular Carcinoma

Buzz Words: Cirrhosis + RUQ discomfort + weight loss + elevated AFP + HBV, HCV, aflatoxin, CCl4 exposure

Clinical Presentation: Patient with previously compensated cirrhosis with decompensation (jaundice, encephalopathy, ascites). May also manifest weight loss, early satiety, expending hepatomegaly, and abdominal pain. Production of ectopic hormones such as EPO, PTH-related protein, and insulin-like factor. Lungs are the most common metastatic site. Males > females. Causes in order of frequency: HCV, alcoholic cirrhosis, HBV. Other minor causes of hepatocellular carcinoma (HCC): hemochromatosis, Wilson disease, aflatoxin-B1 (from *Aspergillus*), primary biliary cirrhosis, and α-1 antitrypsin deficiency. Second most common cause of cancer death worldwide (after lung).

PPx: Ultrasound surveillance (q6 months) in patients with high-risk profiles

MoD: Associated to preexisting cirrhosis and states of constant damage repair. Portal and hepatic vein invasion is common.

Dx:

1. Liver panel (elevated AFP, ALP, and GGT)
2. CT and ultrasound would show a lesion with hypervascularity and venous invasion
3. CEA level to r/o mets from colon
4. Laparoscopic u/s gold standard

Tx/Mgmt: Surgery ± chemoradiation depending on stage

99 AR

Malignant liver tumors video—pathophysiology and symptoms

Peritoneal Cancer

Clinical Presentation: Abdominal pain + ascites + weight loss + palpable abdominal mass

PPx: N/A

MoD: Malignant mesothelioma is the most common primary peritoneal cancer. Nonetheless, metastasis and seeding from other tumors (i.e., ovarian) is common.

Dx: Peritoneal lavage through percutaneous technique or at time of surgical exploration. An ultrasound is the imaging study with the highest sensitivity.

Tx/Mgmt: Multimodal therapy that consists of surgical resection to decrease the tumor load (± hysterectomy and b/l salpingo-oophorectomy), intraperitoneal administration of chemotherapy, and hyperthermia

Pancreas

Neoplasms of the pancreas can be divided into two types. First, there are neoplasms of the exocrine pancreas, which do not produce hormones but lead to symptoms 2/2 mass effect. Second, there are neoplasms of the endocrine pancreas (e.g., VIPoma, gastrinoma), which do lead to disorders of hormonal production (Table 8.7).

Exocrine Pancreas, Pancreatic Carcinoma

Buzz Words:

- **Adenocarcinoma of pancreatic head:** Painless jaundice + recently diagnosed diabetes + weight loss +

TABLE 8.7 Endocrine Pancreatic Tumors

Tumor	Summary
Insulinoma (β cells)	Most common islet cell tumor. Association with MEN1 syndrome (80% of tumors). Fasting hypoglycemia. High levels of insulin and C-peptide. Treatment: surgical excision of mass. Streptozotocin may also be used (highly toxic to β and δ cells)
Glucagonoma (α cells)	Hyperglycemia and rash (**necrolytic migratory erythema**) are the most common manifestations. Treatment: surgical excision. Octreotide may also be used.
Somatostatinoma (δ cells)	Somatostatin inhibits the effects of gastrin, CCK, GIP, and secretin. Manifestation: achlorhydria, cholelithiasis, steatorrhea, and DM. Treatment: surgical excision of mass. Streptozotocin may also be used (highly toxic to β and δ cells).
VIPoma	Excessive secretion of vasoactive intestinal peptide which produces secretory diarrhea (pancreatic cholera) and achlorhydria. Dx: metabolic acidosis due to loss of HCO_3 in stool and hypokalemia Treatment: surgical excision. Octreotide may also be used.
Zollinger-Ellison (Gastrinoma)	Peptic ulcer refractory to PPI and triple therapy + high gastrin even after secretin administration and calcium infusion Dx: (1) CT, (2) somatostatin radionuclide scan Tx/Mgmt: (1) Surgical removal, (2) omeprazole for mets

CCK, Cholecystokinin; *CT*, computed tomography; *DM*, diabetes mellitus; *MEN1*, multiple endocrine neoplasia type 1; *PPI*, proton pump inhibitor.

abdominal pain + gastric outlet obstruction + large, nontender gallbladder + itching + migratory thrombophlebitis
- **Malignant extrahepatic biliary obstruction:** Painless jaundice + palpable nontender gall bladder
- **Cystic adenocarcinoma:** Mass in pancreas + subtle symptoms + elevated CEA + no weight loss or diabetes
  - Cystic cancer of the pancreas can be **resected** and have a much better survival rate!
  - Cystadenoma of the pancreas → distal pancreatectomy

- **Migratory thrombophlebitis (Trousseau sign):** Venous thrombosis in different places+ hypercoagulability + pancreatic mass

Clinical Presentation:
Patient (male > female) in the seventh to eighth decade of life with epigastric pain that radiates to the back and weight loss ± signs of biliary obstruction. Metastasis occurs to Virchow node (left supraclavicular node) and periumbilical region (Sister Mary Joseph sign). Risk factors include smoking, chronic pancreatitis, hereditary pancreatitis, diabetes mellitus, high saturated fat diet, obesity, and cirrhosis.

PPx: N/A

MoD: Adenocarcinoma has a high association with *K-ras* gene mutation and mutation of tumor suppressor genes p16 and p53. Most cases (65%) occur at the head of the pancreas.

Dx:
1. CT scan
2. FNA biopsy
3. CA19-9 tumor marker

Tx/Mgmt: Surgery (Whipple procedure aka pancreaticoduodenectomy) ± chemoradiation

99 AR

Whipple procedure = resection of pancreas, duodenum, common bile duct, and distal stomach

Signs, Symptoms and Ill-Defined Disorders

Upper Gastrointestinal Bleeding

Buzz Words: Bloody vomit + melena

Clinical Presentation: Melena, nausea, vomiting bright red blood, abdominal pain, abdominal distention. Upper GI bleeding is a potential source for massive blood loss and hemorrhagic shock.

PPx: N/A

MoD: Melena is dark, foul-smelling feces, which occur from protein denaturation after having hemoglobin exposed to gastric acid and pepsin. The source of hemorrhage is proximal to the ligament of Treitz. Major causes of upper GI bleed (GIB) are: esophageal varices, esophageal tear, peptic ulcer disease (PUD), AV malformations, and tumors.

Dx: EGD. Rebound tenderness in a patient with upper GIB can suggest bowel perforation.

Tx/Mgmt: Nil by mouth (NPO), provide supportive measures, replace lost intravascular volume, place nasogastric tube to decompress bowel, manage coagulopathies,

QUICK TIPS

Classically any hemorrhage originates proximal to the ligament of Treitz has been considered an upper GI bleed, while any source of hemorrhage has been considered to produce a lower GI bleed.

gg AR

Distinguishing upper and lower GI bleeding review article

and discontinue any anticoagulants or antiplatelets. Provide blood transfusions to maintain adequate oxygen carrying capacity (ideally hemoglobin >7.0 g/dL).

Lower Gastrointestinal Bleeding

Buzz Words: Hematochezia

Clinical Presentation: Blood per rectum. The color of the blood differs from depending on the source of hemorrhage. Blood from the left colon appears bright red once it comes out of the rectum. Blood from the right column gets partially digested by gut flora and portrays a brown color.

PPx: N/A

MoD: Source of hemorrhage distal to the ligament of Treitz. Rarely do patients develop hemorrhagic shock from lower GI bleed.

Dx: Colonoscopy is the best initial test.

Tx/Mgmt: Provide supportive measures, replace lost intravascular volume, manage coagulopathies, and discontinue any anticoagulants or antiplatelets.

Constipation

Clinical Presentation: Lack of defecation or flatus, usually with abdominal distention and pain

PPx: Drugs that can cause constipation are: CCB, opiates, tricyclic antidepressants, and calcium carbonate.

MoD: Decreased intestinal motility

Dx: Rule out hypothyroidism (i.e., serum thyroid-stimulating hormone [TSH]).

Tx/Mgmt: Patient education on most common causes for constipation, behavior modification, dietary modifications, laxatives, and/or enema

Diarrhea

Clinical Presentation: High fecal output (i.e., >250 grams of stool/day)

PPx: N/A

MoD: The three types of diarrhea are synthesized in Table 8.8.

Dx: Severe infectious diarrhea is a combination of blood in stool, volume depletion, abdominal pain/tenderness, and fever.

Tx/Mgmt: Most anti-motility agents can be used if there is no blood and no fever. Antibiotics are indicated in *severe* infectious diarrhea.

TABLE 8.8 Types of Diarrhea

	Osmotic	Secretory	Invasive
Characteristics	Osmotically active substance in the lumen High volume No inflammatory process	GI epithelial cells secrete ions to draw water along with them High volume	Invasion and damage of enterocytes Low volume Blood and leukocytes
Differential	>100 mOsm/kg	<50 mOsm/kg	Stool antigens, culture, and O&P
Common causes	Giardiasis, osmotic laxatives, disaccharidase deficiency	Enterotoxins, increased serotonin levels (carcinoid syndrome)	*Campylobacter*, *Shigella*, *Entamoeba histolytica*

GI, Gastrointestinal; *O&P*, ova and parasite.

Nausea and Vomiting

Buzz Words: Contraction alkalosis

Clinical Presentation: Nausea, vomiting, and rumination

PPx: N/A

MoD:

The physiologic causes of nausea can be synthesized into three different pathways.

- GI tract—$5HT_3$ receptors stimulated by mechanical and chemical irritants
- Chemoreceptor trigger zone (area postrema)—D_2 receptors stimulated by emetogenic substances in the cerebrospinal fluid
- Vestibular system—H_1 and M_1 receptors stimulated by motion

Vomiting produces loss of volume and protons (for every H^+ there is a molecule of HCO_3^- generated in blood), which produces a metabolic alkalosis, commonly referred to as contraction alkalosis, which is responsive to an infusion of saline.

Dx: Symptom referred by the patient

Tx/Mgmt:

1. $5HT_3$ receptor antagonists (-setrons) for nausea produced from the GI tract
2. D_2 receptor antagonists (metoclopramide and domperidone) for nausea produced from the area postrema
3. Antihistamines and antimuscarinic aid in nausea induced by motion sickness

Disorders of the Salivary Gland and Esophagus

Disorders of the Salivary Glands

Stones

Buzz Words: Pain and swelling of the salivary glands

Clinical Presentation: Pain and swelling of the salivary glands

PPx: Avoid dehydration.

MoD: Caused by dehydration. Submandibular glands are the most commonly obstructed (80%–90%) by single stones within Wharton duct. Anticholinergic medications are associated with the development of stones.

Dx:

1. Clinical diagnosis (e.g., palpation)
2. High-resolution CT if too small

Tx/Mgmt:

1. Supportive (hydration, lozenges to stimulate saliva production)
2. NSAIDs
3. Stones less than 2 mm will probably pass on their own

Sialadenitis

Buzz Words: Erythema and purulent drainage of salivary glands

Clinical Presentation: Elderly patient with pain, swelling, and tenderness of the oral cavity. May complain of mouth dryness. On exam erythema and purulent drainage may be identified.

PPx: Same as with stones; avoid dehydration

MoD: Infection of a salivary gland is usually preceded by the formation of a stone causing obstruction and stasis of secretions. The submandibular gland is most often involved. Chronic sialadenitis may cause gland atrophy and a significant decrease in volume of the saliva produced.

Dx:

1. Clinical presentation
2. CT scan

Tx/Mgmt: Dicloxacillin or cephalexin

Suppurative Parotitis

Buzz Words: Discharge of purulent material during examination of the buccal mucosa

Clinical Presentation: Elderly patient with pain and swelling at the angle of the mandible and periauricular region accompanied by fever and chills. During palpation of the parotid gland purulent discharge may be expressed from Stensen duct.

PPx: N/A

MoD: These infections are most commonly polymicrobial, and the pathogens most commonly isolated are *S. aureus*, *S. viridans*, and anaerobes.

Dx: Clinical diagnosis

Tx/Mgmt: Fluid replacement and IV antibiotics (i.e., nafcillin, metronidazole, or vancomycin when MRSA is suspected)

Esophagus

Achalasia

Buzz Words:

- Dysphagia + swallowing liquids harder than solids + Chagas disease + birds beak sign + patient sits straight to swallow liquids
- **Carcinoma:** Dysphagia + swallowing solids harder than liquids
- **Plummer-Vinson** (increased esophageal cancer risk): **Esophageal web** + atrophic oral mucosa + spoon-shaped brittle nails (koilonychia) + Fe deficiency anemia

Clinical Presentation: Usually the patient is less than 50 years old, who has nonprogressive difficulty swallowing for both solids and liquids, has weight loss, and heartburn that is unresponsive to PPI therapy. This can be noticed when there is difficulty passing a scope into the stomach during upper endoscopy.

PPx: N/A

MoD: Degeneration of the Auerbach ganglion cells resulting in failed relaxation of the LES and the absence of peristalsis in the proximal part of the esophagus with food retention

Dx:

1. Barium swallow shows *bird's beak* narrowing in the lower third
2. Manometry (confirms Dx)
3. Chest x-ray (CXR) can show megaesophagus
4. Endoscopy to r/o Plummer-Vinson syndrome (would reveal fibrous web below cricopharyngeus muscle)

Tx/Mgmt:

1. CCBs + nitrates
2. Botox injections
3. Repeat dilatations
4. Heller myotomy
5. Fundoplication if GERD

Bird's beak appearance on x-ray

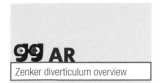

Zenker Diverticulum

Buzz Words: Mucosal outpouching in the hypopharynx + halitosis + elderly patient

Clinical Presentation: Male patient more than 60 years old with oropharyngeal dysphagia, food regurgitation, and halitosis from decomposing food inside the diverticulum

PPx: Avoid nasogastric tube 2/2 high risk of perforation

MoD: Pseudodiverticulum (does not contain *muscularis* layer) within Killian triangle (posterior hypopharyngeal mucosa) secondary to weakness in cricopharyngeal muscles

Dx: Barium swallow

Tx/Mgmt: Cricopharyngeal myotomy, diverticulectomy, flexible or rigid endoscopy

Esophagitis/Esophageal Reflux

Buzz Words: Postprandial "heartburn" or chest discomfort/epigastric pain + chronic cough + symptomatic relief with antacids

Clinical Presentation: The most common symptoms are postprandial retrosternal/epigastric pain, regurgitation, and chronic cough. Alarm symptoms that are concerning for malignancy are weight loss, dysphagia, bleeding, anemia, and recurrent vomiting. Can lead to Barrett esophagus.

PPx:
1. Elevate head of bed
2. Weight loss, smoking cessation, avoidance of caffeine, chocolate, spicy foods, fatty foods, carbonated beverages, and peppermint from the diet

MoD: Abnormally relaxed LES, which allows reflux of stomach contents to cause symptoms and complications. These contents can make way to the pharynx and larynx.

Dx:
1. EKG to r/o myocardial infarction (MI)
2. Esophageal pH monitoring (or nuclear scintigraphy)
3. Endoscopy (when diagnosis is fairly certain)
4. Barium swallow to plan for surgery (looking for location of gastroesophageal junction [GEJ] in relation to diaphragm)
5. Biopsy to r/o complications from esophagitis
6. Manometry to r/o motility d/o
7. Gastric emptying study (to r/o stomach d/o)

Tx/Mgmt:
1. Lifestyle modification
2. PPI
3. Surgery with Nissen fundoplication, resection, or endoscopic therapy

Esophagitis, Pill

Buzz Words: Epigastric pain s/p taking a pill

Clinical Presentation: Patient who lies a lot on their back with complaints of dysphagia, odynophagia, or chest pain. Medications that most frequently produce esophagitis are aspirin, alprenolol, bisphosphonates, iron compounds, NSAIDs, potassium chloride, quinidine, and tetracycline.

PPx: Avoid these medications in patients prone to develop esophageal stasis.

MoD: Produced by prolonged mucosal contact with the contents of the medication. Any condition that prolongs or produces stasis of food in the esophagus is a direct risk of suffering from pill esophagitis.

Dx: EGD with biopsy to rule out other etiologies

Tx/Mgmt: Stop causative medication and use acid suppressants to avoid GERD, which might be exacerbating the injury.

Mallory-Weiss Syndrome

Buzz Words: Repeated painful emesis 2/2 alcohol consumption + hematemesis + epigastric

Clinical Presentation: Mallory-Weiss tears occur is a longitudinal tear of the mucosa in the GEJ 2/2 bouts of emesis from alcohol consumption. Patients typically present with epigastric pain and signs/symptoms of acute upper GIB.

PPx: N/A

MoD: Increased intraabdominal pressure → Longitudinal mucosal tear in the proximal stomach or distal esophagus from severe retching

Dx: EGD to document the tear

Tx/Mgmt:
1. Active bleeding at time of EGD should be attended to (i.e., ligation or thermal coagulation)
2. Most tears will heal with supportive therapy and acid suppression. Hypovolemia should be corrected aggressively
3. Hospitalization for observation

Paraesophageal (Hiatal) Hernia

Buzz Words:
- Retrocardiac air-fluid level + dysphagia + epigastric pain + GEJ displacement on imaging
- Schatzki ring: >65 + dysphagia + lower esophageal stricture + associated with hiatal hernia

Clinical Presentation: Most patients are asymptomatic. Those who do have symptoms may have epigastric or retrosternal pain, nausea, retching, and postprandial fullness.

PPx: N/A

MoD: Often the precise mechanism of development of the hernia is elusive. Paraesophageal hernias are classified depending on the abdominal organs protruding through the hiatus:

- Type I—sliding hernia, fundus remains in place while GEJ is displaced into the thorax. Most common (90%)
- Type II—"true" paraesophageal hernia, GEJ remains in the place while the fundus is displaced into the thorax
- Type III—both the GEJ and fundus are displaced through the hiatus
- Type IV—wider defect where organs other than the stomach are displaced into the thorax

Dx:

1. CXR
2. Flexible endoscopy (r/o Schatzki ring, which is a thin circumferential scar in lower esophagus 2/2 trauma; tx with antireflux surgery)

Tx/Mgmt:

1. Type 1 hiatal hernias → conservative
2. Types 2–4 → surgical management

Diffuse Esophageal Spasm

Buzz Words:

- Mild inflammation of esophagus + prolonged high-amplitude contractions + high lower esophageal sphincter pressure + relaxation on swallowing
- Dysphagia worse with hot and cold liquids + chest pain that feels like MI + no regurgitation

Clinical Presentation: Diffuse esophageal spasm (DES) is a disorder of episodic chest pain and trouble swallowing that is exacerbated by hot and cold liquids.

PPx: N/A

MoD: Inflammation of esophagus → esophageal contractions

Dx:

1. Endoscopy
2. Manometry
3. Barium swallow (corkscrew esophagus)

Tx/Mgmt:

1. CCB + nitrates
2. Myotomy length

Disorders of the Stomach, Small Intestine, Colon, Rectum, Anus

Stomach

Important definitions to know:

- **Gastritis** is inflammation of the gastric mucosa of any etiology, including from *H. pylori* and NSAIDs. Can present with dyspepsia and GI bleeding and is diagnosed with neutrophil infiltration of the glands through endoscope.
- **Gastroparesis** is delayed gastric emptying that leads to bloating, constipation, nausea, and abdominal discomfort. Often seen in conjunction with diabetes. Can be treated with dietary modifications (small, frequent meals, low in fat, and containing soluble fiber), pro-kinetic agents, like metoclopramide or erythromycin (motilin receptor agonist), and anti-emetics. If refractory to medical management, decompression (gastrostomy) and post-pyloric feeding are considered.

Peptic Ulcer Disease

Buzz Words:

- **Gastric ulcer**: Epigastric/retrosternal pain **exacerbated** by eating
- **Duodenal ulcer**: Epigastric/retrosternal pain **improved** by eating

Clinical Presentation: PUD can occur either in the stomach or duodenum. Food exacerbates the pain of the former but relieves the pain of the latter. In general, PUD patients may experience epigastric pain provoked by eating, abdominal fullness, early satiety, and nausea. For gastric ulcers, patients with blood group A have a higher risk.

For duodenal ulcers, when perforation occurs, the gastroduodenal artery is the most commonly injured vessel; the patient will manifest signs and symptoms of acute abdomen and upper GIB. There is an increased risk in patients with MEN1 syndrome.

PPx: Avoid NSAIDs and smoking.

MoD: *H. pylori* (G-tennis racket shaped organism) → impaired mucosal defense (gastric ulcer) or hyperacid secretion (duodenal ulcer) (Table 8.9)

Dx:

1. Urea breath test (increased CO_2 after urea ingestion because *H. pylori* converts urea to CO_2)
2. Blood antibodies to *H. pylori*.

TABLE 8.9 Comparison Between Gastric and Duodenal Ulcers

	Gastric Ulcers	Duodenal Ulcers
Association with *Helicobacter pylori*	Duodenal > gastric	
Postprandial pain	Exacerbated	Relieved
Blood group commonly associated	Group A	Group O
Frequency of ulcer cases	25%	75%
Location	Lesser curvature of antrum	Anterior portion of first part of duodenum
Vessel involved when bleeding	Left gastric artery	Gastroduodenal artery
Diagnosis	EGD + biopsy	EGD alone
Carcinogenic risk	1%–4%	Almost none

EGD, Esophagogastroduodenoscopy.

3. *H. pylori* in feces
4. Direct biopsy (CLO test) to r/o cancer

Tx/Mgmt:

1. If gastric ulcer: biopsy ulcer, *H. pylori* treatment and avoid NSAIDs for simple ulcers, surgery if complicated
2. If duodenal ulcer: *H. pylori* treatment
   - If atypical, test for serum gastrin. If gastrin is high, administer secretin stimulation test to r/o Zollinger-Ellison syndrome (ZES)

Peptic Ulcer Perforation

Buzz Words: Signs of peritonitis (rebound, guarding) + free air on CXR

Clinical Presentation: Sudden, severe, diffuse abdominal pain, and abdominal rigidity, which may be accompanied by syncope. Exam is relevant for tachycardia, low temperature, weak pulse, and clammy skin.

PPx: Early diagnosis of PUD and adequate management

MoD: Most common sites for perforation are duodenal (60%), antral (20%), and body of the stomach (20%). Release of gastric acid into the peritoneal cavity produces an initial vasoplegic response.

Dx:

1. Upright CXR and abdominal films (±free air)
2. Abdominal CT

Tx/Mgmt:

1. Nasogastric tube insertion, IV fluids, and PP
2. If unstable, emergent operation

Small Intestine and Colon

Appendicitis

Buzz Words: Umbilical pain that migrates to RLQ + acute + leukocytosis + peritoneal signs + fever + **refuses to eat** + neutrophils w/ bands

Clinical Presentation: Patient presents with nausea and vomiting, an aversion to food, and epigastric dull pain that migrates to McBurney point and can have positive Rovsing sign, psoas test, and obturator sign. Diameter of appendix greater than 6 mm in imaging studies. Children and elderly patients may have vague symptoms, which make perforation and rupture more common than in adults. Very high yield. Easy to identify in question stem so expect to be tested on mechanism, diagnostic steps, and management. Intermittent right lower quadrant (RLQ) pain may be gastroenteritis instead.

PPx: N/A

MoD: Obstruction of the lumen of the appendix is the most common cause of inflammation. Fecaliths, undigested seeds, pinworm infections, or lymphoid hyperplasia may be the culprits of obstruction. Once occluded, the epithelial lining continues to secrete mucus until the intraluminal pressure occludes venous outflow. Venous congestion and intraluminal stasis set the stage for bacterial overgrowth and progressive inflammation.

Dx:
1. Clinical presentation
2. Abdominal CT
   a. If pregnant or a child, ultrasound or MRI preferred
3. If the patient is a female in reproductive-age, order serum beta-hCG to r/o ectopic pregnancy. Urinalysis to r/o urinary tract infection.

Tx/Mgmt: Appendectomy. If cancer at base of appendix → right hemicolectomy.

Angiodysplasia

Buzz Words: Lower GIB + small, dilated, thin-walled veins in GI tract + more than 50 years old + aortic stenosis

Clinical Presentation: Patients usually don't notice occult blood loss, although signs and symptoms of a lower GIB might manifest (i.e., hematochezia, melena, and sometimes hematemesis). Second leading cause of lower GIB in patients more than 60 years old.

PPx: N/A

FOR THE WARDS

A normal-appearing appendix during surgical exploration should be removed regardless to avoid future complications.

 AR

Appendicitis—signs, symptoms, and causes

MoD: Ectatic, dilated, thin-walled vessels with tortuous submucosal veins. Most common abnormality of the GI tract. Lesions are commonly found in the cecum and ascending colon.

Dx:
1. CBC, iron studies
2. FOBT
3. Colonoscopy and capsule endoscopy

Tx/Mgmt:
1. Self-limited
2. If bleeding does not stop, epinephrine or coagulation from colonoscopy

Diverticulosis and Diverticulitis

Buzz Words:
- **Acute diverticulitis:** Lower left quadrant (LLQ) acute abdomen + fever + leukocytosis + peritoneal pain
- **Diverticulosis:** LLQ chronic abdominal pain + no signs of acute infection ± signs of lower GIB

Clinical Presentation: Diverticula are sac-like protrusion from the colonic wall that occur 2/2 colonic muscular weakening. Diverticulosis refers to the presence of multiple diverticula in the colon. Diverticulitis refers to the inflammation and infection of these diverticula. The classic patient is more than 50 years old with abdominal pain in LLQ.

Diverticulitis would also present with fever, leukocytosis, and sudden manifestation of symptoms. Common complications of diverticulitis are perforation, abscess, fistula, and obstruction.

PPx: Vegetarian and **high-fiber diets**

MoD: Increased intraluminal pressure in the colon, from constant strain (i.e., constipation), produce an outward bulge at points where blood vessels penetrate the bowel wall. Increasing age is a significant risk factor for the development of diverticula. Diverticulitis occurs when bacterial overgrowth happens within these protrusions.

Sigmoid Diverticulosis Video

Dx:
- Diverticulosis: Colonoscopy and barium enema
- Diverticulitis: Abdominal CT (scope may cause perforation), which allows to distinguish between complicated and uncomplicated disease

Tx/Mgmt:
- Diverticulosis
  - High-fiber diet (most are asymptomatic)
  - If persistent bleeding, angiographic/endoscopic treatment

- Diverticulitis
  - Antibiotic therapy (ciprofloxacin + metronidazole, TMP/SMX + metronidazole, or amoxicillin/clavulanate)
  - Bowel rest with slow re-introduction of enteral nutrition

Diverticula, diverticulosis, & diverticulitis

Hirschsprung Disease

Buzz Words: Neonate + to pass meconium + squirt sign

Clinical Presentation: Bilious emesis, abdominal distention, and failure to pass meconium within 48 hours of birth. May be complicated by enterocolitis, which carries a significant morbidity and mortality in newborns. Increased incidence in Down syndrome, neurofibromatosis 1, MEN2 syndromes, and Waardenburg syndrome.

PPx: N/A

MoD: Incomplete migration of ganglion cells from their origin in the neural crest to the distal rectum

Dx: Tight anal sphincter and squirt sign on digital rectal examination. Suction rectal biopsy (gold standard) taken 2 cm above dentate line shows the absence of ganglion cells.

Tx/Mgmt: Surgical resection of the affected segment

Hirschsprung disease (congenital aganglionic megacolon)

Irritable Colon/Irritable Bowel Syndrome

Buzz Words: Alternating diarrhea and constipation + pain decreased after bowel movement

Clinical Presentation: Nonspecific abdominal pain, diarrhea, constipation. Associated with anxiety. Pain is relieved by a bowel movement and symptoms are less intense at night. Patients are rarely admitted to the hospital. Diagnosis made by Rome III criteria, which includes recurrent abdominal pain or discomfort at least 3 days/month in the last 3 months associated with ≥2 of change in frequency of stool, change in appearance of stool, and symptomatic improvement with defecation.

Rome III diagnostic criteria

PPx: Dietary modification, which consists of the exclusion of gas-producing foods, low consumption of fermentable carbohydrates (FODMAPs = fermentable oligo-, di-, and monosaccharides and polyols), and lactose/gluten avoidance

MoD: Pathophysiology remains uncertain and multiple theories and correlations have been postulated: hypersensitization of visceral afferent nerves, mucosal immune system activation, and small bowel bacteria overgrowth to name a few.

Dx: Rome III criteria

Tx/Mgmt: Fiber and osmotic agents, antispasmodic agents, and TCAs.

Ischemic Bowel

Buzz Words: Air in bowel + dead gut + abdominal pain out of proportion to exam

Clinical Presentation: Commonly occurs in terminally ill patients receiving intensive care. High mortality rate (60%–70%).

PPx: N/A

MoD: Reduced perfusion to the intestine from low cardiac output, arterial occlusion, venous congestion, or spasmodic vasoconstriction.

Dx:

1. Abdominal CT scan to identify signs of regional ischemia and intramural gas bubbles (pneumatosis intestinalis).
2. Rising serum lactate is an early indicator of ischemic bowel.

Tx/Mgmt:

1. Urgent exploratory laparotomy to resect injured segment of bowel.
2. If there are no contraindications, anticoagulants should be initiated to prevent further clot formation.

99 AR

Virtual colonoscopy of patient with sigmoid volvulus

Malnutrition

Buzz Words: Cachexia + sunken eyeballs + absent muscle mass + frailty

Clinical Presentation: Common in elderly, institutionalized, bedridden, homeless, or chronic alcoholics

PPx: Most patients can be started on early postoperative enteral feeding (<48 hours).

MoD: Elderly patients usually consume less than half of their recommended dietary allowance (RDA) due to suppressed appetite, diminished sense of smell, depression, social isolation, and low income. Malnutrition sets the stage for impaired wound healing, an increased risk for infections, and a higher risk for perioperative mortality.

Dx: Visceral protein stores in organs (i.e., liver) are evaluated by measurement of serum albumin and transferrin. Somatic protein stores are evaluated by measuring circumference of the arm. Low levels of albumin, prealbumin, transferrin, and retinol-binding protein correlate with malnutrition.

Tx/Mgmt: Any patient who is not able to consume at least 60% of their RDA requires adjunctive nutritional therapy through either enteral or parenteral routes. When selecting the route of access, duration of therapy should be taken into consideration. Naso- and orogastric tubes should not be considered for the patient who will require therapy for more than 4 weeks. Whenever possible, enteral nutrition is preferred over parenteral because it provides better glycemic control, avoids gut bacterial overgrowth, maintains integrity of mucosal barrier, and increases the variety of nutrients absorbed. Parenteral nutrition should be considered for patients who have not been able to tolerate/receive enteral feeds more than 7 days.

Malabsorption

Buzz Words: Oily, greasy, floating stool + CF or chronic pancreatitis patients

Clinical Presentation: Abdominal bloating and steatorrhea ± weight loss. Lipophilic vitamins (ADEK) and vitamin B_{12} will not be absorbed adequately (Table 8.10).

PPx: Adequately manage underlying condition

MoD: Commonly due to defects in pancreatic secretion (i.e., chronic pancreatitis, CF), mucosal disorders (i.e., celiac disease, IBD), bacterial overgrowth (i.e., surgical alterations in GI anatomy, abnormal motility), or parasitic disease (*Giardia* is most common).

Dx: Fecal fat test (Sudan stain)

Tx/Mgmt: Supplement vitamins and pancreatic enzymes.

TABLE 8.10 Common Vitamin Deficiencies in Malabsorption

Vitamin	Normal Function	Findings in Deficient States
A	Vision, epithelial tissue, growth in children	Nyctalopia, xerophthalmia, Bitot spots (conjunctival keratin spots), follicular hyperkeratosis, growth retardation
B_{12}	RBC and neural development	Megaloblastic anemia, hypersegmented PMNs, pancytopenia, posterior column and lateral corticospinal tract demyelination, glossitis
D	Bone mineralization and blood Ca^{2+} regulation	Pathologic fractures, tibial bowing, muscle spasms, tetany, rickets, osteomalacia
E	Antioxidant	Hemolytic anemia, peripheral neuropathy (posterior column degeneration), ataxia, peripheral edema, thrombocytosis
K	Clotting factor synthesis	Ecchymoses, GI bleeding, prolonged PT/INR and PTT

GI, Gastrointestinal, *PMN*, polymorphonuclear leukocytes; *PT/INR*, prothrombin/International normalized ratio; *PTT*, partial thromboplastin time.

Dumping Syndrome

Buzz Words: Bloating + cramping + diarrhea + flushing + weakness/dizziness + palpitations + diaphoresis + recent GI surgery

Clinical Presentation: After GI surgery (particularly post-gastrectomy), patients may get dumping syndrome, which is a disorder characterized by carcinoid-like symptoms occurring after food ingestion. Early dumping syndrome occurs w/in 30 minutes 2/2 rapid gastric emptying of hyperosmolar load. Late dumping syndrome occurs 1–3 hours after eating.

PPx: Avoid large amounts of sugar, eat small meals frequently, and separate ingestion of solids and fluids.

MoD: Rapid influx of fluid can cause a high osmotic gradient. Rapid influx of food and rapid rise in postprandial glucose causes excessive release of insulin and vasomotor symptoms.

Dx: Clinical presentation

Tx/Mgmt:
1. Change diet regimen
2. Octreotide
3. Surgical management if refractory

Lactose Intolerance

Buzz Words: Resolution after 1 day of avoiding milk products

Clinical Presentation: Abdominal distention, bloating, diarrhea. Rare in children less than 6 years old; rates increase with age.

PPx: Avoid dairy products.

MoD: Lactase enzyme nonpersistence. Lactase normally hydrolyzes lactose into glucose and galactose, which can be absorbed by the intestinal epithelium. When lactose reaches the colon, bacteria convert it to short-chain fatty acids, hydrogen gas, and ketones. Could also be secondary to underlying disease (i.e., bacterial overgrowth, giardiasis, celiac disease, etc.).

Dx:
1. Clinical suspicion and improvement with dietary modifications.
2. Stool osmotic gap greater than 125 mOsm/kg and pH < 6.0 secondary to bacterial fermentation.

Tx/Mgmt: Avoid dairy products or use lactase pills.

Short Bowel Syndrome

Buzz Words: Small bowel removed + enteral feeding + large amounts of liquid stool

Clinical Presentation: Patient who underwent extensive resection of intestines and manifests deficiency of macro or micronutrients (see Table 8.11 for specific nutrient deficiencies), and diarrhea. Associated with gastric hypersecretion, liver disease, and cholelithiasis.

PPx: N/A

MoD: Malabsorptive condition caused by the absence of an essential segment of the bowel removed by surgical resection. The bowel becomes incapable of maintaining an individual's nutrient requirements on its own due to a reduction in absorptive surface area.

Dx: Clinical diagnosis

Tx/Mgmt:
1. Replacement of fluids and electrolytes
2. Resuming enteral feeding (intraluminal nutrients are the best stimulant for intestinal adaptation)

Rectum and Anus

Abscess of Anal and Rectal Regions

Buzz Words: Palpable mass at the anal verge

Clinical Presentation: Severe pain in anorectal area ± fever. Four major variants exist, which are classified on their anatomic relationship with the sphincters and muscles of the pelvic floor: intersphincteric, perianal, ischiorectal, and supraelevator. Most patients never seek medical attention.

PPx: N/A

MoD: Obstruction of the anorectal glands, which are located between the internal and external sphincters, leading to bacterial infection

Dx:
1. Clinical presentation
2. MRI to see extent of infection

Tx/Mgmt:
1. Incision and drainage
2. If immunocompromised, give antibiotics

99 AR

Intestinal sites of nutrient absorption

TABLE 8.11 Commonly Tested Nutrient Deficiencies in Short Bowel Syndrome

Segment Missing	Nutrient Deficiencies
Stomach	Vitamin B_{12} (lack of IF)
Duodenum	Minerals: iron, calcium, and others
Ileum	Vitamin B_{12} (no absorption) and bile salts
Cecum	Potassium, short chain fatty acids, and vitamin K

IF, Intrinsic factor.

Anorectal Fistula

Buzz Words:
- Past anorectal abscess + perineal opening in skin + cordlike tract can be palpated + brownish purulent discharge + fecal streaks soiling underwear
- Operation for perianal fistula + area does not heal well + unhealing ulcers/fissures + purulent discharge + no palpable masses

Clinical Presentation: Chronic drainage of pus or stool from a skin opening in the perirectal area ± mention of a prior perirectal abscess. Associated with Crohn disease.

PPx: Treatment of Crohn and avoiding surgeries that weaken the muscular wall

MoD: Almost half of the anorectal abscesses become fistulas, which connect the rectal mucosa with the perirectal skin. **Goodsall rule** allows the examiner to predict the tract of the fistula by drawing an imaginary line between the ischial spines; all fistulas with external openings posterior to this line travel in a curvilinear fashion while those with anterior openings travel in a radial fashion. Can occur 2/2 prior surgeries, anorectal abscess, or Crohn's.

Dx: Fistulas are classified in relationship to their anatomic tract.

Tx/Mgmt:
1. Digital rectal examination (DRE), anoscope, proctosigmoidoscopy to r/o cancer.
2. Biopsy to confirm Crohn's.
3. Elective fistulotomy (marsupialization).
4. If Crohn's, give metronidazole.

FOR THE WARDS

Anorectal fistulas rarely heal spontaneously and require surgical management. The goal is to eradicate the fistula while preserving fecal continence.

Anal Fissure

Buzz Words: Exquisite pain with defecation + bright red blood per rectum (BRBPR) + fear of bowel movements + refuses PE because it is too painful to draw apart buttocks

Clinical Presentation: Severe, localized, anorectal pain, which increases with defecation as accompanied by streaks of blood on fecal matter. Most often located posteriorly.

PPx: Dietary modifications and medication interruption to avoid constipation. Proper anal hygiene.

MoD: Linear tears in the lining of the rectal canal below the level of the dentate line that may be a product of severe straining to defecate from constipation or a tight sphincter.

Dx:
1. Physical exam.
2. If too painful, examine **under anesthesia** using DRE, anoscope, or proctosigmoidoscope to r/o cancer.

Tx/Mgmt:

1. Stool softeners, sitz baths.
2. Topical nitroglycerin.
3. Botulinum toxin (relax sphincter).
4. Forceful dilatation.
5. Lateral internal sphincterotomy if refractory.

Hemorrhoids

Buzz Words:

- **Internal hemorrhoids:** BRBPR + no pain
- **External hemorrhoids:** BRBPR + pain + skin tags

Clinical Presentation: Hemorrhoids are swollen veins in the anus that can present as bright red blood coating fecal matter, anal pruritus, and pain. Risk factors for development of symptomatic hemorrhoids are age, portal hypertension, anal intercourse, pregnancy, straining, constipation, and anticoagulation/antiplatelet therapy. A more than 50-year-old patient with BRBPR should have a colonoscopy to r/o cancer even if s/he has a known history of hemorrhoids.

They are classified as either internal or external hemorrhoids. Internal originate above the dentate line and are usually painless. External originate below the dentate line and produce pain when thrombosis occurs. Internal hemorrhoids are classified in the following manner:

- Grade I—do not prolapse
- Grade II—prolapse with defecation and return spontaneously into the anal canal
- Grade III—prolapse with defecation and require manual reduction
- Grade IV—not reducible

PPx: Fluids, fiber, and prevention of constipation

MoD: Normal vascular structures of the anal canal located in the submucosal layer that arise in three primary locations (L lateral, R anterior, and R posterior)

Dx:

1. DRE
2. Anoscopy, flexible sigmoidoscope, or proctosigmoidoscope to r/o anorectal cancer

Tx/Mgmt:

All patients should be started on prophylactic measures to avoid constipation and straining.

- Grade 1 → Diet change
- Grade 2 → Band ligation
- Grade 3 → Band ligation, hemorrhoidectomy
- Grade 4 → Hemorrhoidectomy

Rectal Prolapse

Buzz Words: Elderly woman + multiple gestation + protruding rectal mass + rectal pain

Clinical Presentation: Thin, frail woman with h/o multiple pregnancies who complains of mucosal mass protruding from rectal region, rectal pain, mild bleeding, fecal incontinence, and a wet anus. The mass may protrude after bowel movements and may be manually reduced. A type of procidentia, which just means an organ displacing downwards from anatomic position

PPx: Dietary modifications and medication interruption to avoid constipation

MoD: Intussusception of a portion of rectum thorough the anal canal

Dx: Clinical diagnosis

Tx/Mgmt: Surgical resection of redundant sigmoid colon with fixation of the rectum (rectopexy) to the sacral fascia

Disorders of the Liver and Biliary System, Noninfectious

Liver

Cirrhosis

Buzz Words: Micronodular pattern in hepatic surface + decreased LFTs (Table 8.12)

Clinical Presentation: Signs and symptoms of hepatic failure, cholestasis, portal hypertension, hepatic encephalopathy, and decreased degradation of estrogens (i.e., gynecomastia, impotence, erectile dysfunction, and spider angiomas)

PPx: Depends on etiologic factor

MoD: Irreversible fibrosis of the liver parenchyma. Regenerative nodules are formed as part of the reaction to injury and contain islands of healthy tissue surrounded by bands of fibrosis. Hydrostatic pressure in the portal system is increased by compression of nodules. See Box 8.1 for most common etiologic factors.

Dx: RUQ is the best initial test under suspicion of cirrhosis. Liver biopsy confirms diagnosis.

Tx/Mgmt:

Determination of etiology
- Consider liver transplantation for end-stage dysfunction
- For cirrhosis + portal hypertension → beta blockers to decrease portal pressure and TIPS/lactulose for refractory portal HTN

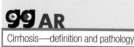
Cirrhosis—definition and pathology

TABLE 8.12 Simplified Meaning of Liver Function Tests

Test	Meaning
Albumin	Talks to the synthetic function of the liver and nutritional status of the patient May be low in malnutrition and nephritic syndrome Low albumin means little-to-none hepatic functional reserve
Alkaline phosphatase	Biliary duct obstruction Caveat: bone can produce and leak the enzyme as well
ALT	Hepatocyte membrane damage and leak ALT > AST think viral hepatitis
AST	Hepatocyte membrane damage and leak AST > ALT think alcohol, or drug toxicity
γ-glutamyl transferase	Biliary duct obstruction Rises immediately after binge drinking
Prothrombin time and international normalized ratio	Talks to the synthetic function of the liver, most accurate marker

ALT, alanine aminotransferase; *AST*, aspartate aminotransferase.

BOX 8.1 Most Common Causes of Cirrhosis

Alcoholic liver disease
Chronic viral hepatitis (i.e., HBV and HCV)
Hemochromatosis
Nonalcoholic fatty liver disease
Autoimmune disease (i.e., primary biliary cirrhosis)
Wilson disease
α_1-Antitrypsin deficiency
HBV, Hepatitis B virus; *HCV*, hepatitis C virus.

Dubin-Johnson Syndrome

Buzz Words: Black liver (dark pigment in hepatocytes) + episodes of self-resolving jaundice + direct (aka conjugated bilirubinemia)

Clinical Presentation: Usually asymptomatic, might present mild jaundice w/o pruritus. Chronic conjugated hyperbilirubinemia not associated with hemolysis. Condition may be exacerbated by illnesses, pregnancy, or use of oral contraceptives. Associated to reduced prothrombin activity secondary to factor VII deficiency in (60% of cases).

PPx: N/A

MoD: Dysfunctional transport of conjugated bilirubin out of the liver. Autosomal recessive mutation in the ABCC2 gene, which codes for MRP2 (multidrug resistance

99 AR
Jaundice video

QUICK TIPS
Conjugated bilirubinemia = direct bilirubinemia; unconjugated = indirect

TABLE 8.13 Interpretation of Urinary Coproporphyrin Excretion Patterns for Direct Bilirubinemia

	Healthy	Dubin–Johnson Syndrome	Rotor Syndrome
Total amount excreted	Normal	Normal	Elevated
Predominant type	Coproporphyrin III	Coproporphyrin I	Coproporphyrin I
Hepatocytes with dark pigment	No	Yes	No

protein 2), used in the hepatocellular excretion of bilirubin glucuronides into bile canaliculi. Dense pigments composed of epinephrine metabolites accumulate in lysosomes making the liver appear grossly black.

Dx:
1. Liver panel: Total bilirubin 2–5 mg/DL range, of which 50% is usually conjugated with normal LFTs.
2. UA: Bilirubinuria is common; may see urinary coproporphyrin I > corpoporphyrin II.

Tx/Mgmt: No treatment required

Rotor Syndrome

Buzz Words: Normal-appearing liver (no black pigment) + episodes of self-resolving jaundice + direct (aka conjugated) bilirubinemia)

Clinical Presentation: Asymptomatic, chronic conjugated, and unconjugated hyperbilirubinemia w/o evidence of hemolysis. Normal liver histology (absent melanin pigments).

PPx: N/A

MoD: Defect in hepatic storage of conjugated bilirubin, which leaks into plasma. Autosomal recessive inheritance.

Dx: Similar labs to DJS. Urinary coproporphyrin excretion pattern allows to distinguish between DJS and Rotor syndrome (Table 8.13)

Tx/Mgmt: No treatment required.

Gilbert Syndrome

Buzz Words: Adult + jaundice in s/o stress (e.g., fasting, exertion) + unconjugated hyperbilirubinemia

Clinical Presentation: Recurrent episodes of jaundice due to unconjugated hyperbilirubinemia. Most common inherited disorder of bilirubin glucuronidation.

PPx: N/A

MoD: Defect in the promoter of the gene that encodes UDP-glucoronosyltransferase 1A1

Dx: Unconjugated (indirect) hyperbilirubinemia, total bilirubin is usually less than 3 mg/dL. Normal LFTs. Rifampin test: UGB rises after administration of drug.

Tx/Mgmt: No treatment required. Avoid irinotecan (it requires bilirubin-UGT and these patients are at increased risk for toxicity).

Crigler-Najjar Syndrome

Buzz Words:
- **Type 1:** Indirect bilirubinemia + jaundice + kernicterus/bilirubin in basal ganglia + infant/kid (does not live to adulthood)
- **Type 2:** Indirect bilirubinemia + normal LFTs + adult (survives into adulthood)

QUICK TIPS
Crigler Type 1 is worse than Crigler Type 2

Clinical Presentation: Crigler-Najjar syndrome is an autosomal recessive disorder where metabolism of bilirubin is impaired leading to a buildup of indirect bilirubin. Two subtypes exist: type 1 has severe hyperbilirubinemia (20–50 mg/dL) due to absent bilirubin UGT activity and leads to kernicterus, while type 2 has total bilirubin levels less than 20 mg/dL, only has reduced bilirubin UGT activity, and rarely leads to kernicterus. Type 1 dies before adulthood while type 2 lives into adulthood.

PPx: N/A

MoD: Autosomal recessive. Decreased UGT activity → hyper unconjugated bilirubinemia

Dx: Liver panel (total bilirubin is higher than in Gilbert; normal LFTs)

Tx/Mgmt:
- If type 1 → phototherapy + plasmapheresis + liver transplant (only cure)
- If type 2 → no Tx needed in many cases but phenobarbital and clofibrate if needed

End-Stage Liver Disease (Including Indications for Transplantation)

Buzz Words: Cirrhosis + cholestasis + portal HTN

99 AR
Liver cholestasis—definition and pathology

Clinical Presentation: Important to recognize indications for transplantation on the medicine shelf (Table 8.14). The Model for End-stage Liver Disease (MELD) score is used in this regard.

PPx: Treat cirrhosis.

MoD: Natural progression of cirrhosis to liver failure

Dx: The MELD score is a risk stratification tool which uses bilirubin, creatinine, and INR and has been strongly correlated with 3-month survival. A MELD score of 30 correlates with a 50% 3-month survival.

TABLE 8.14 Indications for Liver Transplantation

Indication	Observations for Consideration
Acute liver failure (<26 weeks)	Receive highest priority for transplantation Severe liver injury + encephalopathy or impaired synthetic function (international normalized ratio ≥ 1.5)
Cirrhosis	Complications of portal hypertension Manifestations of compromised liver function (i.e., hepatorenal syndrome)
Alcoholic liver damage	Patients are required to have >6 months of abstinence, enrollment in rehabilitation, and adequate social support Transplantation offers a significant 5-year survival rate for these patients and only 5%–7% return to excessive drinking
Neoplasms	Hepatocellular carcinoma (single lesion <5 cm), epithelioid hemangioendothelioma, and large hepatic adenomas
Metabolic disorders	Cystic fibrosis, α_1-antitrypsin deficiency, von Gierke disease, Andersen disease, hemochromatosis, Wilson disease, acute intermittent porphyria

Tx/Mgmt: Evaluation for transplantation should be obtained when MELD ≥ 10 and patient candidacy should be considered when MELD ≥ 15. Management should be directed to slowing the progression of disease, preventing further insults to the liver, preventing complications of cirrhosis, and adjusting dosing of medications according to preserved liver function.

Hepatic Coma/Encephalopathy

Buzz Words: Flapping tremor + inability to sustain outstretch arms posture (asterixis)

Clinical Presentation: Irritability, confusion, altered mental state, asterixis (flapping of extended wrists), coma, and death.

PPx: The goal is to decrease the amount of available ammonia (NH_3) in the colon by decreasing the amount of amino acids for bacteria to metabolize (protein-restricted diet), wiping out the gut flora (rifaximin), or converting ammonia into ammonium (NH_4), which cannot be absorbed by the colon (lactulose).

MoD: Reversible metabolic disorder due to increased serum NH_3 level. The urea cycle is defective in the setting of advanced liver dysfunction, allowing for abnormally high levels of NH_3 to accumulate. Factors that may precipitate encephalopathy are:

- GIBs may precipitate encephalopathy due to increased nitrogen load in the lumen
- Portosystemic shunting
- Diuretics (thiazide/loop) which incite metabolic alkalosis keeping ammonia in the NH_3 state

Dx: Clinical presentation and ammonia levels (hyperammonemia)

Tx/Mgmt: Identify any precipitating causes. Continue preventative measures to decrease gut absorption of NH_3. Provide supportive therapy and nutritional support. Admit any patient with moderate–severe levels of confusion, which might not be able to adhere to treatment.

Fatty Liver, Alcoholic Hepatitis

Buzz Words: Steatosis + steatohepatitis + yellow discoloration of the liver

Clinical Presentation: Patients may be asymptomatic or manifest hepatomegaly and abdominal distention. Usually 10%–20% of patients will progress to develop cirrhosis if alcohol consumption is not interrupted.

PPx: Alcohol abstinence

MoD: Substrates of alcohol metabolism (i.e., glycerol 3-phosphate) are used to synthesize triglycerides (TGL), which accumulate in the cytosol of hepatocytes. Alcohol also activates hormone sensitive lipase, which increases TGL availability in blood and indirectly inhibits β-oxidation.

Dx:

1. Liver panel with gamma-glutamyl transferase (GGT) (to quantify alcohol consumption)
2. Ultrasound shows increased echogenicity, CT shows decreased hepatic attenuation, MRI shows increased fat signal.

Tx/Mgmt:

1. Supportive therapy.
2. Treatment for alcohol substance use disorder (e.g., 12-step program, naltrexone, disulfiram).

Hepatorenal Syndrome

Buzz Words: H/o liver dysfunction + acute kidney injury w/o renal organic dysfunction + poor response to fluid therapy (i.e., ascites resistant to diuretics)

Clinical Presentation: Presentation of kidney injury is usually insidious and labs will probably provide identification

QUICK TIPS

Increased production of NADH accelerates conversion of DHAP to G3-P which leads to formation of TGL.

of disease process before any clinical manifestations become evident. Any patient with liver dysfunction and no known renal dysfunction who develops oliguria should be considered.

It is a diagnosis of exclusion with poor prognosis (mortality rate of 80%). Increased creatinine and blood urea nitrogen. Renal tubular function is preserved, therefore a random urine Na^+ should be less than 20 mEq/L, also proteinuria and hematuria should be absent. Biopsy would show normal renal parenchyma.

PPx: N/A

MoD: Loss of renal autoregulation as a complication of end-stage liver disease, which results in intense renal vasoconstriction and reversible ischemic injury (i.e., decreased glomerular filtration rate in the absence of shock or renal dysfunction). Poor response to fluid therapy. Usually precipitated by hypovolemia (GIB) or a bacterial infection.

Dx:
1. BMP
2. Liver panel
3. UA
4. BNP
5. Echo to r/o heart failure

Tx/Mgmt:
1. Treat etiology of liver failure
2. Supportive therapy
3. Norepinephrine, vasopressin, midodrine
4. Albumin
5. Dialysis
6. Liver transplant

Hepatopulmonary Syndrome

Buzz Words: Hypoxemia + history of liver disease

Clinical Presentation: Pulmonary dysfunction 2/2 primary liver dysfunction. Patient present with symptoms of hypoxemia in the setting of liver disease and/or portal hypertension. Work-up of the disease will show poor arterial hemoglobin saturation (<96%). Arterial oxygen tension (P_aO_2) while on room air determines severity of disease (mild >80 mm Hg, moderate 60–80 mm Hg, and severe <60 mm Hg). Evaluation for shunting is best done by getting a transthoracic contrast echocardiography. Chest imaging has nonspecific results. PFTs might indicate reduced diffusion capacity (low DLCO).

PPx: N/A

MoD: Pathogenesis is poorly understood. Intrapulmonary vascular dilations cause blood shunting leading to an increased alveolar-arterial oxygen gradient (≥15 mm Hg). Associated with increased levels of NO, endothelin-1.

Dx:
1. O_2 sat
2. CXR
3. Arterial line
4. PFTs

Tx/Mgmt:
1. O_2 supplementation
2. Liver transplant

Jaundice

Buzz Words: Icterus

Clinical Presentation: Yellow pigmentation in skin and eyes. UGB is lipophilic and can cross the BBB, leading to kernicterus (accumulation in basal ganglia). Leakage of bile salts, bile acids, and cholesterol into the blood would manifest pruritus and xanthomas.

PPx: Depends on the mechanism

MoD: Accumulation of bilirubin, the end product of heme degradation. Table 8.15 briefly depicts the distinct mechanisms in which jaundice may be produced.

Dx: Adequate identification of risk factors for disease and interpretation of LFTs (see Table 8.12) are key to narrowing down on the mechanism for the presentation.

Tx/Mgmt: Phototherapy is a safe method to treat severe unconjugated hyperbilirubinemia in newborns by increasing the solubility of UGB and allowing it to be excreted in urine. Administration of calcium carbonate modestly enhances the effect of phototherapy.

99 AR

Jaundice—definition and pathology

Nonalcoholic Fatty Liver Disease

Buzz Words: Yellow liver + liver fat signal on MRI + echogenicity on ultrasound

Clinical Presentation: Hepatic steatosis in absence of causes for secondary fat accumulation (i.e., alcohol consumption, infection, medications, metabolic derangements). Patients are usually asymptomatic. Ultrasound shows increased echogenicity, CT shows decreased hepatic attenuation, MRI shows increased fat signal. Yellow discoloration of the liver.

PPx: Avoid alcohol consumption.

MoD: The primary pathophysiologic component is insulin resistance because it leads to increased TGL synthesis, hepatic uptake of free fatty acids, and lipolysis.

TABLE 8.15 Mechanisms of Hyperbilirubinemia

Mechanism	Bilirubinemia	Causes
Increased bilirubin production	UCB > CB	Hemolytic anemia, Wilson disease, extravasation of blood
Decreased conjugation	UCB > CB	Physiologic jaundice of the newborn, breast milk jaundice, Gilbert syndrome, or Crigler-Najjar syndrome
Defective conjugation of UCB and secretion of CB	UCB ≈ CB	Viral hepatitis, pregnancy, or TPN
Decreased intrahepatic bile flow	CB > UCB	Primary biliary cirrhosis, drug-related (i.e., oral contraceptives and anabolic steroids), Dubin-Johnson syndrome, or Rotor syndrome
Decreased extrahepatic bile flow	CB > UCB	Gallstone, structural pancreatic anomalies (i.e., cancer, pancreas divisum, strictures), structural biliary anomalies (i.e., cholangiocarcinoma, primary sclerosing cholangitis), *Clonorchis sinensis* (Chinese liver fluke)

CB, Conjugated bilirubin; *TPN*, total parenteral nutrition; *UCB*, unconjugated bilirubin.

Important regulators of hepatic insulin sensitivity are leptin, adiponectin, and resistin. Activation of stellate and hepatic progenitor cells leads to fibrosis of zone 3.

Dx:
1. Liver panel
2. Liver ultrasound
3. MRI

Tx/Mgmt:
1. Weight loss ± orlistat for patients who fail to lose weight through diet and exercise alone
2. Avoid alcohol consumption

Portal Hypertension/Esophageal Varices

Buzz Words: Massive hematemesis + painless upper GIB + strange vascular markings around umbilicus

Clinical Presentation: Usually asymptomatic until complications develop. Varices at sites of portosystemic shunting (esophageal, umbilical, and hemorrhoidal), ascites, and congestive splenomegaly. Complications of portal hypertension are variceal hemorrhage, ascites, and SBP.

PPx: Treat the underlying cause to prevent progression and increased risk of variceal bleeds.

MoD: Resistance to hepatic blood flow from intrasinusoidal hypertension, which is secondary to regenerative nodule compression. Anastomosis from portal tributaries (i.e., esophageal, paraumbilical, and inferior rectal veins) to the cava system occur to shunt blood away. Resistance may also develop in the pre-hepatic (i.e., portal vein thrombosis) or posthepatic circulation (i.e., Budd-Chiari syndrome).

Dx:

1. Clinical presentation
2. Ultrasound or CT
3. Measurement of hepatic venous pressure gradient with transjugular catheter (rarely done)

Tx/Mgmt:

1. Management of ascites (fluid and Na^+ restriction + spironolactone, drain if breathing becomes impaired)
2. Prevention of variceal hemorrhage with nonselective β-blockers, octreotide, and endoscopic ligation
3. Active hemorrhage may be managed with intraluminal compression (i.e., Sengstaken-Blakemore tube) or portocaval shunting (i.e., transjugular intrahepatic portosystemic shunt placement)

Biliary System

Cholestasis

Buzz Words: "*Bile lakes*" inside hepatocytes

Clinical Presentation: Jaundice with pruritus, malabsorption, cholesterol deposition in the skin (i.e., xanthomas), and light-colored stool (lack of stercobilin)

PPx: N/A

MoD: Hepatocellular cholestasis can be caused by drugs (i.e., oral contraceptives or anabolic steroids), neonatal hepatitis, or pregnancy-induced (estrogen inhibits bile secretion). Obstructive cholestasis is usually due to blockage of the common bile duct (CBD): gallstone, primary sclerosing cholangitis, biliary atresia, or neoplasm at the head of the pancreas.

Dx: Hyperbilirubinemia, conjugated bilirubin greater than 50%, bilirubinuria, hypercholesterolemia, increased serum ALP and GGT, absent urobilinogen in the urine

Liver cholestasis—definition and pathology

Tx/Mgmt: Discontinue causative agent, remove source of obstruction, ursodiol

Ascending Cholangitis

Buzz Words:
- Charcot triad = fever + abdominal pain + jaundice
- Reynold pentad (suppurative cholangitis) = Charcot triad + confusion + hypotension

Clinical Presentation: Fever, chills, RUQ abdominal pain, and jaundice. Elder or immunosuppressed patients may manifest hypotension only.

PPx: N/A

MoD: Infection of the biliary tract secondary to obstruction and stasis. Most common pathogens are *E. coli*, *Pseudomonas*, and *Enterobacter.*

Dx:
1. Elevated liver enzymes (especially ALP and GGT)
2. Ultrasound or CT (biliary dilation and a source of obstruction)

Tx/Mgmt:
1. Antibiotic therapy and biliary drainage (endoscopic sphincterotomy with stone extraction ± stent placement)
2. Preferred antibiotics are those with Gram-negative and anaerobic coverage: pip/tazo, ampicillin/sulbactam, or ceftriaxone + metronidazole
3. Narrow-spectrum once blood cultures and sensitivities are available
4. Urgent (open) biliary decompression is required in patients with failed ERCP or signs of acute suppurative cholangitis

Cholelithiasis and Acute Cholecystitis

Buzz Words: Double wall sign on ultrasound + Murphy sign

Clinical Presentation: RUQ pain (prolonged, steady, and severe), fever, nausea, vomiting, anorexia, and tenderness on palpation. Risk factors for stone formation are increasing age, obesity, excessive bile salt loss (terminal ileum disease), and female sex. Cholecystectomy is the preferred treatment for patients with symptomatic gallstones, porcelain gall bladder, cholecystitis, and asymptomatic gallstones in patients with sickle cell. No surgery for healthy asymptomatic patients. Antibiotic therapy should be initiated and continued until surgical removal with pip/tazo, ampicillin/sulbactam, or ceftriaxone + metronidazole. Patients refusing surgery or with high surgical risk can receive medical management with a bile acid supplement (ursodeoxycholic acid), which reduces biliary cholesterol secretion and increases biliary bile acid concentration. Medical management confers a high rate of recurrence.

PPx:
1. Weight loss.
2. Avoid fibrates in patients with risk factors because they increase cholesterol content in bile, therefore increasing the risk of stone formation.
3. Ursodeoxycholic acid

MoD: Cholesterol stones form in the setting of supersaturation of cholesterol in bile salts, which allows precipitation or gallbladder stasis. Pigmented stones are made of bilirubin and form when UGB precipitates with calcium. Acute cholecystitis (inflammation of gallbladder wall) occurs with stone impaction in the cystic duct leading to gallbladder distention and bacterial overgrowth.

Dx:
1. Ultrasound is the best initial test (gallbladder wall >5 mm or edema)
   a. CT has lower sensitivity for small stones.
2. Liver panel (normal bilirubin and LFTs)
3. Abdominal x-ray: pigmented gallstones can be visualized on abdominal films (cholesterol stones are radiolucent)

Tx/Mgmt:
1. Ursodeoxycholic acid
2. Antibiotics
3. Cholecystectomy

Choledocholithiasis

Buzz Words: CBD > 1 cm + stone in biliary tree
Clinical Presentation: RUQ or epigastric abdominal pain, jaundice, nausea, and vomiting
PPx: Weight loss and avoidance of fibrates in patients at risk to develop gallstones
MoD: Intermittent obstruction of the CBD by a gallstone. Progression of obstruction might lead to acute cholangitis or acute pancreatitis.
Dx:
1. Ultrasound
2. Patients with prior cholecystectomy should undergo MRCP or endoscopic ultrasound to better assess possibility of choledocholithiasis
Tx/Mgmt: Anytime that the abdomen is entered to perform a cholecystectomy, a cholangiography or CBD exploration may be performed to better assess risk.
- High-risk: ERCP with sphincterotomy + elective laparoscopic cholecystectomy

- Intermediate-risk: MRCP or elective laparoscopic cholecystectomy + intra-op evaluation of CBD
- Low-risk: direct cholecystectomy w/o additional imaging

Cholestasis Due to Parenteral Nutrition

Clinical Presentation: Hepatocellular and cholestatic injury that occurs after prolonged TPN (usually >2 weeks). Low birth weight, prematurity, duration of TPN, and intestinal stasis are significant risk factors.

PPx: Frequently assess the plausibility of re-initiating enteral nutrition to avoid prolonged periods of TPN.

MoD: Injury may vary widely between steatosis and mild hepatocellular damage to cirrhosis. Hepatic changes are related to prolonged rest of the enterohepatic circulation, changes in the nutritive composition, and the administration of nutrients from the hepatic artery rather than the portal vein.

Dx: Increase in serum conjugated bilirubin (>2 mg/dL), spike in liver enzymes, and exclusion other causes of hepatotoxic injury

Tx/Mgmt: Cessation of TPN and treat small bowel bacterial overgrowth (metronidazole)

Gallstone Ileus

Buzz Words: Pneumobilia + intestinal obstruction

Clinical Presentation: Elderly woman with episodic subacute bowel obstruction. High rate of morbidity and mortality.

PPx: Weight loss and avoidance of fibrates in patients at risk of developing gallstones

MoD: Mechanical bowel obstruction caused by impaction of a gallstone (usually >2 cm) at the ileocecal valve. These larger stones usually make their way to the bowel by way of a biliary-enteric fistula.

Dx: Abdominal CT is the preferred imaging study and would show intestinal obstruction with gallstone(s) in the ileum. Pneumobilia (air in the gallbladder) may be an associated finding secondary to the biliary-enteric fistula.

Tx/Mgmt: Surgery

Mirizzi Syndrome

Buzz Words: Obstructive jaundice + fever + RUQ pain

Clinical Presentation: Mirizzi syndrome occurs when a gallstone is lodged in the cystic duct. Same risk factors as for cholecystolithiasis.

PPx: Weight loss and avoidance of fibrates

MoD: Hepatic duct obstruction by an extrinsic compression from an impacted stone in the cystic duct. Associated with higher frequency of gallbladder cancer.

Dx: Elevated ALP + hyperbilirubinemia + RUQ ultrasound showing intrahepatic biliary dilatation and sludge in the cystic duct

Tx/Mgmt: Laparoscopic cholecystectomy

Primary Biliary Cirrhosis

Buzz Words: Pruritus that does not improve with antihistamines

Clinical Presentation: Middle-aged woman with Northern European descent who presents with pruritus, fatigue, and xanthelasma. Abdominal exam shows hepatomegaly and RUQ tenderness to palpation. It may be associated with osteopenia, hyperlipidemia, and other autoimmune conditions (i.e., autoimmune hepatitis and Sjögren syndrome). May progress to cirrhosis.

PPx: N/A

MoD: T-cell mediated cholangiocyte damage, which allows bile leakage into the blood stream. The etiology of pruritus is uncertain, perhaps due to the increased production of endogenous opioids and retained bile salts.

Dx:
1. Anti-mitochondrial antibodies (against PDC-E2 protein)
2. ALP and GGT are elevated
3. Biopsy shows inflammation around bile ducts

Tx/Mgmt:
1. Ursodeoxycholic acid
2. In refractory disease, cholestyramine may reduce pruritus and slow down disease progression
3. Liver transplant in end-stage liver dysfunction

Primary Sclerosing Cholangitis

Buzz Words: *Beading* of the bile ducts + *"onion-skin"* fibrosis of the bile ducts

Clinical Presentation: Young adult male patient with jaundice, pruritus, and hepatosplenomegaly. Associated to IBD in 70% of cases (**ulcerative colitis** > Crohn disease). May progress to portal hypertension, liver cirrhosis, and cholangiocarcinoma.

PPx: N/A

MoD: Obliterative, interrupted fibrosis of bile ducts (both intra- and extrahepatic). Association with HLA-DR52a (100% of the time), HLA-B8, HLA-Dr3, and HLA-Cw7 subtypes. These patients also have elevated IgM and perinuclear

QUICK TIPS

Extrinsic compression of the HEPATIC duct, not the common bile duct.

99 AR

Primary biliary cholangitis— causes, symptoms, diagnosis, treatment, and pathology

99 AR

Primary sclerosing cholangitis—
pathophysiology and symptoms

antineutrophil cytoplasmic antibodies (80% of the time). Pruritus occurs due to bile salt deposition into the skin.

Dx:

1. Labs consistent with cholestasis (conjugated bilirubin >50%, bilirubinuria, absent urine urobilinogen, increased ALP and GGT).
2. ERCP (narrowing and dilation of the bile ducts [*beading*]).

Tx/Mgmt: Immunosuppressants (steroids, azathioprine, and MTX) and liver transplant

Disorders of the Pancreas

Acute Pancreatitis

Buzz Words:

- **Acute pancreatitis:** epigastric pain + acute abdomen (<24 hours pain) + radiating straight through back + N/V + amylase/lipase (lipase is more specific) + **hypocalcemia**
- **Edematous pancreatitis:** Alcohol + gallstones + pancreatitis + **high hematocrit**
- **Hemorrhagic pancreatitis:** Edematous pancreatitis + **low hematocrit** + refractory to treatment + **flank bruising**
- **Pancreatic abscess:** Persistent fever + leukocytosis 10 days s/p pancreatitis + pus collection
- **Pancreatic pseudocyst:** Mass in pancreas + **5 weeks s/p pancreatitis** + upper abdominal trauma + early satiety/vague discomfort 2/2 fluid around pancreas

Clinical Presentation: Acute and severe epigastric abdominal pain that irradiates posteriorly; nausea and vomiting. Tenderness on palpation. Might also manifest signs of volume depletion. Classically described signs are Grey-Turner (flank hemorrhage) and Cullen (periumbilical hemorrhage).

Increased serum amylase and lipase; lipase more specific. Imaging studies (CT/ultrasound) are necessary to determine if a stone is the culprit and if removal is needed. MRCP gives the best image of the ductal structure of both pancreas and biliary systems. In the setting of necrosis, sampling by aspiration is warranted to rule out superinfection.

Replete intravascular volume! Dehydration is the most common cause of mortality. Rest the pancreas (NPO) and provide pain management. ERCP allows for

FOR THE WARDS

Know the Ranson criteria

QUICK TIPS

In pancreatitis, serum amylase is normal if (1) hyperlipidemia (interferes with amylase production), (2) there is increased urinary excretion of amylase, or (3) near destruction of pancreatic parenchyma.

removal and dilation of strictures. Surgical debridement is indicated in the setting of infected necrosis that does not improve with broad-spectrum antibiotics.

PPx: Avoidance of alcohol

MoD: Many causes exist for pancreatitis (Box 8.2); identifying the cause allows for adequacy in management. There must be activation of enzymes within the pancreatic ductal system that will produce pancreatitis (i.e., obstruction, activation by calcium, drug toxicity, etc.). This event will initiate a systemic inflammatory response, which may set the setting for DIC, shock, and sepsis. A significant amount of peri-pancreatic fluid accumulates (*third-space*) as the pancreas autodigests itself. Splenic vein thrombosis may occur since most of the pancreatic venous drainage goes to the splenic vein (classic finding: antral varices w/o esophageal varices).

Dx:
1. Lipase/amylase
2. CT
3. Ultrasound

Tx/Mgmt:
1. NPO
2. Nasogastric suction
3. IV fluids
4. Drain if pancreatic abscess

Chronic Pancreatitis

Buzz Words: Radiographic dyes show a "chain of lakes" appearance in the major duct + dystrophic calcifications + repeated episodes of past pancreatitis + steatorrhea + hypocalcemia + diabetes + constant epigastric pain

Clinical Presentation: Patient (men > women) with debilitating abdominal pain and h/o repeated episodes

---

BOX 8.2 Common Causes of Acute Pancreatitis

Gallstone obstruction
Alcohol
Drugs: azathioprine, furosemide, thiazides, TMP-SMX, valproate
Hypertriglyceridemia
Hypercalcemia
Structural pancreatic anomalies: cancer, pancreas divisum, strictures
Recent endoscopic retrograde cholangiopancreatography, gastric, or biliary surgery
Infection: *Coxsackie*, mumps, *Mycoplasma pneumoniae*
Trauma (i.e., seatbelt injury)
TMP-SMX, Trimethoprim/sulfamethoxazole.

of pancreatitis. Patient may manifest deficiency in any of the following vitamins: A, B_{12}, D, E, or K (see Table 8.10 for manifestations). Amylase and lipase will probably be within normal range (no enzymes left to release). Dystrophic calcifications may be seen on abdominal films or CT scans. Most accurate test is the secretin stimulation test (given IV). The bentiromide test assesses the ability of chymotrypsin to cleave orally administered bentiromide to para-aminobenzoic acid (measured in urine). Oral supplementation of pancreatic enzymes and fat-soluble vitamins. Simple analgesics or NSAIDs. Refractory pain management may be mediated with ganglion block with injection guided by endoscopic ultrasound. Poor prognosis 50% mortality within 10 years. Can lead to splenic vein thrombosis

PPx: Treatment of acute pancreatitis, avoidance of alcohol

MoD: Repeated attachment of acute pancreatitis produce duct obstruction. Calcification and dilation of the major ducts occur. Type 1 DM may develop in 70% of cases of chronic pancreatitis.

Dx:
1. CT abdomen
2. ERCP

Tx/Mgmt:
1. Insulin for diabetes
2. Pancreatic enzymes for steatorrhea
3. Pain control
4. Surgery to drain pancreatic duct

Hereditary Pancreatitis

Buzz Words: Pancreatitis in child, family history of similar episodes

Clinical Presentation: Pancreatitis before 20 years of age. One-third of patients develops pancreatic insufficiency and are at a greater risk for pancreatic cancer.

PPx: Avoid alcohol, smoking, limit dietary fat intake, and supplement with daily multivitamins and antioxidants.

MoD: Mutations in the serine protease 1 gene (PRSS1) may promote premature activation of trypsinogen or interfere with the inactivation of trypsin. Other genes which may be implicated are SPINK1, CFTR, CPA1, or CLDN2. There is autosomal dominant inheritance.

Dx: Genetic testing should be done for young patients in which a discernable cause is not identified.

Tx/Mgmt: Management is identical to previously discussed for acute pancreatitis. Pancreatectomy with islet autotransplantation may be considered for patients with opioid addiction due to chronic pancreatitis.

Pancreatic Cyst/Pseudocyst

Buzz Words: Persistent increase in serum amylase greater than 10 days + walled-off pancreatic necrosis

Clinical Presentation: Development of a fluid-filled abdominal mass in a patient recovering from acute pancreatitis (20% of cases) associated with amylase levels, which have remained elevated for a prolonged period of time. Amylase should return to normal levels in 2–4 days. These cysts can suffer spontaneous infection. Involvement of adjacent vessels could result in pseudoaneurysm, which may rupture and produce a GIB (hemosuccus pancreaticus).

PPx: N/A

MoD: The amount of amylase in the fluid surpasses the renal clearance of amylase.

Dx: Abdominal CT scan

Tx/Mgmt: Depends on diameter. Less than 5 cm f/u with more scans will most likely resolve on its own. Greater than 5 cm or symptomatic lesion requires guided drainage (endoscopic ultrasound or CT).

Pancreatic Insufficiency

Buzz Words: N/A

Clinical Presentation: Mild insufficiency might manifest abdominal discomfort and bloating while severe insufficiency would manifest malabsorption with steatorrhea, fat-soluble vitamin deficiency, and vitamin B_{12} deficiency.

PPx: N/A

MoD: Chronic pancreatitis, cystic fibrosis, hemochromatosis, and Shwachman-Diamond syndrome. Malabsorption occurs when greater than 90% of the exocrine function has been destroyed.

Dx: Decreased fecal elastase-1

Tx/Mgmt: Similar management as described for chronic pancreatitis.

Traumatic and Mechanical Disorders

Postgastric Surgery Syndromes

Blind Loop Syndrome

Buzz Words: N/A

Clinical Presentation: Patient who had a gastrectomy (Billroth II or Roux-en-Y procedure) in the past who presents with foul-smelling diarrhea, weight loss, and weakness. Patients may present with megaloblastic anemia (secondary to folate and B_{12} deficiency), peripheral neuropathy (B_{12} deficiency), and steatorrhea (from deconjugation of bile salts)

PPx: N/A

MoD: Bacterial overgrowth in the segment of bowel that is excluded from the pass of chyme. These bacteria might interfere with folate absorption, vitamin B_{12} absorption, and/or enterohepatic circulation.

Dx: B12 levels

Tx/Mgmt:
1. Broad-spectrum antibiotics to halt bacteria overgrowth.
2. Definitive treatment requires a second procedure to avoid having a blind loop of bowel present.

Adhesions

Clinical Presentation: Most commonly asymptomatic. Symptomatic patients may present with signs and symptoms of bowel obstruction, multiple miscarriages, or failure to conceive.

PPx: Meticulous surgical technique with minimal manipulation of peritoneal surfaces. Solid or liquid barriers can be used to prevent adhesion formation after abdominal surgery.

MoD: Adhesions form after any sort of manipulation of the intraabdominal organs during surgery. It is the normal peritoneal response to surgical injury. A common cause of bowel obstruction.

Dx: Clinical suspicion + confirmation on surgical exploration

Tx/Mgmt: Surgical lysis of adhesions is indicated in patients who manifest bowel obstruction or with the purpose of aiding in conception and improvement of fertility.

Hernias

Direct Inguinal Hernia

Buzz Words: The defect in the abdominal wall is inside Hesselbach triangle (i.e., medial to the inferior epigastric vessels).

Clinical Presentation: Older male patient with a bulge in the groin that protrudes during abdominal straining. These hernias rarely occur in women and children.

PPx: Dietary habits that prevent constipation and excessive straining

MoD: These lesions tend to be acquired over time as a result of excessive pressure and tension on the abdominal wall.

Dx: Clinical presentation

Tx/Mgmt: Surgical repair of the defect. Patients with signs of incarceration or bowel obstruction should be taken to the operating room (OR) urgently.

Indirect Inguinal Hernia

Buzz Words: Defect in the abdominal wall is outside of Hesselbach triangle, through the inguinal canal and **lateral to the inferior epigastric vessels**

Clinical Presentation: Young patient with a bulge in the groin that protrudes during abdominal straining. These hernias occur more commonly on the right side. It is the most common groin hernia in men and women.

PPx: Dietary habits which prevent constipation and the excessive straining

MoD: Congenital defect in which the processus vaginalis remains patent. Intra-abdominal organs protrude through both the internal and external inguinal rings.

Dx: Clinical presentation

Tx/Mgmt: Surgery. Patients with signs of incarceration or bowel obstruction should be taken to the OR urgently.

Femoral Hernia

Buzz Words: Reducible bulge in the groin

Clinical Presentation: Bulge in the groin (usually lower than inguinal hernias) that protrudes during abdominal straining. These hernias occur most commonly in women. Femoral hernias are highly susceptible to incarceration due to the rigid structures that surround the femoral canal.

PPx: N/A

MoD: Similar to direct inguinal hernias, these are acquired defects secondary to laxity in the abdominal wall. The defect usually occurs near the attachment of the transversus abdominis muscle onto Cooper ligament (i.e., through the femoral ring) with abdominal organs going into the femoral canal.

Dx: The defect in the abdominal wall is inferior to the inguinal ligament.

Tx/Mgmt: Surgical repair. The femoral hernia can be repaired from different approaches (i.e., inguinal, thigh, laparoscopic, or abdominal) if the femoral canal becomes occluded.

Umbilical Hernia

Buzz Words: Periumbilical bulge that protrudes with straining

Clinical Presentation: Periumbilical bulge that protrudes with straining. Rare hernias in adults, most commonly present

---

QUICK TIPS

Hesselbach triangle = inguinal ligament + rectus abdominis + inferior epigastric vessels

MNEMONIC

Remember the contents of the femoral triangle from lateral to medial with the mnemonic **NAVEL**: femoral **N**erve, **A**rtery, **V**ein, **E**mpty space (where femoral hernias occur), and **L**ymph nodes in newborns. Females > males. Associated to obesity, ascites, and pregnancy.

PPx: Dietary habits which prevent constipation and excessive straining

MoD: Dilatation of the umbilical ring and protrusion of the omentum (most commonly) into the hernia sac. Ascites in the setting of preexisting umbilical hernia produces thinning of the skin and increases the risk of spontaneous rupture.

Dx: Clinical presentation

Tx/Mgmt: Asymptomatic hernias do not require repair. Small symptomatic hernias can be repaired quickly through an open approach, while larger defects are better handled through a laparoscopic approach.

Penetrating Wounds, Abdominal

Buzz Words: Hemodynamic instability s/p abdominal trauma (knife or gunshot)

Clinical Presentation: Emergent condition that requires immediate laparotomy. Depending on the awareness and neurologic status of the patient, obtaining a description of the mechanisms of injury may be a possibility.

PPx: N/A

MoD: Penetrating abdominal trauma

Dx:
1. FAST (focused abdominal sonography for trauma) can be done at the bedside to evaluate for hemoperitoneum
2. CT scan

Tx/Mgmt:
1. Emergent laparotomy if indicated (Box 8.3)
2. Adequate fluid resuscitation, initiate broad-spectrum antibiotics, provide adequate pain management

Perforation of Hollow Viscus and Blunt Abdominal Trauma

Buzz Words: Free abdominal air + pneumoperitoneum + mesenteric air + fecal matter in peritoneal cavity

---

BOX 8.3 Indications for Emergent Exploratory Laparotomy

Evisceration of intraabdominal organs
Signs of gastrointestinal hemorrhage
Hemodynamic instability
Signs of peritonitis
Impalement

Clinical Presentation: Emergent condition that requires immediate laparotomy. H/o abdominal trauma (penetrating or blunt) + signs and symptoms of acute abdomen.

PPx: N/A

MoD: Trauma

Dx:

1. Abdominal CT scans, to be performed only in stable patients, would show discontinuity in the wall of hollow viscus, mesenteric hematoma, free intra-abdominal fluid, signs of active bleeding, or extravasation of intravenous contrast.

Tx/Mgmt: Emergent exploratory laparotomy

99 AR

AATS Injury Scoring Scale (For the Wards!)

Perforation/Rupture of Esophagus (Boerhaave Syndrome)

Buzz Words: Pneumomediastinum + L pneumothorax in a patient who was vomiting earlier that day

Clinical Presentation: Acute and intense retrosternal pain that begins during vomiting and is aggravated by swallowing. May be accompanied by hoarseness, back pain, subcutaneous emphysema, and dyspnea. Often associated with alcoholic intoxication or bulimia in young patients. Can also occur during endoscopic examinations.

PPx: N/A

MoD: Spontaneous full-thickness rupture of the esophagus after forceful retching. Results in contamination of the mediastinal cavity.

Dx:

1. CXR may show left-sided pneumothorax, pneumomediastinum, or esophageal thickening
2. Barium should NOT be used as a contrast medium for fluoroscopy

Tx/Mgmt:

1. NPO and nutritional support
2. Broad-spectrum antibiotics
3. IV proton-pump inhibitor
4. Surgical repair w/in 24 hours for patients with perforation

Congenital Disorders

Intussusception

Buzz Words: Colicky abdominal pain + kids have to squat to relieve pain + 6–12 months old + vague mass on right side of abdomen + empty RLQ + currant jelly stools + preceded by viral infection + bull's eye sign on ultrasound

Clinical Presentation: Child with intermittent abdominal pain, distention, cramping, vomiting, and bloody stools. Some cases have been associated with the **rotavirus** live-attenuated vaccine. Can also have an association with a recent viral infection.

PPx: N/A

MoD: Three quarters of cases are idiopathic, while the other quarter has an underlying condition that creates a nidus for intussusception. Meckel diverticulum a common cause of intussusception. The overlying bowel loop entraps the mesentery, occluding blood flow to the inner loop.

Dx:

1. Abdominal ultrasound may detect layers of intestine within another loop of bowel, often described as *coiled spring* lesion or *bull's eye* sign
2. Barium or air enema

Tx/Mgmt:

1. Barium or air enema
2. Surgery if reduction not achieved by edema

Necrotizing Enterocolitis

Buzz Words:

- Premature infants + first feed + feeding intolerance + abdominal distention + **bleeding stools** + rapidly dropping platelet count (a sign of sepsis in babies)
- Abdominal x-ray with air in bowel wall and portal veins + preemie + vomiting + leukocytosis
- Non-preemie + heart condition (e.g., DiGeorge) + any condition that predisposes to hypoperfusion + poor feeding + bloody stools

Clinical Presentation: Necrotizing enterocolitis (NEC) is the destruction of colon by infection. Occurs in **premature** infant who develops abdominal distention, tenderness, vomiting, rectal bleeding, and diarrhea. Associated with pneumatosis intestinalis on abdominal x-ray. A 5-day-old former 33-week preemie develops bloody diarrhea.

PPx: N/A

MoD: Ischemic necrosis of the mucosa, which allows bacterial invasion (e.g., staph epidermidis) with subsequent dissection of gas into the muscularis and portal system. Immaturity of GI tract appears to be a significant risk factor.

Dx:

1. Clinical diagnosis
2. Abdominal films show pneumatosis intestinalis
3. Labs show thrombocytopenia, metabolic acidosis, and blood in stool samples

gg AR

Pneumatosis intestinalis
abdominal XR

Tx/Mgmt:
1. NPO
2. Broad spectrum antibiotics
3. IV fluids/nutrition (i.e., TPN)
4. If abdominal wall erythema, air in biliary tree, pneumatosis intestinalis, or pneumoperitoneum → surgery

Volvulus

Buzz Words:
- *Coffee-bean* shaped bowel on abdominal film, *whirl* sign (twisting of mesentery), loss of haustral markings
- Elderly patient + tympanic air-fluid levels + distended colon/abdomen + tenderness + air-filled loop in RUQ that tapers down toward the LLQ with a parrot's beak

Clinical Presentation: Elderly patient with slowly progressive abdominal pain who finally develops signs and symptoms of bowel obstruction (discussed previously) and significant abdominal distention

PPx: N/A

MoD: Bowel twists around its own mesentery. Common cases are chronic constipation, laxative abuse, fiber-rich diet, and Chagas disease.

Dx:
1. Abdominal x-ray (air-filled coffee bean shape RUQ)
2. CT abdomen
3. Proctosigmoidoscopy

Tx/Mgmt:
1. Rectal tube
2. Proctosigmoidoscopic exam
3. Flexible sigmoidoscopy in attempt to untwist the segment of bowel followed by rectal tube placement
4. Exploratory laparotomy is reserved for failed endoscopic correction

Abdominal film of patient with sigmoid volvulus

Annular Pancreas

Buzz Words: Pancreas around the duodenum on imaging

Clinical Presentation: Most patients are asymptomatic but some infants may manifest abdominal distention, vomiting, and feeding intolerance. This malformation predisposes to pancreatitis and duodenal obstruction from subsequent fibrosis. Associated with Down syndrome, esophageal/duodenal atresia, polyhydramnios, and Meckel diverticulum.

PPx: N/A

MoD: Failure of the ventral bud to rotate around the duodenum, forming a ring around the second portion of the duodenum

Dx:

1. Abdominal x-ray
2. Abdominal ultrasound

Tx/Mgmt: Surgery to bypass the annulus

Biliary Atresia

Buzz Words: Neonatal conjugated hyperbilirubinemia

Clinical Presentation: Jaundice in newborn accompanied by alcoholic stools and dark-colored urine. Abdominal exam is notable for splenomegaly and a firm liver. Associated with lateralization anomalies (i.e., situs inversus and asplenia).

PPx: N/A

MoD: Inflammatory process that causes obstruction or absence of bile duct. Mutations of the CFC1 gene (regulates L–R distribution in embryonic development) have been associated with biliary atresia.

Dx:

1. Conjugated hyperbilirubinemia
2. Cholangiogram is gold standard for confirmation

Tx/Mgmt: Kasai procedure (hepatoportoenterostomy) may confer palliation of obstruction initially. Nonetheless, most patients (60%–80%) will eventually require liver transplantation.

99 AR

Biliary atresia—definition and pathophysiology

Cleft Lip and Palate

Buzz Words: Complicated breastfeeding + nasal speech + communication between nasal and oral cavities

Clinical Presentation: Incidence 1:800 live births. Cleft lip and palate is the most common presentation occurring in 50% of cases. Cleft lip alone occurs in 25% of cases and is more common in males. Cleft palate alone occurs in 25% of cases and is more common in females.

Complications from cleft lip/palate: inadequate suction during breastfeeding, malocclusion, speech problems, and Eustachian tube dysfunction (i.e., chronic otitis media).

PPx: Avoid smoking and drugs known to cause this malformation during pregnancy.

MoD: Failure in fusion of facial processes. Associated to teratogenic drug exposure during pregnancy (e.g., phenytoin, valproic acid, thalidomide). Defect is present in 60%–80% of patients with Patau syndrome (trisomy 13), Potter sequence (think oligohydramnios), and CATCH-22.

Dx: Clinical presentation

Tx/Mgmt: Cleft lip is usually closed at 3 months of age; cleft palate closure follows usually before 1 year of age. Surgical closure if cleft lip/palate doesn't close.

Esophageal Atresia

Buzz Words: Polyhydramnios + drooling and cyanosis with feeds

Clinical Presentation: Newborn with excessive drooling. Breastfeeding attempt produces coughing, perioral cyanosis, and a drop in hemoglobin saturation. Commonly, this will present in association with a tracheoesophageal fistula (85% of cases). TEF/EA form part of the VACTERL association.

PPx: N/A

MoD: Polyhydramnios develops due to the inability of the fetus to swallow amniotic fluid.

Dx: X-ray showing nasogastric tube in the atretic esophageal pouch after an attempt to pass the tube into the stomach

Tx/Mgmt:
1. Primary anastomosis when the distance between the proximal and distal esophageal segments allows.
2. In the case of significant distance of separation a staged procedure is used, which might require elongation of the esophagus, gastric transposition, or interposition of the jejunum or colon.

> **MNEMONIC**
> **VACTERL** association: **V**ertebral anomalies, **A**nal atresia, **C**ardiac defects, **T**racheoesophageal fistula, **E**sophageal atresia, **R**enal anomalies, and **L**imb defects

Malrotation Without Volvulus

Buzz Words: Bands of peritoneum attaching the cecum to the lateral abdominal wall + duodenum with a *corkscrew* appearance + incomplete rotation around the superior mesenteric artery (SMA)

Clinical Presentation: Vomiting, abdominal distention, and tenderness. Usually occurs in patients with other congenital anomalies.

PPx: N/A

MoD: Incomplete rotation of the cecocolic limb around the SMA, which means that the cecum ends in the mid-upper abdomen and is attached to the R lateral abdominal wall by bands of peritoneum (Ladd bands). These bands cross the duodenum causing intrinsic obstruction and compression. In malrotation, the third portion of the duodenum does not pass in between the abdominal aorta and the SMA.

Dx: Contrast enema shows a high, medially directed cecum.

Tx/Mgmt: Ladd procedure consists in division of Ladd bands + widening of the mediastinum + appendectomy + fixation of the cecum and colon in their correct anatomic location.

Meckel Diverticulum

Buzz Words: Failed obliteration + blind pouch connected to ileum + pancreatic acini in mucosa + ectopic gastric mucosa + fecal matter in umbilical area at birth

Clinical Presentation: Painless melena and iron deficiency anemia during the first years of life. Another presentation could be bowel obstruction secondary to small bowel intussusception (diverticulum functions as nidus). Most common congenital anomaly of the small bowel. A ligament between the terminal ileum and umbilicus may be identified during surgical exploration of the abdomen.

PPx: N/A

MoD: Omphalomesenteric (vitelline) duct remnant, which usually obliterates by the seventh week of embryonic development. The pouch may contain retained gastric (most common), pancreatic, colonic, jejunal, duodenal, or endometrial tissues. Ectopic gastric acid produces mucosal ulceration and bleeding.

Dx: ^{99m}Tc nuclear scan to identify gastric mucosa

Tx/Mgmt: Segmental bowel resection in all symptomatic patients or young patients due to potential for complications.

Pyloric Stenosis

Buzz Words: Projectile vomit + palpable *"olive-like"* RUQ abdominal mass

Clinical Presentation: Baby (3–5 weeks of age) w/ forceful nonbilious vomiting, which occurs after feeding. Abdominal exam is notable for hyperperistalsis and palpable pyloric sphincter.

PPx: N/A

MoD: Hypertrophy of the pyloric sphincter, usually not present at birth but develops over the first 3–5 weeks of life. NO synthase deficiency precipitates the disease.

Dx: Abdominal ultrasound shows increased pyloric muscle thickness, length, and diameter.

Tx/Mgmt:

1. Laparoscopic pyloromyotomy
2. Correction of electrolyte abnormalities and fluid repletion
3. Early re-initiation of feeding

Gastric Outlet Obstruction

Buzz Words: Enlarged gastric bubble in abdominal film

Clinical Presentation: Epigastric abdominal pain, nausea, and vomiting after eating. Also related to early satiety, weight loss, and abdominal distention.

PPx: N/A

MoD: Mechanical obstruction of the stomach and duodenum. Common causes of compression are pancreatic cancer, gastric lymphoma, Crohn disease, PUD, fibrosis after caustic injury, gastric bezoars, and percutaneous endoscopic gastrostomy tube migration.

Dx: Metabolic derangements from excessive vomiting are hypokalemia and hypochloremic metabolic alkalosis. Abdominal CT scan will most likely point out the cause of compression.

Tx/Mgmt:

1. Medical management consists in NPO + nasogastric tube, address electrolyte and metabolic imbalances, fluid replacement, and IV PPI.
2. Causes with etiologies with potential surgical correction should undergo the procedure.

Tracheoesophageal fistula

Buzz Words: Cyanosis during breastfeeding

Clinical Presentation: Coughing and cyanosis after feeding in newborn. If the defect is not corrected, aspiration pneumonia will ensue.

PPx: N/A

MoD: Cyanosis is secondary to laryngospasm to protect airway after aspiration of milk/formula.

Dx: Fistula can normally be identified in a lateral chest film. Fluoroscopic imaging studies be performed with water-soluble contrast agents (DO NOT USE BARIUM) to avoid chemical pneumonitis.

Tx/Mgmt: Surgical ligation of the fistula through a cervical approach when the fistula is isolated. In cases with

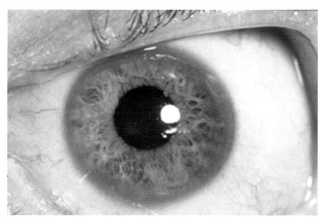

FIG. 8.1 Kayser-Fleischer ring. (From Wikimedia Commons. https:// en.wikipedia.org/wiki/Kayser%E2%80%93Fleischer_ring#/media/ File:Kayser-Fleischer_ring.jpg. Created by Herbert L. Fred, MD and Hendrik A. van Dijk. Used under Creative Commons Attribution 3.0 Unported license.)

esophageal atresia (EA), resection and primary anastomosis of the esophageal segments is preferred.

Wilson Disease

Buzz Words: Hepatic dysfunction between 8 and 16 years + young kid + Kayser Fleischer ring (Fig. 8.1) + Wing-beating tremors + seizures + ataxia + dysarthria + tremor + dystonia + Parkinsonism + tics

Clinical Presentation: Wilson disease is a disorder of copper regulation, whereby a mutation on chromosome 13 leads to accumulation of copper in hepatocytes, cornea, basal ganglia, and kidneys. This leads to many unique signs and symptoms, such as Kayser-Fleischer ring and wing-beating tremor.

The diagnostic lab results are also classically tested. Know that Wilson disease is present when ceruloplasmin is low and urine copper is high.

PPx: Low copper diet

MoD: AR mutation in ATP7B gene (chromosome 13) → copper accumulates in hepatocytes, then cornea, basal ganglia, and kidneys

Dx:
1. Serum ceruloplasmin (low)
2. Urine copper (high)
3. Liver biopsy

Tx/Mgmt:
1. Chelation with penicillamine, trientene, and zinc
2. Liver transplant in advanced disease

Adverse Drug Effects

Drug-Induced Changes in Motility

Chronic Laxative Abuse

Buzz Words: Factitious diarrhea + contraction alkalosis

Clinical Presentation: A classic patient is a woman who works in healthcare with profuse watery diarrhea associated with cramping abdominal pain. Signs of dehydration may be present.

PPx: N/A

MoD: Voluntary abuse of osmotic laxatives (i.e., magnesium, sorbitol, lactulose, polyethylene glycol)

Dx: Hypokalemia and metabolic (contraction) alkalosis. Those abusing magnesium cathartics will have hypermagnesemia. Stool osmotic gap usually exceeds 75 mOsm/kg. Diagnosis of exclusion after ruling out organic causes of diarrhea.

Tx/Mgmt:
1. Electrolyte and fluid replacement
2. Referral to psychiatric evaluation

Opioids

Clinical Presentation: A patient with chronic pain managed with opioids or substance abuse disorder who complains of abdominal distention, failure to pass flatus, and diffuse abdominal pain

PPx: Prophylactic laxative therapy for patients requiring chronic pain management

MoD: Opioids inhibit bowel motility through direct and anticholinergic mechanisms. Longer transit times allow for excessive reabsorption of fluids from feces, creating rock-solid fecal matter, and impaction. In the setting of chronic opioid abuse, tolerance does not develop to constipation (or miosis either).

Dx: Clinical diagnosis

Tx/Mgmt: Stool softener or osmotic laxatives to rehydrate fecal matter and allow for uneventful passing

Drug-Induced Gastritis, Duodenitis, and Peptic Ulcer

Clinical Presentation: The same presentation as that described previously for gastritis, duodenitis, and PUD

PPx: Use of selective cyclo-oxygenase-2 (COX-2) inhibitors (i.e., celexocib)

MoD: The arachidonic acid degradation pathway allows the formation of pro-inflammatory and physiologically active molecules, which aid in platelet aggregation, vasoconstriction, and protection of gastric mucosa. Nonselective inhibition of COX from NSAIDs reduces the stimulus to maintain mucus production and mucosal perfusion, and increase gastric acid production.

Dx: Clinical suspicion

Tx/Mgmt: Avoid nonselective COX inhibitors

Drug-Induced Hepatitis

Buzz Words: Symptoms or abnormal labs that appear to have a time relationship with the initiation of a drug

Clinical Presentation: Most patients are asymptomatic; within those who do manifest symptoms the most common would be nausea, vomiting, RUQ pain, jaundice, malaise, low-grade fever, acholic stools, and choluria.

PPx: Awareness of marginal liver function and avoidance of hepatotoxic drugs in these patients

MoD: Drug-induced injury may be classified in several ways, perhaps the most useful is by clinical presentation: hepatocellular, cholestatic, or mixed injury. Table 8.16 presents the most common causative agents by method injury.

Dx: Hepatocellular injury will be characterized by elevation in ALT and AST greater than 3× the upper limit of normal (ULN). Cholestatic injury will be characterized by elevation of ALP greater than 2× ULN. Hyperbilirubinemia will be present in both injuries.

Tx/Mgmt: Withdrawal of drug

Drug-Induced Pancreatitis (e.g., Thiazides)

Buzz Words: Elevated serum amylase and lipase after initiating a new drug

TABLE 8.16 Causative Agents of Drug-Induced Hepatitis by Injury

Injury	Agents
Hepatocellular	Acetaminophen, isoniazid, halothane, methyldopa
Cholestasis	Amoxicillin-clavulanate, amiodarone, oral contraceptives, anabolic steroids, rifampin
Mixed	Captopril, ibuprofen, phenytoin

Clinical Presentation: Similar to the presentation mentioned above for acute pancreatitis. Patients have excellent prognosis with a low risk of mortality once the drug is stopped.

PPx: Awareness of drug prescription in patients with marginal pancreatic function

MoD: Pathogenesis of drug-related insult is poorly understood. Some drugs that cause pancreatitis are: azithromycin, furosemide, thiazides, TMP-SMX, and valproate.

Dx: Clinical suspicion

Tx/Mgmt: Management of acute pancreatitis (described above) + cessation of drug use

GUNNER PRACTICE

1. A 78-year-old man is brought to the Emergency Department with bright red blood per rectum. He lives in a nursing home and was noted in the morning to be fatigued and slow to respond. His adult diaper revealed a pool of blood. He has a history of hypertension, atrial fibrillation, and osteoarthritis. His medications include amlodipine, aspirin, hydrochlorothiazide, naproxen, and warfarin. In the emergency department, his vital signs (VS) are T 97.3, HR 120, BP 87/41, and RR 18, SpO$_2$ 97% on room air. Labs show a Hgb 6.8, PLT 301, BUN 35, Cr 1.1, and INR 2.6. He is given 2 units packed RBCs (PRBCs), vitamin K (IM), and fresh frozen plasma. He continues to have significant hematochezia. What is the next best step in management?
   A. Administer protamine sulfate
   B. Give bowel preparation for colonoscopy tomorrow
   C. Urgent upper endoscopy
   D. Give platelet transfusion
   E. Wait for bleeding to cease and restart warfarin with goal INR 2.0–2.5

2. A 66-year-old woman comes to the emergency department after her husband notices that her eyes are looking yellow. She has a history of hypertension and chronic obstructive pulmonary disease (COPD). She quit smoking last year. She takes albuterol, amlodipine, fluticasone-salmeterol, and tiotropium. On further questioning, she notes several weeks of weight loss, anorexia, and low energy. Her vital signs are T 98.3, HR 84, BP 147/89, and RR 16 SpO$_2$ 98% on room air. On exam, she is thin with temporal wasting, and she has a painless but palpable gallbladder in the abdominal RUQ. Labs reveal white blood cell count of 7.4, Hgb

11.1, normal electrolytes, normal coagulation studies, total bilirubin 5.9, direct bilirubin 5.1, and ALT of 15. What is the best next step in management?

A. Surgical consult for cholecystectomy tomorrow

B. Intravenous piperacillin-tazobactam

C. Emergent laparotomy

D. Endoscopic retrograde cholangiopancreatography

E. CT scan of the abdomen and pelvis

F. Transvaginal ultrasound

3. A 49-year-old male immigrant from Poland comes to the emergency department after his friend notices that his eyes look yellow. On further questioning, he reports vague RUQ abdominal aching for several months. He has a history of Trisomy 21, the metabolic syndrome, and Long QT syndrome. His medications include propranolol and sertraline. His vital signs are T 98.8, HR 69, BP 138/88, and RR 18 SpO_2 97% on room air. An RUQ abdominal ultrasound shows concern for a cystic liver mass, and CT abdomen/pelvis reveals an 8 cm multiloculated "popcorn" cyst in the right lobe of the liver. Surgery is consulted and advises additional antimicrobial treatment targeting the causative organism. What antimicrobial should best prescribed?

A. Piperacillin-tazobactam

B. Albendazole

C. Vancomycin

D. Amikacin

E. Metronidazole

Notes

ANSWERS: What Would Gunner Jess/Jim Do?

1. WWGJD? A 78-year-old man is brought to the emergency department with bright red blood per rectum. He lives in a nursing home, and was noted in the morning to be fatigued and slow to respond. His adult diaper revealed a pool of blood. He has a history of hypertension, atrial fibrillation, and osteoarthritis. His medications include amlodipine, aspirin, hydrochlorothiazide, naproxen, and warfarin. In the emergency department, his VS are T 97.3, HR 120, BP 87/41, RR 18, SpO$_2$ 97% on room air. Labs show a Hgb 6.8, PLT 301, BUN 35, Cr 1.1, and INR 2.6. He is given 2 units PRBCs, vitamin K IM, and fresh frozen plasma. He continues to have significant hematochezia. What is the next best step in management?

Answer: C, urgent upper endoscopy

Explanation: Patient has acute, ongoing hematochezia leading to significant hemodynamic instability and anemia. Massive upper GI bleed is possible, especially in the setting of elevated INR and multiple NSAIDs (which can cause and exacerbate gastric ulcers). The BUN/Cr ratio above 30 is further evidence of possible upper GI source. EGD can both establish a diagnosis and provide intervention if this is the case. This answer also can be reached by a process of elimination, as none of the other answers are acceptable.

A. Administer protamine sulfate → Incorrect. Protamine sulfate would reverse aPTT elevation 2/2 heparin, which the patient has not received.

B. Give bowel preparation for colonoscopy tomorrow → Incorrect. Should EGD not reveal a source of bleeding, other testing (including CT angiogram, flexible sigmoidoscopy, or colonoscopy) may be warranted. However, given the ongoing bleeding and hemodynamic instability at presentation, waiting until tomorrow and not including upper GI evaluation is not appropriate.

D. Give platelet transfusion → Incorrect. The patient's platelets are of adequate quantity and we are provided no history of qualitative platelet dysfunction. Platelet transfusion would likely not fix the bleeding and would expose the patient to unnecessary transfusions.

E. Wait for bleeding to cease and restart warfarin with goal INR 2.0–2.5 → Incorrect. The patient continues to bleed, and there is concern for a massive upper GI source. Waiting would be inappropriate.

2. WWGJD? A 66-year-old woman comes to the emergency department after her husband notices that her eyes are looking yellow. She has a history of hypertension and **COPD**. She quit smoking last year. She takes albuterol, amlodipine, fluticasone-salmeterol, and tiotropium. On further questioning, she notes several weeks of weight loss, anorexia, and low energy. Her vital signs are T 98.3, HR 84, BP 147/89, and RR 16 SpO2 98% on room air. On exam, she is thin with temporal wasting, and she has a painless but palpable gallbladder in the abdominal RUQ. Labs reveal WBC 7.4, Hgb 11.1, normal electrolytes, normal coagulation studies, total bilirubin 5.9, direct bilirubin 5.1, and ALT of 15. Which of the following is the best next step in management?

Answer: E, CT scan of the abdomen and pelvis

Explanation: This elderly woman's presentation, with a significant smoking history, weight loss, asthenia, Courvoisier sign, and direct hyperbilirubinemia, raises concern for a pancreatic head mass (likely 2/2 pancreatic ductal adenocarcinoma). While there is no current emergency, she requires imaging of the abdomen for characterization of the mass and staging, which will guide treatment.

A. Surgical consult for cholecystectomy tomorrow → Incorrect. This would be appropriate in the setting of cholecystitis. However, she is not having pain or fever, and there is evidence to support another diagnosis as more likely. She would need a RUQ ultrasound to evaluate before jumping to surgery.

B. Intravenous piperacillin-tazobactam → Incorrect. The concern with biliary obstruction is for ascending cholangitis, for which this would be an appropriate treatment. However, this is heralded by Charcot triad (fever, RUQ pain, and jaundice), and she is afebrile and not in pain.

C. Emergent laparotomy → Incorrect. This would be inappropriate management, as the patient does not have peritonitis and the resectability of a pancreatic head mass must be determined by staging/imaging before a planned surgical procedure.

D. ERCP → Incorrect. While she might need endoscopic ultrasound with FNA and possibly an ERCP-guided intervention in the future, it would not be appropriate to jump to a procedure before the identification and staging of the pancreatic head mass, which is still undiagnosed.

F. Transvaginal ultrasound → Incorrect. The question should alert the reader that there is biliary obstruction, likely from some sort of mass, which would not be identified on transvaginal ultrasound, which surveys pelvic organs.

3. WWGJD? A 49-year-old male immigrant from Poland comes to the emergency department after his friend notices that his eyes look yellow. On further questioning, he reports vague RUQ abdominal aching for several months. He has a history of Trisomy 21, the metabolic syndrome, and Long QT syndrome. His medications include propranolol and sertraline. His vital signs are T 98.8, HR 69, BP 138/88, RR 18 SpO_2 97% on room air. A RUQ abdominal ultrasound shows concern for a cystic liver mass, and CT abdomen/pelvis reveals an 8 cm multiloculated "popcorn" cyst in the right lobe of the liver. Surgery is consulted and advises additional antimicrobial treatment targeting the causative organism. What antimicrobial should best prescribed?

Answer: B, albendazole

Explanation: This is a hydatid cyst, caused by *Echinococcus granulosus*, a tapeworm frequently acquired from dogs. It is causing cholestasis and pain, likely due to mass effect. Albendazole, an anti-helminthic with a broad range of activity, is the appropriate antimicrobial medication for *E. granulosus.*

A. Piperacillin-tazobactam → Incorrect. This is a beta-lactam and anti-beta lactamase combination with broad coverage for Gram +, Gram −, and anaerobic bacteria. *E. granulosus* is not a bacterium.

C. Vancomycin → Incorrect. This antibiotic inhibits bacterial wall synthesis and is used for Gram + bacterial infections.

D. Aztreonam → Incorrect. This antibiotic is an aminoglycoside used largely for Gram − bacterial infections.

E. Metronidazole → Incorrect. This antibiotic is used for anaerobic bacterial infections.

Gynecologic Disorders

Hao-Hua Wu, Leo Wang, Rebecca Gao,
and Wanda Ronner

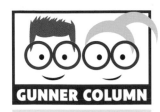

GUNNER COLUMN

Introduction

A little-known fact about the Medicine Shelf is that it includes up to five questions that specifically address gynecologic disorders. These disorders are either on the differential of common chief complaints (e.g., ectopic pregnancy for lower-right-quadrant [LRQ]/lower-left-quadrant [LLQ] abdominal pain) or are important care issues (e.g., breast cancer patients undergoing chemo). Learning these disorders well will also help you ace both the ob/gyn and Medicine Shelf, as many of these (e.g., Fitz-Hugh-Curtis syndrome, sexually transmitted infections) are high-yield and multidisciplinary.

Study this chapter by focusing on buzz words and clinical presentation. Prophylaxis (PPx) will be important to know only for the neoplasms (e.g., breast). mechanisms of disease (MoD), diagnostic steps (Dx), and treatment/management (Tx/Mgmt) are less high-yield for medicine and more likely to appear on ob/gyn. Anticipate spending 3 to 5 hours perusing content and answering questions. Pay particular attention to the subsection on sexually transmitted infections, which includes extremely high-yield topics like syphilis. This chapter is divided into (1) Menopause, (2) Gynecologic Neoplasms, (3) Sexually Transmitted Infections, (4) Multisystem Processes, and (5) Gunner Practice. As always, disorders are presented in the Buzz Words, Clinical Presentation, PPx, MoD, Dx, and Tx/Mgmt format.

Menopause

Questions about menopause will likely focus on the endocrine disturbance and medical sequelae of the disorder. Remember the basic structure of the hypothalamic-pituitary-gonadal (HPG) axis: gonadotropin-releasing hormone (GnRH) from hypothalamus → upregulates luteinizing hormone/follicle stimulating hormone (LH/FSH) in the anterior pituitary → upregulates estrogen in the ovaries → estrogen downregulates GnRH and LH/FSH. Menopause is a disorder of decreased estrogen. Thus, menopausal patients have decreased estrogen levels but increased FSH, LH, and GnRH because of lack of a feedback mechanism.

99 AR

Hormone Therapy and Heart Disease

99 AR

Estrogen inhibits bone resorption by decreasing RANKL and thereby downregulating osteoclast activity. A hypoestrogenic state thereby increases risk of osteopenia/porosis

Buzz Words: >45-year-old female + hot flashes + dyspareunia + osteoporosis + cardiovascular disease + insomnia/sleep disturbance + no menses for ≥12 months

Clinical Presentation: Menopause is defined as a point when women no longer experience menstrual cycles; it marks the end of the reproductive years. The formal diagnosis is made when it has been 12 months since the last menstrual cycle. On the Medicine Shelf, it is unlikely that you will be tested on amenorrhea or abnormal menstrual patterns. Instead, you may see an elderly female with a chief complaint related to menopause (e.g., trouble sleeping, fear of breaking a bone) come in for a well visit and be asked for the next best step in prophylaxis. This is the highest-yielding of the four physician tasks. Dx and Tx/Mgmt are included for the sake of completeness but are unlikely to be tested.

PPx: Calcium for osteoporosis

MoD: No more ovarian follicles → ovaries no longer making estrogen → hypoestrogenic state

Dx:
1. Pelvic exam
2. TSH and FSH to rate of (r/o) other pathology
3. UA/UCx

Tx/Mgmt:
1. Vaginal estrogen replacement
2. Hormone replacement therapy (estrogen + progestin)
3. Calcium supplementation

Gynecologic Neoplasms

The two most common gynecologic neoplasms on the Medicine Shelf are breast and ovarian cancer. Both are treated by oncology-trained physicians and can present with multidisciplinary chief complaints (e.g., abdominal pain in ovarian cancer). For breast cancer, be aware of the buzz words for fibroadenoma and intraductal papilloma (unrelated to neoplasm) as well as Paget disease of the breast (concurrent underlying breast cancer).

Fibroadenoma

Buzz Words: Firm, rubbery, nontender round mass + freely movable + well-circumscribed + often solitary and unilateral + *no* fluctuation in size with menstrual cycle + slow or no growth (vs. phyllodes tumors, which grow rapidly)

Clinical Presentation: A young female (late teens to 20s) has a breast mass on routine exam. The mass is firm, rubbery, and nontender to palpation. She did not notice any changes in the size of the mass over the past year.

PPx: N/A

MoD: Benign proliferation of breast epithelium and stroma

Dx:

1. Mammogram to visualize lesion
2. Ultrasound to differentiate solid versus cystic components
3. Fine-needle aspiration (FNA) to confirm

Tx/Mgmt:

1. If asymptomatic: Observation. Most fibroadenomas will be reabsorbed
2. If mass enlarges or is persistent for >3 months: excisional biopsy
3. If mass is very large (>5 cm): FNA to rule out cystosarcoma phyllodes.

Intraductal Papilloma

Buzz Words: Unilateral bloody or serosanguinous nipple discharge

Clinical Presentation: A female (20s–40s) complains of unilateral bloody nipple discharge. There are no breast masses on physical exam.

PPx: N/A

MoD: Benign growth of epithelial lining (papilloma) arises within the lactiferous ducts (intraductal). Large papillomas blocks duct, causing infarction → bloody discharge.

Dx:

1. Cytology of discharge to rule out invasive papillary cancer
2. Mammogram to rule out other lesions. Mammogram will not show the papilloma due to its small size

Tx/Mgmt: Surgical excision of involved duct

Breast Cancer

Buzz Words: Irregular fixed breast mass + spiculated mass on imaging + asymmetric + architectural distortion + retraction of overlying skin and/or nipple + "orange peel" skin texture (*peau d'orange*) + eczematous lesion of nipple/areola + palpable axillary lymph nodes

Clinical Presentation: Most commonly postmenopausal females. Key elements of the history to watch out for:

- History of ductal carcinoma in situ (DCIS) or lobular carcinoma in situ (LCIS)

QUICK TIPS

The two primary causes of bloody nipple discharge are intraductal papilloma (benign) and papillary breast cancer (malignant).

- Increased lifetime estrogen exposure due to younger age at menarche, nulliparity, older age of first live birth, older age at menopause, obesity, and long-term (>5 years) use of hormone replacement therapy
- Prior exposure to ionizing radiation (e.g., treatment of Hodgkin lymphoma during childhood)
- Family history of gynecologic malignancies
- First-degree relatives with breast cancer. Risk increases with number of first-degree relatives and early age at time of Dx
- *BRCA1/BRCA2* genes are associated with bilateral premenopausal breast cancer and ovarian cancer.

PPx: USPSTF: Biennial mammograms from ages 50–74

American Cancer Society: Annual mammograms from ages 45–54, then annually or biennially for as long as the woman is in good health

Prophylactic mastectomy for *BRCA*-positive

MoD: Different depending on the type and genetic abnormality, but *BRCA* is recognized as a common genetic cause of breast cancer.

Dx:
1. Screening mammography
2. Needle core biopsy or FNA for definitive diagnosis
3. Determination of ER-, PR-, and Her2/neu-responsive cancer
4. Staging workup for metastatic disease

Tx/Mgmt (Table 9.1): Lumpectomy + axillary sampling

Neoadjuvant therapy (e.g., radiation, tamoxifen for premenopausal ER-positive, aromatase inhibitors like anastrozole for postmenopausal ER-positive, trastuzumab for Her2/neu-positive, selective estrogen receptor modulator)

Radical mastectomy

Treatment can vary depending on type of breast cancer (Fig. 9.1)

Paget Disease of the Breast

Buzz Words: Eczema (scaling, crusting, ulceration) of the nipple/areolar complex + unilateral + malignant intraepithelial cells (Paget cells) ± concurrent underlying breast cancer (~90% of cases; Fig. 9.2)

Clinical Presentation: A postmenopausal female presents with erythema, scaling, and crusting surrounding her left nipple.

PPx: N/A

TABLE 9.1 Breast Neoplasms

	Description	Classic Presentation	Treatment
LCIS	**Noninvasive** proliferation of malignant epithelial cells in breast **lobules**	Asymptomatic Incidental finding on biopsy for an unrelated indication	Observe Selective estrogen-receptor modifiers
DCIS	**Noninvasive** proliferation of malignant epithelial cells in breast **ducts**	Asymptomatic Found on screening mammography showing clustered microcalcifications	Lumpectomy + radiation therapy Simple mastectomy for extensive multicentric lesions
Invasive cancer	—	Ill-defined fixed breast mass Irregular asymmetric mass with spiculations mass and architectural distortion on imaging	Lumpectomy + radiation therapy Simple mastectomy for larger lesions Radical mastectomy for disease with axillary node involvement
Lobular carcinoma	Invasive proliferation of malignant epithelial cells in breast **lobules**	Less common than ductal carcinoma Frequently bilateral	—
Ductal carcinoma	Invasive proliferation of malignant epithelial cells in breast **ducts**	More common that lobular carcinoma	—

DCIS, ductal carcinoma in situ; *LCIS,* lobular carcinoma in situ.

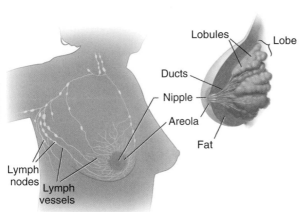

FIG. 9.1 Anatomic origins of breast neoplasms. (From National Cancer Institute, National Institutes of Health.)

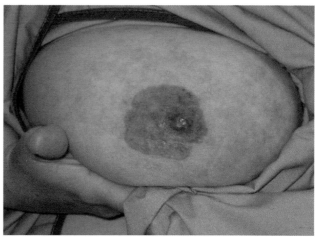

FIG. 9.2 Paget disease of the breast. Photo demonstrating classic physical exam findings with Paget disease (scaling, crusting, ulceration near the nipple/areolar complex). (From radiopaedia.org. Used under Creative Commons Attribution-Share Alike 3.0 Unported license.)

MoD: Malignant cells invade epidermis of the nipple → inflammation of the nipple → spread to areola → eczematous changes of the nipple/areolar complex

Dx: You must remember to evaluate for breast cancer because Paget disease of the breast is almost always associated with an underlying neoplasm.

    a. Diagnostic biopsy of skin demonstrating presence of intraepithelial adenocarcinoma cells (Paget cells) within the nipple

    b. Mammography to identify the breast mass

Tx/Mgmt: Surgical resection of the lesion. The type of surgery and adjuvant therapy will depend on the stage of the concurrent underlying breast cancer.

Ovarian Cancer

Buzz Words: Ascites + abdominal distention + abdominal pain + early satiety + constipation + elevated CA-125

Clinical Presentation: A postmenopausal female presents with early satiety, constipation, weight loss, and bloating. Risk factors relate to increased number of ovulatory cycles: nulliparity and older age. Oral contraceptives (OCPs) are protective because they decrease the number of ovulatory cycles. Other risk factors include family history of breast or ovarian cancer or mutations: *BRCA1/BRCA2*, hereditary nonpolyposis colorectal cancer (HNPCC), Turner syndrome.

PPx: Screening for ovarian cancer is not indicated except in select high-risk subgroups (e.g., patients with known *BRCA1/BRCA2* mutations).

MoD: The ovary consists of three primary tissue types: epithelial cells, germ cells, and stromal tissue. Malignant neoplasms can arise from each of these.

Dx:
1. Physical exam
2. Transvaginal ultrasound
3. **Elevated CA-125** (elevated in epithelial-derived neoplasms
4. Biopsy

Tx/Mgmt:
1. Surgical resection including total abdominal hysterectomy, bilateral salpingo-oophorectomy, and removal of pelvic and para-aortic lymph nodes
2. Chemotherapy
3. Radiation for palliation or persistent disease

Sexually Transmitted Infections

The highest-yielding sexually transmitted infection (STI) is syphilis, also known as "the great imitator"; it can be included in the differential for most chief complaints. Another important concept is Fitz-Hugh-Curtis syndrome, a perihepatitis that arises from chlamydia and gonorrhea. For STIs, focus on buzz words and know the gold standard for diagnosis/treatment (e.g., RPR and VDRL to diagnose syphilis; doxycycline/ceftriaxone to treat chlamydia/gonorrhea, respectively). Also, be sure to differentiate painful ulcers (e.g., herpes and chancroid) from painless ulcers (e.g., syphilis and granuloma inguinale).

Most of the STIs discussed in the following paragraphs can affect **both men and women** (e.g., syphilis, chlamydia/gonorrhea). However, these are listed as gynecologic disorders because they are more commonly presented in female patients on the shelf exams.

Herpes Simplex Virus

Buzz Words: Genital herpes simplex virus (HSV): Painful ulcer + solitary/grouped vesicles on erythematous base + inguinal adenopathy + can evolve to **shallow,** punched-out ulcerations/erosions

HSV prodrome: Cold 10 days ago + vulvar burning, irritation + new sexual partner/no birth control + no painful lesions

QUICK TIPS

CA-125 is a tumor marker for ovarian tumors derived from epithelial cells. It is used to monitor treatment effectiveness over time rather than as a primary screening tool.

Temporal lobe encephalitis due to HSV: Seizures + altered mental status + hyponatremia + RBCs in cerebrospinal fluid (CSF) + temporal lobe lesion on magnetic resonance imaging (MRI).

Clinical Presentation: HSV-1 and 2 can both be transmitted sexually, although HSV-2 is classically more associated with STIs. The key on the Medicine Shelf is to know that genital/mouth ulcers from HSV are painful. Patients have single or grouped vesicles with an erythematous base and have associated inguinal adenopathy. If it is a primary HSV lesion (first time patient exhibits symptoms), there is vulvar pain associated with constitutional symptoms of fever or malaise. If the HSV lesion is recurrent, it will present only as a painful ulcer. The only other STI with painful ulcers tested on the shelf is chancroid, which can be differentiated by irregular/ragged borders and matted lymph nodes (e.g., buboes) that can suppurate or rupture.

HSV can also have a prodrome whereby the patient has a cold a few days after sexual contact, with no painful lesions but burning/irritation in area of transmission. Lastly, HSV can also cause a form of encephalitis that occurs in the temporal lobe. This is a point frequently tested on the Neurology Shelf, but it can also appear on Medicine.

Differentiate HSV-1 versus HSV-2 based on site of infection. Most cases of oral herpes are caused by HSV-1. Most cases of genital herpes are caused by HSV-2.

PPx:
1. Avoid routes of transmission (e.g., kissing, sexual contact)
2. Avoid vaginal delivery if mom has active HSV lesions on vagina (C-section to avoid congenital herpes)

MoD: Transmission/infection through mucosal epithelium (e.g., kissing, sexual contact) → virus lodged in nerve ganglion → remains latent until activated by event (e.g., stress, immunodeficiency).

Dx:
1. Tzanck smear (from ulcer base scrapings); multinucleated giant cells are characteristic of herpes and varicella
2. If cultures negative → polymerase chain reaction (PCR)

Tx/Mgmt: Acyclovir

Neisseria Gonorrhea

Buzz Words: Yellow, mucopurulent cervical discharge + gram-negative diplococci

Clinical Presentation: Gonorrhea is a one of the most common STIs. Many patients are asymptomatic or may present with abnormal discharge. However, it is very important to treat gonorrhea to avoid important sequelae such as pelvic inflammatory disease and Fitz-Hugh-Curtis syndrome. Gonorrhea is one of the only infections (the other being chlamydia) where treatment is given **before** the definitive diagnosis is made. Patients with gonorrhea are often coinfected (46%) with chlamydia; therefore the treatment of choice should always be dual treatment for gonorrhea (ceftriaxone) and chlamydia (azithromycin/doxycycline). Untreated gonorrhea or chlamydia can lead to pelvic inflammatory disease (PID) and infertility.

PPx:
1. Barrier contraception
2. Screen from when patient begins to be sexually active until age 25
3. Ceftriaxone if exposure to gonorrhea

MoD: Transmission/infection through sexual contact (vaginal, oral, anal).

Dx:
1. Positive Gram stain (gram-negative diplococcic)
2. Nucleic acid amplification test
3. Test for syphilis and HIV

Tx/Mgmt: Ceftriaxone AND azithromycin/doxycycline (assume concurrent chlamydia)

Chlamydia Trachomatis

Buzz Words: Yellow, mucopurulent cervical discharge + nothing on Gram stain.

Clinical Presentation: Chlamydia is the most common STI in the world and is spread through unprotected sexual intercourse. Many patients are asymptomatic or may present with abnormal discharge. However, it is very important to treat chlamydia to avoid sequelae such as pelvic inflammatory disease and Fitz-Hugh-Curtis syndrome. Like gonorrhea, chlamydia is common and can be treated easily, so definitive treatment is provided before diagnostic tests are complete.

PPx:
1. Barrier contraception
2. Screen from when patient begins to be sexually active until age 25.

MoD: Transmission/infection through sexual contact (vaginal, oral, anal). *Chlamydia trachomatis* serovars L1–3 can lead to lymphogranuloma venereum (LGV); but these strains of chlamydia are not the same as the one that causes chlamydia transmission/infection through sexual contact (vaginal, oral, anal).

Dx:
1. Negative Gram stain (chlamydia is intracellular)
2. Nucleic acid amplification test (aka DNA probe test)
3. Test for syphilis and HIV

Tx/Mgmt: Azithromycin or doxycycline

Fitz-Hugh-Curtis Syndrome

Buzz Words: Acute right-upper-quadrant (RUQ) pain + elevated liver function test (LFT) + history of STI or unprotected sex + other disease pathology ruled out

Clinical Presentation: Fitz-Hugh-Curtis syndrome is an inflammation of the liver caused by chlamydia or gonorrhea. It is a relatively rare disease but common on the shelf because it is less well known as a cause of RUQ pain. The classic presentation is a sexually active young female who has a history of unprotected sex or untreated STI who presents with RUQ pain, elevated values on the LFT, as well as constitutional symptoms (e.g., fever, chills, night sweats). Can be associated with PID. Definitive diagnosis is made after other causes are ruled out.

PPx:
1. Barrier contraception
2. Treat chlamydia and gonorrhea early.

MoD: Unknown

Dx:
1. Beta human chorionic gonadotropin (hCG)
2. Complete blood count (CBC)/basic metabolic panel (BMP)
3. LFT (elevated indicative of inflammation)
4. Abdominal ultrasound
5. MRI/computed tomography (CT)
6. Diagnostic laparoscopy (perihepatic adhesions)

Tx/Mgmt:
1. Antibiotics (e.g., doxycycline, tetracycline)
2. Laparotomy (lysis of adhesions)

Pelvic Inflammatory Disease (Acute Salpingitis)

Buzz Words: PID: Lower abdominal pain + N/V + fever + adnexal, cervical motion tenderness + vaginal discharge + chandelier sign

99 AR

Theories as to development of Fitz-Hugh-Curtis syndrome

PID + sepsis: N/V + lower abdominal pain + no contraception + >38°C + tachycardic + copious yellow discharge + exquisite uterine tenderness + peritoneal signs

Clinical Presentation: PID is an infection of the uterus, fallopian tubes, and ovaries in a female; it is due to untreated STIs. Patients with PID present with lower abdominal pain, purulent cervical discharge, elevated ESR, leukocytosis, and fever. Untreated PID can lead to infertility, tubo-ovarian abscess, pelvic peritonitis, sepsis, and ectopic pregnancy. It is important to treat suspected PID before receiving culture or diagnostic results.

PPx:
1. Barrier contraception
2. Treat STIs (e.g., chlamydia and gonorrhea) early.

MoD: Inflammation caused by bacterial STIs such as chlamydia, gonorrhea, or mycoplasma spp.

Dx:
1. Beta Hcg
2. CBC/BMP
3. LFTs (r/o Fitz-Hugh–Curtis)
4. Pelvic ultrasound (r/o ectopic pregnancy)

Tx/Mgmt:
1. Admit to hospital if patient is unable to take medication PO
2. Treat with cefotetan/doxycycline, cefoxitin, or clindamycin/gentamycin
3. If outpatient → IM cefoxitin + PO probenecid or doxycycline or ceftriaxone

Tubo-ovarian Abscess (TOA)

Buzz Words: Acute lower abdominal pain + tender adnexal mass + vaginal discharge + systemic symptoms (fevers, chills) + history of PID

Clinical Presentation: A 40-year-old woman with a history of PID and multiple sexual partners presents with sudden lower abdominal pain, fever, and purulent vaginal discharge. On physical exam, you palpate a tender adnexal mass.

PPx:
1. Barrier contraception
2. Appropriate early treatment of STIs

MoD: Ascending infection originates within lower genital tract → migrates into upper genital tract → transforms into localized collection of pus and associated tissue destruction within the fallopian tube ("tubo") and ovary ("ovarian"). TOAs are often polymicrobial. Common organisms include *Escherichia coli and Bacteroides fragilis.* Although *Neisseria gonorrhoeae* and *C. trachomatis* are often responsible for the preceding upper genital tract infection, they are rarely found within the abscess cavity.

Dx:
1. History and physical (H&P) (PID symptoms)
2. Labs (elevated WBC, positive gonorrhea or chlamydia tests)
3. Pelvic ultrasound (multiloculated locally destructive adnexal mass with inflammatory debris)

Tx/Mgmt:
1. If patient is premenopausal, hemodynamically stable, and abscess is small (<9 cm): antibiotics alone
2. If patient is postmenopausal and abscess is small: surgical exploration, given high rate of concurrent gynecologic malignancy
3. If patient does not respond to antibiotics or is worsening: surgical drainage (open or laparoscopic)
4. If patient appears septic or has an acute abdomen: suspect abscess rupture. Immediate surgical exploration with abscess drainage and/or abdominal washout.

Syphilis

Buzz Words: Primary syphilis: Sexually active + painless papule + lymphadenopathy + RPR/VDRL-positive

Secondary syphilis: Brown macular rash on palms and soles (copper penny lesions) + condylomata lata + lymphadenopathy + constitutional symptoms (fever/myalgias/malaise) + painless ulcers

Tertiary syphilis: Pupil constricts with accommodation but unreactive to light (Argyll Robertson pupil) + granulomas + broad-based ataxia due to tabes dorsalis) + inflammation of the aorta

Congenital syphilis: newborn + rhinitis + hepatosplenomegaly + skin lesions + interstitial keratitis + Hutchinson teeth (smaller teeth, widely spaced, with notches on biting surfaces) + saddle nose + saber shins + deafness

Clinical Presentation: Syphilis is the highest-yielding STI and one of the most commonly tested topics on the shelf because it has four different presentations: primary, secondary, tertiary, and congenital syphilis.
- Primary syphilis = only a painless lesion on the genitals.

- Secondary syphilis = systemic constitutional signs/ symptoms and characterized by rashes on the palms and soles.
- Tertiary syphilis = most severe sequelae, such as Argyll Robertson pupil, tabes dorsalis, and aortitis.
- Congenital syphilis presents in a newborn with constant rhinitis and Hutchison incisors.

Syphilis will not only be on the Medicine Shelf but also potentially on every other shelf (e.g., Pediatrics, Neurology, Psychiatry, Family Medicine, Ob/Gyn, and Surgery). The key is to recognize both buzz words and how to differentiate syphilis from diseases with similar presentations (e.g., vs. granuloma inguinale and LGV for painless ulcers; vs. Rocky Mountain spotted fever and hand-foot-mouth disease from Coxsackie A virus for rash on palms/soles of foot). In addition, know that definitive diagnosis is made by dark-field microscopy and penicillin is used for treatment. Lastly, be mindful that congenital syphilis is unlikely to be tested on the medicine shelf but is included here for the sake of completeness.

PPx: Barrier contraception

MoD: Syphilis is an STI caused by *Treponema pallidum*, a spirochete that disseminates infection widely throughout the body.

Dx:

1. Rapid plasma regain (RPR)
2. VDRL (may be false-positive with lupus, rheumatic fever, and viral infections)
3. If VDRL-positive at 1:4 → progress to fluorescent treponemal antibody absorption test (FTA-A)
4. Definitive diagnosis = dark-field microscopy
5. If newborn, test for concomitant human immunodeficiency virus (HIV) and hepatitis B virus (HBV).

Tx/Mgmt:

1. Penicillin
2. If allergic to penicillin, desensitize by incremental doses of PO penicillin V.

Granuloma Inguinale

Buzz Words: Red, beefy ulcers + painless ulcers + face ulcers + smelly ulcers + NO lymphadenopathy + Donovan bodies

Clinical Presentation: Granuloma inguinale is an STI caused by *Klebsiella granulomatis*. It is on the differential for painless ulcers and has a characteristic diagnostic feature (Donovan bodies). Learn the buzz words for

QUICK TIPS

Argyll Robertson pupil is known as "prostitute's pupil" because it accommodates but never reacts.

QUICK TIPS

Patients with syphilis can experience flu-like symptoms such as muscle aches and fever after taking antibiotics. This is known as the Jarisch Herxeimer reaction and is a result of toxin release by spirochetes.

QUICK TIPS

Can differentiate granuloma inguinale painless ulcers from syphilis because there is no concomitant lymphadenopathy.

99 AR

Stages of LGV

99 AR

Painful and painless genital ulcers mnemonic

granuloma inguinale and don't worry about PPx, MoD, Dx, and Tx/Mgmt for the Medicine Shelf.

Lymphogranuloma Venereum

Buzz Words: Painless ulcers + small, shallow ulcers (often asymptomatic) + matted lymph nodes (adjacent lymph nodes that become stuck together) + large, **painless**, fluctuant "buboes" + sinus tracts

Clinical Presentation: LGV should be on the differential for any patient with painless ulcers. The characteristic physical exam feature is its buboes, and it can occur in three stages:
a. An asymptomatic skin lesion appears.
b. Two weeks later, buboes (fluctuant masses) appear.
c. Scarring from inflammation may obstruct lymphatic vessels and cause swelling. Late-stage complications include pericarditis and arthralgias.

Learn the buzz words for LGV and don't worry about PPx, MoD, Dx, and Tx/Mgmt for the Medicine Shelf.

PPx: Barrier contraception

MoD: Infection with *C. trachomatis* serovars L1–3, which are different from serotypes that cause vaginitis, conjunctivitis, and cervicitis. L1–3, unlike the others, can invade lymph nodes.

Dx: Enzyme-linked immunosorbent assay (ELISA) to look for antibodies to chlamydia endotoxin.

Tx/Mgmt: Tetracyclines (e.g., doxycycline)

Chancroid

Buzz Words: Small, **painful** papules 3–7 days, followed by breakdown to shallow, soft, painful ulcers + ragged undetermined edges + red border + tender lymphadenopathy (LAD) + formation of swollen, inflamed lymph node (bubo) with pus inside
• Chancroid versus LGV: Chancroid buboes are **painful**; LGV buboes are **painless.**
• Chancroid versus HSV: Both are painful. Chancroid has associated buboes; HSV has only recurring, isolated painful lesions.

Clinical Presentation: Chancroid is an STI caused by *Haemophilus ducreyi.* It is on the differential for painful.

PPx: Barrier contraception and testing of sexual partners

MoD: Infection caused by *H. ducreyi* (gram-negative bacillus with rounded ends).

Dx:
1. Clinical diagnosis
2. Culture (difficult to culture) or polymerase chain reaction (PCR)

3. Test for other STIs such as HIV and syphilis.

Tx/Mgmt:
1. Azithromycin
2. Ceftriaxone
3. Aspirate buboes.

Treatment of chancroid

Trichomoniasis

Buzz Words: Vaginal discharge + pruritus + dysuria + dyspareunia + thin, malodorous yellow discharge + erythematous patches on cervix ("strawberry cervix") or vagina + erythema of vulva/vagina (possibly due to itching)

Clinical Presentation: Trichomoniasis is an STI caused by flagellated protozoa. Patients can present with erythematous patches on the cervix, known as strawberry cervix. For the Medicine Shelf, know the buzz words and treatment (e.g., metronidazole for patient and partner).

PPx: Barrier contraception

MoD: Infection by trichomonads, which are unicellular flagellated protozoans.

Dx:
1. Pelvic exam
2. Culture and wet mount (see flagellated protozoa)
3. pH test (pH of 5)

Tx/Mgmt: Metronidazole (treat sexual partner as well).

Strawberry cervix

Bacterial Vaginosis (BV)

Buzz Words: Clue cells on wet mount + foul odor + vaginal pH >4.5 + **thin** gray-white vaginal discharge + clue cells + pH > 4.5 + fishy odor with KOH

Clinical Presentation: A reproductive-age woman presents with white-gray vaginal discharge with a fishy odor that worsens after sexual intercourse. Commonly confused with trichomoniasis. For the Medicine Shelf, just learn the Buzz Words.

PPx: Counsel patient to avoid vaginal douching, which alters normal vaginal flora.

MoD: Imbalance in normal vaginal bacteria leading to the proliferation of anaerobic bacteria, such as *Gardnerella vaginalis.* NOT an STI.

Dx: Vaginal discharge with a pH > 4 (alkaline)

Clue cells under the microscope (see Fig. 4.1)

Positive whiff test (fishy odor when adding KOH to sample of discharge)

Tx/Mgmt: Metronidazole or clindamycin. Treatment is indicated for pregnant women because untreated BV can cause preterm birth (Table 9.2).

TABLE 9.2

	Trichomoniasis	Candidiasis	Bacterial Vaginosis
Symptoms	Discharge, itch or asymptomatic	Itch, discomfort or dysuria	Odor, discharge, itch
Discharge	Gray to yellow	"Cottage cheese"	Milky white, "fishy"
Exam findings	Strawberry cervix	Inflammation and erythema	—
pH	>4.5	<4.5	>4.5
KOH test	+	−	+
Wet mount	Motile flagellated protozoa, many WBCs	Few WBCs	Clue cells, no WBCs
KOH wet mount	Pseudohyphae		

Multisystem Processes

The three most important multisystem gynecologic disorders are polycystic ovarian syndrome, endometriosis, and ectopic pregnancy. All three can make female patients come in with chief complaints (e.g., hirsutism, abdominal pain) that are not obviously of gynecologic origin.

Polycystic Ovarian Syndrome (PCOS, Stein-Leventhal Syndrome)

Buzz Words: Hirsutism + acne + male-pattern baldness + amenorrhea/oligorrhea + multiple cysts in ovaries + acanthosis

Clinical Presentation: PCOS is a disorder of unknown etiology that is a common cause of secondary amenorrhea. It is diagnosed if patients meet two of the three Rotterdam criteria: (1) laboratory or clinical signs (e.g., male-pattern baldness, acne, or hirsutism) due to presence of high serum androgen, (2) amenorrhea or oligomenorrhea, (3) cystic ovaries seen on pelvic ultrasound ("string of pearls"). Because insulin resistance is a characteristic of PCOS, patients with PCOS are at increased risk for diabetes, dyslipidemia, cardiovascular disease, and metabolic syndrome. In addition, patients have an increased risk of endometrial hyperplasia and endometrial cancer.

PPx: None to prevent PCOS. Once patient has PCOS, PPx diabetes and cardiovascular disease

MoD: Unknown but associated with insulin resistance, cystic ovaries, and hyperandrogenism

Dx:

1. Clinical evaluation (Rotterdam criteria)
2. Pelvic ultrasound of ovaries
3. Testosterone levels (should be elevated)
4. FSH/LH (should be elevated, LH >FSH, so higher LH:FSH ratios)
5. Glucose tolerance test (>140 on 2-hour GTT → insulin resistance; >200 on 2-hour GTT → diabetes mellitus)
6. Fasting lipid panel → for all newly diagnosed patients

Tx/Mgmt:

1. Metformin
   - Prevents type 2 diabetes mellitus (T2DM); helps with weight loss.
   - Helps induce ovulation in PCOS (mechanism unknown but likely by altering insulin levels to allow for more favorable ovulation).
   - Suppresses androgen production by decreasing ovarian gluconeogenesis (helps correct hirsutism).
2. Lifestyle/diet to control diabetes/weight
3. Clomiphene citrate
   - An estrogen analog that improves GnRH/FSH release. Used to induce ovulation.
4. Ketoconazole
5. Spironolactone

Endometriosis

Buzz Words:

- **Chronic pelvic pain** (worsens before menses) + dyspareunia + dysmenorrhea for 2 years + regular menses + nodularity over uterosacral area + 27-year-old with retroverted uterus + tender adnexa that are normal in size
- Thickening of uterosacral ligaments + decreased uterine mobility + infertility + homogeneous cystic-appearing mass in left ovary

Clinical Presentation: Endometriosis is a condition that results from the appearance of endometrial tissue outside the uterus, causing pelvic pain. Ectopic endometrial tissue can implant in a variety of places, including the ovaries, appendix, sigmoid colon, round ligaments, and broad ligaments. About half of all patients with endometriosis are infertile.

99 AR

ACOG PCOS practice bulletin

MNEMONIC

The 3 Ds of endometriosis: **dyschezia** (pain when defecating) + dysmenorrhea + dyspareunia → endometriosis

QUICK TIPS

The 3 Ds of endometriosis: **Dyschezia** (pain when defecating) + Dysmenorrhea + Dyspareunia

A common cause of secondary dysmenorrhea. Exam will show nodularity of the uterus and tenderness of the adnexa. Pain is from bleeding coming from ectopic endometrium. Almost half of all patients with endometriosis are infertile.

PPx: None

MoD: Ectopic endometrial tissue forms on or beneath pelvic mucosal/serosal surfaces → cyclic hyperplasia and degeneration due to response to female sex hormones → chronic hemorrhaging → fibrotic pelvic adhesions → **infertility**

Dx:

1. Pelvic exam (clinical diagnosis)
2. Beta-hCG
3. CBC, BMP
4. Transvaginal ultrasound (TVUS) to r/o abnormal anatomy.
5. Laparoscopy (will show chocolate-like material representing old blood) to confirm diagnosis

Tx/Mgmt:

1. Nonsteroidal antiinflammatory drugs (NSAIDs) ± combined OCPs
2. Progestins, GnRH agonists for those who don't respond to NSAIDs and OCPs
3. If no improvement → laparoscopy to biopsy, ablate or excise implants
4. Danazol if refractory to laparoscopy
5. Hysterectomy + bilateral salpingoophorectomy = definitive treatment

Ectopic Pregnancy

- **Ectopic pregnancy:** Abdominal pain + amenorrhea + vaginal bleeding + palpable adnexal mass → ectopic pregnancy
- **Ectopic pregnancy:** Beta-hCG >2000 + thin endometrial stripe + "no adnexal masses" + no fetal pole in uterus → ectopic pregnancy
- **Ruptured ectopic pregnancy:** Abdominal pain + amenorrhea + vaginal bleeding + orthostatic changes + hypovolemic shock

Clinical Presentation: Ectopic pregnancy occurs when a fertilized egg matures outside of the uterus (e.g., in the fallopian tube). This can present as RLQ or LLQ abdominal pain and may be mistaken for a gastrointestinal disorder. A patient with hypotension or vital signs that suggest hypovolemic shock likely has a ruptured ectopic pregnancy and requires admission and surgery.

APGO video ectopic pregnancy

Patients with a history of previous pelvic/tubal surgery, PID, intrauterine device (IUD) use, multiple sexual partners, infertility, and/or in utero exposure to diethylstilbestrol (DES) are more at risk.

PPx: Risk factors are often unavoidable and may include ectopic/pelvic/tubal surgery, in utero DES exposure, infertility treatments, IUD use, PID, and multiple sexual partners

MoD: Ectopic pregnancy is caused by failure of a fertilized egg to implant in the endometrium. Most often occurs in the ampulla of the fallopian tube.

Dx:
1. Pelvic exam
2. Beta-hCG (lower than expected)
3. Pelvic ultrasound.

Tx/Mgmt:
1. If hemodynamically stable, methotrexate
2. If unstable, surgery

FOR THE WARDS

A young woman of childbearing age presenting with abdominal pain should ALWAYS be suspected of having an ectopic pregnancy.

GUNNER PRACTICE

1. A 32-year-old female comes to the emergency room for abdominal pain, nausea, and vomiting that have been ongoing for the last 24 hours. She said that she ate a slice of pizza before the pain started but has been unable to keep anything down since then. Her past medical history is notable for a year of "pain in my lower belly," for which she has refused to see a doctor. She has not had surgery and currently takes only a multivitamin. She is sexually active with multiple partners but does not smoke cigarettes or drink alcohol. Her vitals are 100°F, 100/70 mm Hg, 100 bpm, 20 rpm, and 98% on room air. On exam, she appears uncomfortable and guards to palpation of the RLQ. Aside from a quickening heart rate, the rest of her exam is normal. She is given intravenous (IV) fluids and made NPO. What is the next best step in management?
   A. Abdominal ultrasound
   B. Abdominal CT scan
   C. Abdominal MRI
   D. beta hCG
   E. Urinalysis

2. A 28-year-old woman comes to the physician's office because of right-sided abdominal pain. She states that it started about 6 days ago and has not gotten better despite taking six extra-strength acetaminophens a day. Pain is not associated with meals and she has not

noticed any changes in her bowel movements. She also reports having fever, chills, and muscle aches during this time. A year ago, she had surgery to remove her appendix. Five years ago, she had her last visit with her family doctor but did not return even though she was advised to come back for treatment of pelvic pain at the time. Her vital signs are 99°F, 120/80 mm Hg, 90 HR, 16 RR, and 100% on room air. On exam, she has mild tenderness to palpation of the RUQ. The rest of the exam is normal. What is the best next step to treat the patient's abdominal pain?

A. Doxycycline
B. Discontinue acetaminophen
C. Surgery to remove gallbladder
D. Morphine
E. Liver biopsy

3. A 20-year-old woman comes to the student health office at her university looking for advice about her menstrual cycle. She reports never having had a period despite learning about it in her woman's health course. She appears mildly anxious, although she states that perhaps it is a good thing since she does not experience cramping or bloating every month. Her time at university has been very enjoyable, although she complains that she could not smell the food she eats "for as long as I can remember." Her vitals are 98.7°F, 120/80 mm Hg, 80 bpm, 12 RR, and 100% on room air. Her pubic hair is Tanner stage 2. Pelvic exam is normal. What is the most likely diagnosis?

A. Delayed puberty
B. Pituitary adenoma
C. Kallman syndrome
D. Normal development
E. Alcohol use disorder

Notes

ANSWERS: What Would Gunner Jess/Jim Do?

1. WWGJD? A 32-year-old female comes to the emergency room for abdominal pain, nausea, and vomiting that has been ongoing for the last 24 hours. She said that she ate a slice of pizza before the pain started but has been unable to keep anything down since then. Her past medical history is notable for a year of "pain in my lower belly," for which she has refused to see a doctor. She has not had surgery and currently takes only a multivitamin. She is sexually active with multiple partners but does not smoke cigarettes or drink alcohol. Her vitals are 100°F, 100/70 mm Hg, 100 bpm, 20 rpm, and 98% on room air. On exam, she appears uncomfortable and guards to palpation of the RLQ. Aside from a quickening heart rate, the rest of her exam is normal. She is given IV fluids and made NPO. What is the next best step in management?

Answer: D. beta hCG

Explanation: In any female of reproductive age who presents with belly pain, beta-hCG should done first to rule out pregnancy. The patient here has a chief complaint of RLQ abdominal pain that could be anything from appendicitis to bowel obstruction to ectopic pregnancy. In this case, ectopic pregnancy is suggested owing to her long history of "pain in my lower belly," which connotes chronic pelvic pain possibly due to pelvic inflammatory disease. Her history of multiple sexual partners is also a risk factor for STIs. There is an elevated risk of ectopic pregnancy in patients with a history of STIs and PID.

A. Abdominal ultrasound → Incorrect. Could be used to r/o appendicitis, but not the next best step. More likely that this would be done after beta-hCG and labs are done.

B. Abdominal CT scan → Incorrect. Definitely not the correct answer since we have yet to rule out pregnancy in this patient.

C. Abdominal MRI → Incorrect. Again, imaging is not the correct next step in a woman of reproductive age who has yet to have a beta-hCG.

E. Urinalysis → Incorrect. Although a UA could be used to help look for a source of infection, it is not the next best step in this case.

2. WWGJD? A 28-year-old woman comes to the physician's office because of right-sided abdominal pain.

She states that it started about 6 days ago and has not gotten better despite taking six extra-strength acetaminophens a day. Pain is not associated with meals and she has not noticed any changes in her bowel movements. She also reports having fever, chills, and muscle aches during this time. A year ago, she had surgery to remove her appendix. Five years ago, she had her last visit with her family doctor but did not return even though she was advised to come back for treatment of pelvic pain at the time. Her vital signs are 99°F, 120/80 mm Hg, 90 HR, 16 RR, and 100% on room air. On exam, she has mild tenderness to palpation of the RUQ. The rest of the exam is normal. What is the best next step to treat the patient's abdominal pain?

Answer: A. Doxycycline

Explanation: As a reproductive-age female with a history of chronic pelvic pain and acute RUQ pain, this patient likely has Fitz-Hugh–Curtis syndrome, which is a perihepatitis caused by gonorrhea/chlamydia. Often, patients with this syndrome also present with constitutional symptoms, such as "fever, chills, and muscle aches." It is likely that if LFTs were ordered, the patient's aspartate transaminase (AST) and alanine transaminase (ALT) would be found to be elevated. The first line treatment of Fitz-Hugh-Curtis is antibiotics directed at the causal organism (e.g., chlamydia/gonorrhea). Thus, doxycycline would be a good first choice.

B. Discontinue acetaminophen → Incorrect. Acetaminophen toxicity can present as RUQ pain with constitutional symptoms but is not likely in this case. Patient appears to be taking 3000 mg/day of acetaminophen (given that one extra-strength tablet is 500 mg) which is under the daily limit of 4000 mg/day. Patients with acetaminophen toxicity present with an AST:ALT ratio of >1000.

C. Surgery to remove gallbladder → Incorrect. It is unlikely that the RUQ pain is coming from inflammation or pathology of the gallbladder, since RUQ pain is not associated with food intake.

D. Morphine → Incorrect. Although morphine may help with the pain, the effect of the opiate will only be temporary and would not cure the underlying infectious etiology.

E. Laparotomy → Incorrect. Laparotomy can be used to treat Fitz-Hugh–Curtis syndrome, especially by removing perihepatic adhesions. However, antibiotics targeted at gonorrhea and chlamydia, such as tetracyclines, would still be first line.

3. WWGJD? A 20-year-old woman comes to the student health office at her university looking for advice about her menstrual cycle. She reports never having had a period despite learning about it in her woman's health course. She appears mildly anxious, although she states that perhaps it is a good thing since she does not experience cramping or bloating every month. Her time at university has been very enjoyable, although she complains that she could not smell the food she eats "for as long as I can remember." Her vitals are 98.7°F, 120/80 m mHg, 80 bpm, 12 RR, and 100% on room air. Her pubic hair is Tanner stage 2. Pelvic exam is normal. What is the most likely diagnosis?

Answer: C. Kallman syndrome

Explanation: Kallman syndrome is a hypothalamic disorder in which females or males fail to complete puberty. During fetal development, GnRH cells fail to migrate to the hypothalamus, leading to decreased levels of the hormones needed for pubertal development, such as LH, FSH, GnRH, and testosterone. The most important buzz word to easily distinguish Kallman syndrome is anosmia, which occurs due to a failure of olfactory bulb formation. Thus males with infertility and anosmia or females with amenorrhea and anosmia should immediately be considered to have this disorder until proven otherwise.

A. Delayed puberty → Incorrect. Although patient has not achieved pubertal maturity (e.g., amenorrhea, Tanner stage 2 pubic hair), her anosmia points to a different etiology for her disorder.

B. Pituitary adenoma → Incorrect. The signs and symptoms of pituitary adenoma would reflect whichever hormone is being excessively released as well as the absence of other hormones. In this case, there appears to be a global decrease in reproductive hormones without any sign of other endocrine dysfunction.

D. Normal development → Incorrect. Females typically have their first menstrual cycle by age 16. Breast and pubic hair development should be Tanner stage 5 by the age of 20.

E. Alcohol use disorder → Incorrect. Alcohol does not lead to primary amenorrhea.

Renal, Urinary, and Male Reproductive System

Jacques Greenberg, Hao-Hua Wu, Leo Wang, Rebecca Gao, and Nadia Bennett

Introduction

Although renal physiology and fluid and electrolyte balance were highly tested on the USMLE Step 1, the Medicine Shelf tends to focus much more heavily on the management of renal diseases and the identification of various genitourinary pathologies. Fortunately there are several high-yield buzz words for the various genitourinary disorders, and a mastery of these topics is easily achievable once the commonly tested associations are committed to memory. With a solid understanding of the pathophysiology at work—for example, understanding whether a glomerular disease is primary (intrinsic to the kidney) or secondary (to systemic disease)—one has a framework for which to approach questions addressing the genitourinary system.

This chapter is divided into (1) Organizing Principles and Key Terms, (2) The Upper Urinary Tract, (3) The Lower Urinary Tract, (4) Development of the Genitourinary System and Congenital Disorders, (5) Adverse Effects of Drugs on the Renal, Urinary, and Male Reproductive System, and (6) Gunner Practice. Each disease process is divided into the four physician tasks that the shelf exam will test you on: (1) Prophylactic Management, (2) Mechanism of Disease, (3) Diagnostic Steps, and (4) Treatment/Management.

Organizing Principles and Key Terms

Renal Failure

Acute Kidney Injury/Acute Renal Failure

Acute renal failure (ARF), also known as an acute kidney injury (AKI), occurs when there is a rapid decline in renal function, as represented by a rapid increase in BUN and Cr. ARF can be divided into three phases:

- Phase 1: The oliguric phase, which lasts between 10 and 14 days and is defined as urine output of less than 500 mL/day.
- Phase 2: The diuretic phase, when urine output can increase significantly and there can be massive diuresis of retained fluids and electrolytes.

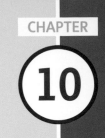

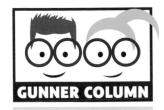

AR

Acute kidney injury overview

- Phase 3: The recovery phase, when there is recovery of tubular function.

Prerenal Renal Failure

Buzz Words: Elevated urine osmolarity (body is attempting to retain water and will concentrate the urine) + decreased urine Na + BUN:Cr ratio > 20:1 + low FeNa <1% + hyaline casts on urinalysis (UA)

Clinical Presentation: A patient has a sudden rise in his BUN to 80 after an 8-hour surgery in which the patient was frequently hypotensive and did not receive adequate fluids. Creatinine bumped up from 1.0 to 1.5. Other risk factors include: congestive heart failure (CHF), cirrhosis, and hepatorenal syndrome.

PPx: Maintain renal perfusion via medications or fluid. Avoid nonsteroidal anti-inflammatory drugs (NSAIDs) and angiotensin-converting enzyme (ACE) inhibitors.

MoD: Blood flow to kidney decreases, leading to a decrease in glomerular filtration rate (GFR).

Dx:
1. Basic metabolic panel (BMP)
2. UA
3. Urine electrolytes
4. Kidney ultrasound

Tx/Mgmt:
1. Maximize renal perfusion by treating underlying cause
2. Swan–Ganz catheter

Intrinsic Renal Failure

Buzz Words: Glomerulonephritis + elevated FENa > 1%

Clinical Presentation: A patient with lupus develops bilateral lower leg edema and his creatinine increases from 1.1 to 1.9. Other risk factors include vascular diseases and hypersensitivity reactions.

PPx: N/A

MoD: Damage to the renal parenchyma from inflammation, ischemia, NSAIDs, or nephrotoxins (e.g., vancomycin, aminoglycosides, contrast material, myoglobin/hemoglobin, chemotherapy)

Dx:
1. BMP (BUN: Cr 10–20:1) due to inability to properly reabsorb BUN
2. UA
   - Low urine osmolarity due to kidney unable to properly concentrate urine, less than 350
   - Urine Na elevated (<20)
   - Elevated FeNa (>2%)

Tx/Mgmt: Eliminate offending agents and treat underlying cause.

Postrenal Acute Renal Failure

Buzz Words: Low urine osmolarity (<350) + elevated urine Na (>40) + BUN:Cr >15:1

Clinical Presentation: Suspect postrenal etiology when you encounter acute renal failure in the setting of benign prostatic hyperplasia (most common), bilateral nephrolithiasis, neoplasm, or retroperitoneal fibrosis.

PPx: N/A

MoD: Increased tubular pressure inhibits the kidney's ability to concentrate urine.

Dx:
- BMP (BUN:Cr >15:1)
- UA/urine electrolytes
  - Low urine osmolarity (<350)
  - Elevated urine Na (>40)
  - Elevated FeNa
- Postvoid residual bladder ultrasound
- Kidney ultrasound

Tx/Mgmt: Bladder catheterization

When a patient has an AKI, think about the *next step* in obtaining your diagnosis. An ultrasound is a quick and easy way to assess for obstruction or hydronephrosis and should be ordered in almost anyone with AKI *unless* the etiology is clearly prerenal. All patients in whom you suspect an AKI should also receive a UA. Look for various casts (these will be covered with their associated intrarenal pathology). Calculate the FeNa *unless* the patient is taking a diuretic. *Get a basic chemistry panel.* In the early phase of renal failure, complications can (rarely) include *hyperkalemia, cardiac arrest,* and *pulmonary edema.*

Treat volume disturbances by balancing diuretic administration against the administration of intravenous (IV) fluids. Keep in mind that both an anion gap and non–anion gap metabolic acidosis can also occur because of the kidney's inability to excrete excess hydrogen ions. Dialysis should be ordered when AEIOU symptoms are present.

Chronic Kidney Disease/Chronic Renal Failure

Buzz Words: GFR <15 or patient on dialysis + small kidneys on ultrasound

Clinical Presentation: Patients will present with insidiously increasing BUN and Cr. They may also have uremic

AR

Hyperkalemia ECG Review

MNEMONIC

AEIOU
  Acidosis (severe metabolic)
  Electrolytes (severe hyperkalemia)
  Intoxication (methanol, ethylene glycol, lithium, aspirin)
  Overload (severe hypervolemia)
  Uremia (severe uremia, pericarditis, BUN >150)

symptoms (nausea/vomiting, pericarditis, encephalopathy, abnormal bleeding from platelet dysfunction, asterixis). They may be anemic from decreased erythropoietin (EPO) production from the kidneys and have painful necrotic skin lesions from vascular calcifications (calciphylaxis).

PPx: N/A

MoD: Greater than 3 months of insult to the kidneys

Dx:

1. UA
2. BMP
3. Complete blood count (CBC)
4. Kidney ultrasound

Tx/Mgmt:

- Decrease in GFR that accompanies chronic kidney disease (CKD) leads to electrolyte retention and increases incidence of hypertension (HTN) and CHF. Manage these carefully.
- Manage infections. These are a major cause of mortality in patients with uremia as CKD inhibits humoral and cellular immunity.
- ACE inhibitors are first-line
- EPO when hemoglobin (Hgb) is less than 10 (may worsen HTN)

Dialysis

Although an astonishing number of Americans receive dialysis, this is a surprisingly sparsely tested topic. The indications for dialysis, however, are extremely high-yield. The mnemonic AEIOU is key to memorize. Note that creatinine level is *not* an absolute indication for dialysis. There are two general methods of dialysis: hemodialysis and peritoneal dialysis. Of the options for hemodialysis, arteriovenous fistula is the preferred method, although the majority of Americans initiate dialysis via a tunneled catheter.

When a patient undergoes hemodialysis, know that blood must be heparinized to prevent it from clotting within the dialyzer. Also, due to the dissimilarities between dialysis and the natural kidney, hypotension during dialysis is a common complication. Patients may also suffer from a "first-use syndrome," characterized by back pain and, occasionally, anaphylaxis.

Peritoneal dialysis, which does not predispose patients to either hypotension or first-use syndrome, requires a high-glucose filtrate that may lead to hyperglycemia and hypertriglyceridemia. Peritonitis may also occur.

Neither peritoneal dialysis nor hemodialysis will replace a kidney's synthetic function. EPO and vitamin D deficiencies are very common. Make sure that a patient has sufficient iron levels when supplementing EPO. Also be sure to differentiate between osteodystrophy secondary to low vitamin D from hemodialysis-associated amyloidosis in bones and joints.

Hematuria

Buzz Words: Blood in urine + blood on dipstick + dipstick-positive

Clinical Presentation: Microscopic hematuria is defined as greater than 3 RBC/HPF, and gross hematuria is visible to the naked eye. Watch out for dipstick-positive blood in the absence of hematuria. This may be due to myoglobin or hemoglobin in the urine.

PPx: N/A

MoD:
- Microscopic hematuria is usually due to glomerular disease.
- Gross hematuria likely has a postrenal etiology. If present at the beginning of the urine stream, it is likely urethritis. If present at the end of the stream, it may be bladder cancer or a prostatic disorder.

Dx:
1. Urine dipstick and UA
   - Assess for renal disease (glomerular or tubular), infection, and non-RBC markers of dipstick positivity (hemoglobin or myoglobin).
   - Watch out for dipstick-positive blood in the absence of hematuria. This may be due to myoglobin or hemoglobin in the urine.
2. Cystoscopy, rarely indicated, except as below:
   - Gross hematuria without evidence of glomerular disease or infection
   - Microscopic hematuria without evidence of glomerular disease but with high risk of infection
   - Recurrent urinary tract infections (UTIs)
   - Obstruction
   - Abnormal bladder imaging

Tx/Mgmt: Address underlying cause.

Proteinuria

We define proteinuria as urinary excretion of protein greater than 150 mg/day. Nephrotic-range proteinuria occurs when urinary excretion exceeds 3.5 g/day. Urinary protein is initially detected by dipstick test. The dipstick is sensitive for albumin; therefore it will not detect globulins (for example, as seen in myeloma).

Any abnormal dipstick test must be followed up by a UA and 24-hour collection. If the patient is asymptomatic and the proteinuria is transient, reassurance will suffice. However, if the patient is asymptomatic but the proteinuria is persistent, further testing is required. *Assess blood pressure and examine the urine sediment.* Treat the underlying condition. When a patient becomes symptomatic, the underlying disease must be addressed and ACE inhibitors should be started. *ACE inhibitors minimize the loss of urinary albumin. They should always be started in diabetics with HTN to prevent microalbuminuria.* Patients with proteinuria have weakened immune systems. They should therefore be vaccinated against influenza and pneumococcus.

Nephritic Versus Nephrotic Syndrome

99 AR
Nephrotic vs Nephritic video

The shelf exams will expect you to differentiate between nephritic and nephrotic syndrome. This is generally straightforward and can allow you to easily rule out certain answer choices. Nephritic syndrome arises secondary to glomerular inflammation. Therefore patients with nephritic syndrome will show symptoms of hematuria, oliguria, HTN, and azotemia, with some proteinuria (<3.5 g/day). Memorize the number 3.5! It should be the first thing you look for in differentiating nephritic syndrome from *nephrotic syndrome, which is due to*

99 AR
Nephrotic vs Nephritic quick overview

the loss of negative charge on the glomerular basement membrane (GBM). Like charges repel. Proteins are full of negative charges. Because of the loss of negative charges on the basement membrane, it is less able to repel the negative charges on the proteins, so you get massive proteinuria (>3.5 g/day).

You will also see edema, hypoalbuminemia, hyperlipidemia, and hypercoagulability. *Watch out for renal vein thrombosis (or any thrombosis for that matter) in patients with nephrotic syndrome.* The hypercoagulability arises due to the loss of anti–thrombin III. Whereas the glomeruli in patients with nephritic syndrome are hypercellular and produce RBC casts, normo-/hypocellular glomeruli are seen in patients with nephrotic syndrome, and they develop fatty casts in their urine.

The Upper Urinary Tract

Inflammatory and Immunologic Disorders of the Upper Urinary Tract
Primary Glomerular
Minimal Change

Buzz Words: Foot process effacement + normal microscopy

Clinical Presentation: Nephrotic syndrome (edema, proteinuria) in children. Associated with viral syndromes, Hodgkin, and Non-Hodgkin lymphoma

PPx: N/A

MoD: Systemic T-cell dysfunction, causing effacement of foot processes

Dx: No need for biopsy
   a. UA
   b. BMP

Tx/Mgmt: Steroids

Focal Segmental Glomerulosclerosis

Buzz Words: Steroid resistant + HIV + heroin

Clinical Presentation: An HIV-positive IV drug user presents with anasarca and nephrotic-level proteinuria (>3.5 g).

PPx: Avoid illicit drugs and HIV risk factors.

MoD: Fibrotic scarring and thickening of the glomerular basement membranes, causing leakage

Dx:
   1. BMP
   2. UA
   3. Renal biopsy

Tx/Mgmt: Generally resistant to steroids, but steroids still used with immunosuppressive agents, cytotoxic agents, and ACE inhibitors/angiotensin receptor blockers (ARBs).

Membranous Glomerulosclerosis

Buzz Words: Steroid resistant + hepatitis B + diffuse GBM thickening + EM "spike and dome"

Clinical Presentation: A adult with systemic lupus erythematosus (SLE), hepatitis B, and syphilis presents with anasarca and nephrotic-level proteinuria (>3.5 g).

PPx: Avoid illicit drugs and high-risk sexual behavior.

MoD: Thickening of glomerular capillary walls

Dx:
   1. UA
   2. BMP
   3. Renal biopsy

Tx/Mgmt: Steroid-resistant. Supportive management with ACE inhibitors/ARBs. Eventual renal failure in about 1/3.

IgA Nephropathy/Berger Disease

Buzz Words: purpura + LM-mesangial deposits + IF-IgA stain

Clinical Presentation: A 12-year-old boy presents and is noted to have proteinuria following a viral syndrome (URI/gastroenteritis).

PPx: NA

MoD: Mesangial deposition of IgA and C3

Dx:
1. BMP
2. UA
3. Renal biopsy

Tx/Mgmt: Steroids questionably beneficial

Alport Syndrome

Buzz Words: deafness + ocular defects + proteinuria

Clinical Presentation: A nephritic or nephrotic syndrome in patients with deafness, blindness. Light microscopy of the renal biopsy shows a split GBM. The patient's father and uncle also experienced similar symptoms.

PPx: N/A

MoD: X-linked recessive or autosomal dominant mutations in type IV collagen.

Dx:
1. BMP
2. UA
3. Renal biopsy
4. Genetic testing

Tx/Mgmt: Supportive

Secondary Glomerular

Diabetic Glomerulonephropathy

Buzz Words: Kimmelstiel-Wilson nodules + microalbuminuria + LM-mesangial expansion

Clinical Presentation: Nephrotic syndrome in diabetic patients

PPx: Glucose control

MoD: Glomerular hyperfiltration is the earliest renal abnormality seen in diabetes mellitus, but thickening of the basement membrane is the first to be quantitated.

Dx:
1. BMP
2. UA
3. Renal biopsy

Tx/Mgmt: ACE inhibitors and diabetes management

Hypertensive Glomerulonephropathy

Buzz Words:
- Benign: thickening of afferent arterioles in patients with long-standing HTN

- Malignant: rapid decrease in renal function and increase in blood pressure

Clinical Presentation: Nephrotic syndrome in hypertensive African American males

PPx: Optimal blood pressure control

MoD: Increased hydrostatic pressure in glomeruli

Dx:
1. BMP
2. UA
3. Renal biopsy

Tx/Mgmt: Optimal blood pressure control

Lupus Nephritis

Buzz Words: Butterfly rash + discoid lesions + malar rash + Libman-Sacks endocarditis + LM-wire loops + EM-subendothelial deposits + IF – full-house staining

Clinical Presentation: Nephritic syndrome in SLE patients, fatigue, malaise, fever, weight loss, progressing to nephrotic-level hematuria. More common in women and African Americans.

PPx: Antimalarial agents (hydroxychloroquine). Remember to get annual eye exam because of retinal toxicity.

MoD: Antigen-antibody deposition in the glomerulus

Dx:
1. BMP
2. UA
3. Renal biopsy

Tx/Mgmt: Treat underlying lupus. Know that renal failure and opportunistic infections from immune suppression are the most common causes of death.

Membranoproliferative Glomerulonephritis

Buzz Words: Hepatitis C + cryoglobulinemia + reduced C3 and C4 + dense intramembranous deposition of immune complexes + IF- and C3-positive + EM "tram tracks"

Clinical Presentation: Nephrotic syndrome in hepatitis C patients. Less commonly, patient may have hepatitis B, syphilis, lupus, or malignancy.

PPx: N/A

MoD: Immune complex deposition

Dx:
1. BMP
2. UA
3. Renal biopsy

Tx/Mgmt: Rarely effective; poor prognosis

Poststreptococcal Glomerulonephritis

Buzz Words: Coke-colored urine + periorbital edema + strep throat, cellulitis + LM-"lumpy bumpy" + antigen-antibody complexes with subendothelial IgG and IgM deposition + elevated ASO + decreased complement

Clinical Presentation: Nephritic syndrome 10–14 days after impetigo or URI in a child or young adult

PPx: N/A

MoD: Antigen-antibody complex with subepithelial deposition of IgG, IgM, and C3, leading to "lumpy bumpy" appearance on light microscopy

Dx:
1. BMP
2. UA
3. Renal biopsy

Tx/Mgmt: Use of antibiotics controversial; supportive measures

Goodpasture Syndrome

Buzz Words: IgG anti-GBM antibody + hemoptysis + hematuria, +LM-crescentic proliferation + IF-linear staining

Clinical Presentation: Renal failure in a patient with lung disease (often manifested by cough, but also hemoptysis). Lung disease precedes renal disease.

PPx: N/A

MoD: IgG antibodies against the GBM

Dx:
1. BMP
2. UA
3. Renal biopsy

Tx/Mgmt:
1. Plasmapheresis
2. Cyclophosphamide
3. Steroids

Thin Basement Membrane Disease

Buzz Words: Persistent hematuria (often microscopic) + mild proteinuria + NO HTN + LM-normal + EM-thin basement membrane

Clinical Presentation: Benign familial hematuria; renal function unaffected

PPx: NA

MoD: Autosomal dominant genetic disorder

Dx:
1. BMP
2. UA

3. Renal biopsy
4. Genetic testing

Tx/Mgmt: None

Tubuluar Interstitial Disease

Acute Tubular Necrosis

Buzz Words: Oliguria + heart failure + normal BUN:Cr ratio + elevated BUN + elevated Cr + muddy brown casts in urine

Clinical Presentation: Renal failure in setting of low cardiac output states such as heart failure, shock, or hypotension

PPX: Maintaining urinary perfusion in a low-cardiac-output state

MoD: Most commonly due to ischemic/hypoxic injury. May also occur secondary to toxic injury (mercury). Does not involve the glomeruli; involves the tubules. **Straight portion of proximal tubule and thick ascending limb of medullary segment are most at risk.**

Dx:
1. BMP
2. UA
3. BNP

Tx/Mgmt:
Improve cardiac output or improve blood flow to kidney

Acute Interstitial Nephritis

Buzz Words: Drug allergy + eosinophilia + known exposure to offensive agent (gentamycin, IV contrast, Hb/Mb, *many other drugs*) + rash, fever, renal insufficiency

Clinical Presentation: Acute renal failure (ARF) after exposure to a new medication or after a recent infection

PPx: Avoidance of predisposing agents

MoD: Allergic reaction

Dx:
1. BMP
2. UA

Tx/Mgmt: Discontinue the offending agent.

Papillary Necrosis

Buzz Words: NSAIDs, Tylenol + sickle cell + transplant rejection

Clinical Presentation: ARF in a patient with diabetes, sickle cell disease, or renal transplant

PPx: Avoid nephrotoxic substances.

MoD: N/A

Dx:
1. Excretory urogram
2. BMP
3. UA

Tx/Mgmt: Treat underlying cause

Human Immunodeficiency Virus Nephropathy

Buzz Words: Nephrotic syndrome + AIDS + slowly progressing

Clinical Presentation: Nephrotic syndrome in a patient with AIDS; similar to focal segmental glomerulosclerosis, slowly progressing

Dx:
1. VMP
2. BMP

Tx/Mgmt: HIV/AIDS management

Renal Tubular Acidosis

Buzz Words: Non–anion gap hyperchloremic metabolic acidosis

Clinical Presentation:
- Type 1 (distal) RTA = fluid contraction, hypokalemia, nephrolithiasis, rickets, non–anion gap hyperchloremic metabolic acidosis
- Type 2 (Proximal) RTA = alkaline urine, hypokalemia, hypophosphatemic rickets, non–anion gap hyperchloremic metabolic acidosis
- Type 4 RTA = **hyperkalemic**, alkaline urine
- Be on the lookout for multiple myeloma and other systemic illnesses

PPx: N/A

MoD:
- Type 1 (distal) RTA = collecting duct cannot excrete H+, with subsequent increased excretion of Na, Ca, K, Su, Phos
- Type 2 (proximal) RTA = proximal tubule cannot reabsorb HCO_3-, with subsequent loss of K+ and Na+
- Type 4 RTA = distal tubule cannot absorb Na and has decreased H and K secretion; secondary to any condition associated with hypoaldosteronism

Dx:
1. BMP
2. UA
3. Urine phosphate and ammonia

Tx/Mgmt:
- Type 1 (distal) RTA = HCO_3 and phosphate salts.
- Type 2 (proximal) RTA = Do NOT give HCO_3. Treat underlying cause (Fanconi, cystinosis, Wilson, lead, multiple myeloma, etc.)
- Type 4 RTA = fludrocortisone

99 AR

Renal tubular acidosis types review sheet

Infectious Disorders of the Upper Urinary Tract

Pyelonephritis

Buzz Words: WBC casts + costovertebral angle (CVA) tenderness + vesiculoureteral reflux (VUR)

Clinical Presentation: Dysuria, ± hematuria, frequency/urgency, suprapubic tenderness (all symptoms of cystitis, may or may not be present), fevers/chills, flank pain, CVA tenderness

Kidney Anatomy

PPx: A vesicoureterogram is indicated to rule out VUR in all young males with a UTI to prevent chronic pyelonephritis. If VUR is found, treat low grade with long-term antibiotics until child "grows out" of it or with surgical reimplantation if high grade.

MoD: *Escherichia coli* most common, but other gram-negative bugs including *Proteus, Klebsiella, Enterobacter*, and *Pseudomonas*, especially in those with Foley or those living in nursing homes.

Dx:
- UA/urine culture (UCx) (pyuria, WBC casts, nitrites, leukocyte esterase)
- Imaging if treatment fails after 48–72 hours or in *any* patient with complicated pyelonephritis, a history of nephrolithiasis, or unusual findings

Tx/Mgmt:
- Uncomplicated: trimethoprim/sulfamethoxazole (TMP/SMX) or ciprofloxacin (outpatient).
- Complicated (very ill, elderly, pregnant, unable to tolerate PO meds, significant comorbidities, or uroseptic): Admit to hospital + IV ampicillin/gentamicin or ciprofloxacin.
- Recurrent with same organism: treat for 6 weeks.

Xanthogranulomatous Pyelonephritis

Buzz Words: Lipid-laden foamy macrophages

Clinical Presentation: A 58-year-old woman with CHF, HTN, diabetes, and chronic obstructive pulmonary disease (COPD) who lives in a nursing home has frequent, recurrent UTIs and nephrolithiasis. A unilateral renal mass is palpated on physical exam. Biopsy of the mass shows lipid-laden foamy macrophages.

PPx: N/A

MoD: Long-term renal obstruction and infected renal stones, usually associated with *Proteus* or *E. coli*.

Dx:
1. BMP/CBC
2. UA (indicates UTI)
3. Biopsy (often indistinguishable from renal cell carcinoma [RCC])

Tx/Mgmt: Surgical removal

Perinephric and Renal Abscess

Buzz Words: Flank pain and CVA tenderness despite treatment

Clinical Presentation: A patient on ciprofloxacin for pyelonephritis has a persistent fever and CVA tenderness on day 5 despite treatment.

PPx: Treatment of pyonephritis

MoD: Abscess formation occurs secondary to urinary tract obstruction and/or hematogenous spread for other sites.

Dx: Both renal ultrasound and CT are useful, but CT is more sensitive.

Tx/Mgmt: Percutaneous drainage of pus and targeted antibiotic therapy

Renal Tuberculosis

Buzz Words: Sterile pyuria

Clinical Presentation: A patient from Cambodia presents with hemoptysis, night sweats, recurrent hematuria, fever, weight loss, and renal failure. A tuberculin skin test is positive.

PPx: Treatment of tuberculosis (TB) before renal seeding

MoD: Development of lesion on the renal cortex with eventual ulceration into renal pelvis

Dx: Examination of *three* early-morning urine specimens for acid-fast bacilli

Tx: TB treatment

Renal Stones

Hematuria occurs in over 90% of patients with nephrolithiasis, or kidney stones. There are a number of high-yield stone types that you should know; these are reviewed here. But first, let's review some big-picture facts. Urinary stones generally become symptomatic when they lead to urinary tract obstruction. In the acute setting, this may present as colicky flank pain with (or without!) radiation to the groin, hematuria, and nausea and vomiting. However, if the stone develops over a long period of time and leads to chronic urinary tract obstruction, a patient may be asymptomatic. *Obstruction happens at junctions.* Recall that the ureters cross anteriorly to the iliac vessels at the bifurcation of the common iliac into the internal and external iliac arteries.

The *most common and preventable* risk factor for stones is low fluid intake. Other risk factors include a family history or stones, predisposing diseases (Crohn disease, gout, hyperparathyroidism, RTAs), certain medications, male gender, UTIs with urease-producing bacteria (*Proteus* species), and a *low-calcium, high-oxalate* diet. Therefore someone with kidney stones should drink plenty of fluids (*the most important intervention*) and have a low-sodium, low-protein, low-oxalate diet. Counterintuitively, such an individual should follow a *high-calcium* diet.

The diagnosis of all stones is done similarly. A UA should be performed to assess for hematuria, the presence of a UTI or bacteriuria, and the presence of crystals within the urine. A kidneys-ureters-bladder (KUB) radiograph is first-line for imaging, but a CT is more sensitive and is the gold standard for diagnosing a stone. An intravenous pyelogram (IVP) is necessary only in planning for intervention, and ultrasound is used only to assess for hydronephrosis or hydroureter and in pregnant women.

Most stones can be treated with analgesics and fluids. A patient should generally be admitted only if his pain is not controlled on oral analgesics, if he is anuric (obstruction + solitary kidney = bad news), if there is an accompanying fever, and if the stone is larger than 1 cm. Such a stone will not pass spontaneously and will therefore require intervention. Conversely, stones less than 0.5 mm generally pass spontaneously. Small, uncomplicated stones may also be treated with alpha blockers. Shock-wave lithotripsy may be used for stones 0.5–1 cm, while a percutaneous nephrolithotomy is required for stones greater than 2 cm.

Calcium Stones

Buzz Words: Radio-dense + bipyramidal/biconcave ovals

Clinical Presentation: Calcium stones are the most common types of renal stones and are composed of calcium oxalate (most commonly) and calcium phosphate. Patients with Crohn disease, steatorrhea, sarcoidosis, malignancy, or hyperparathyroidism are at increased risk for developing calcium stones.

PPx: Hydrochlorothiazide (HCTZ; causes calcium reabsorption, thus decreasing the amount of calcium in urine)

MoD:
- Hypercalciuria (anything that elevates urinary calcium causes hypercalciuria)
- Hyperoxaluria
  a. Drinking too much iced tea!
  b. B6 deficiency
  c. **Crohn disease** (steatorrhea leads to oxalate absorption)

Dx: See Renal Stones

Tx/Mgmt: See Renal Stones

QUICK TIPS

Dx for all stones: (1) UA, (2) ultrasound (in pregnancy), (3) KUB, (4) CT, (5) IVP

QUICK TIPS

Tx/Mgmt for all stones: (1) fluids, (2) analgesics, (3) alpha blockers, (4) shock-wave lithotripsy, (5) percutaneous nephrolithotomy

QUICK TIPS

Which cancers lead to tumor lysis syndrome? Blood dyscrasias!

Uric Acid Stones

Buzz Words: Radiolucent + flat square plates

Clinical Presentation: A patient with gout or tumor lysis syndrome (e.g., from chemotherapy for leukemia/lymphoma).

PPx: Allopurinol

MoD: Low urine pH allows formation of uric acid stones.

Dx: See Renal Stones

Tx/Mgmt: See Renal Stones. Add potassium citrate to alkalinize the urine.

Struvite Stones

Buzz Words: Radiodense + staghorn calculi + rectangular prisms + *Proteus*

Clinical Presentation: A patient has recurrent UTIs with *urease*-producing organisms, most commonly *Proteus mirabilis.*

PPx: Timely antibiotic treatment

MoD: Urease organisms split urea into ammonia → alkalize urine → precipitation of struvite stones.

Dx: See Renal Stones

Tx/Mgmt: See Renal Stones. Be careful if the patient has a fever, as this may be an indication for hospitalization.

Cystine Stones

QUICK TIPS

Other amino acids affected by cystinuria include lysine, arginine, ornithine.

Buzz Words: Radiolucent + "stop sign" stones

Clinical Presentation: Patients who have cystinuria from inborn errors of metabolism

PPx: Acetazolamide

MoD: Defective amino acid transport at brush border

Dx: See Renal Stones. Urinary sodium nitroprusside test

Tx/Mgmt: Recurrence is common.

Neoplastic Disorders and Cysts of the Upper Renal Tract

Simple Renal Cyst

Buzz Words: Incidental finding on CT + cyst + tubular obstruction

Clinical Presentation: A 70-year-old patient on dialysis for several years has an abdominal CT scan that incidentally shows several small cysts on both kidneys.

Dx: CT scan

Tx/Mgmt: Leave it alone!

Autosomal Dominant Polycystic Kidney Disease

Buzz Words: Berry aneurysm + refractory HTN + liver cysts + parathyroid hyperplasia

Clinical Presentation: Patients often don't exhibit symptoms until middle age. They may present with hematuria, refractory hypertension, palpable kidneys, or recurrent pyelonephritis. Autosomal dominant polycystic kidney disease (ADPKD) is a major contributing cause to chronic kidney disease, and renal failure is expected in 50% of patients, most commonly from recurrent pyelonephritis or nephrolithiasis. The main extrarenal manifestation is a *hepatic cyst*. Patients may also have berry aneurysms in the brain, which may rarely rupture, causing a subarachnoid hemorrhage. Associated endocrine abnormalities occur due to the kidney's inability to produce vitamin D or to properly excrete phosphate, leading to secondary hyperparathyroidism. Patients may have a family history of ADPKD, presented in a question as undiagnosed renal disease.

PPx: N/A

MoD: Autosomal dominant transmission with polycystin-1 and polycystin-2 gene mutation found in renal tubules.

Dx: Renal ultrasound showing bilateral cysts that envelope the entire kidney

Tx/Mgmt: Treat symptomatically.

- Antihypertensives
- Antibiotics for infections
- Cyst drainage *only* if symptomatic
- Dialysis and renal transplant

Autosomal Recessive Polycystic Kidney Disease

Buzz Words: Cysts in renal collecting ducts + hepatic fibrosis → portal HTN and cholangitis, Potter sequence

Clinical Presentation: A fetus presents bilateral, symmetrically enlarged kidneys in utero with renal failure at birth and pulmonary hypoplasia. Neither parent has a history of renal problems.

PPx: N/A

MoD: *PKHD1* gene mutation that encodes for the fibrocystin in the kidney, liver, and pancreas

Dx: Neonatal or prenatal ultrasound showing renal cysts with hepatomegaly.

Tx/Mgmt: The main contributing cause of death is pulmonary disease (hypoplasia) due to enlarged kidneys. Treat with kidney transplant and respiratory support.

Medullary Sponge Kidney Disease

Buzz Words: Cystic dilation of collecting ducts in a patient with hematuria + recurrent UTIs + recurrent kidney stone

Clinical Presentation: A 30–40-year-old patient with hyperparathyroidism from a parathyroid adenoma presents with recurrent hematuria, kidney stones, and UTIs.

PPx: Adequate hydration

MoD: N/A

Dx: IV pyelogram revealing sponge-like calyx

Tx/Mgmt: Prevent stones and treat UTIs

Renal Cell Carcinoma

Buzz Words: Clear cell carcinoma + polycythemia + abdominal mass + phenacetin + ADPKD + heavy metals + von Hippel-Lindau

Clinical Presentation: A 55-year-old male presents with an abdominal mass, flank pain, weight loss, and painless hematuria. His labs show anemia.

PPx:

Avoid risk factors: cigarette smoking (greatest risk factor), phenacetin, dialysis, heavy metals, hypertension, dialysis.

MoD: Loss of *both* VHL genes in bilateral RCC

Dx: CT (to be performed if ultrasound shows a mass or numerous cysts)

Tx/Mgmt: Radical nephrectomy

Wilms Tumor/Nephroblastoma

More highly tested on the Pediatrics Shelf.

Buzz Words:

- Wilms tumor: childhood renal tumor + unilateral flank mass + constipation + hematuria
- WAGR: unilateral flank mass + aniridia + mental retardation

Clinical Presentation: Wilms tumor presents as renal masses and/or abdominal pain in child. It is the main renal neoplasm in children and is associated with WAGR syndrome (deletion of short arm of chromosome 11), Beckwith-Wiedemann syndrome (Wilms hemihypertrophy, adrenal cytomegaly).

PPx: N/A

MoD: Loss of Wilms tumor suppressor gene (*WT1*)

Dx: Microscopic pattern resembling fetal kidney nephrogenic zone

Tx/Mgmt: Surgery, chemo, and radiation lead to a high cure rate

Vascular Pathology Affecting the Upper Urinary Tract

Renal Artery Stenosis

Fibromuscular Dysplasia

Buzz Words: Sudden-onset HTN + HTN nonresponsive to medical therapy + malignant hypertension + "string of beads" + young woman

Clinical Presentation: A 25-year-old otherwise healthy woman presents with hypertension refractory to several medication regimens.

PPx: N/A

MoD: Decreased renal blood flow to the juxtaglomerular apparatus leads to activation of the renin-angiotensin-aldosterone system. Noninflammatory, nonatherosclerotic. May involve the carotid artery and lead to ischemic brain symptoms.

Dx:
1. Duplex ultrasound (elevated flow velocities)
2. Renal arteriogram ("string of beads," gold standard)
   a. Do not use in patients with renal insufficiency. Use magnetic resonance angiogram (MRA) instead.

Tx/Mgmt:
1. Percutaneous transluminal angioplasty
2. Surgical bypass if angioplasty fails
   - Various trials have failed to show benefit for renal artery stenting.

Renal Vein Thrombosis

Buzz Words: Renal failure + flank pain + HTN + hematuria + proteinuria

Clinical Presentation: A patient with nephrotic syndrome presents with flank pain and hematuria. Risk factors include hypercoagulable states (e.g., cancer, nephrotic syndrome), trauma, or external compression.

PPx: N/A

MoD: Intrinsic clot or extrinsic compression leads to decreased renal blood flow.

Dx: Elevated lactate dehydrogenase (LDH). Renal venography (gold standard) or IV pyelogram.

Tx/Mgmt: Anticoagulation and treatment of underlying cause

Renal Infarction

Buzz Words: Flank pain + hematuria + coronary artery disease (CAD)

Clinical Presentation: A patient with a history of CAD, hypertension, diabetes, atrial fibrillation, and an unknown vasculitis presents with acute onset flank pain and hematuria.

PPx: N/A

MoD: Embolization (atherosclerotic or otherwise) is the most common cause. Vasculitis is a less common cause.

Dx:
1. Serum creatinine and LDH (elevated)
2. UA and urine culture
3. Electrocardiogram to evaluate for atrial fibrillation
4. Spiral CT without contrast

Tx/Mgmt: Reestablish flow to the kidney. A nephrectomy may be necessary for an infarcted kidney.

The Lower Urinary Tract

Infectious Processes

Cystitis

Buzz Words: Honeymoon + catheter + dysuria (burning on urination), frequency, urgency + suprapubic tenderness

Clinical Presentation: A 30-year-old female presents with burning on urination and increased urinary frequency. On physical exam, she is afebrile and has suprapubic tenderness. Risk factors include pregnancy, indwelling catheters, structural abnormalities, and diabetes (increases risk of ascension to kidneys).

PPx: None

MoD:

Usually ascending infection from the urethra
- *E. coli*: most common cause
- *Staphylococcus saprophyticus*: sexually active young woman
- *Enterococcus, Klebsiella, Proteus, Pseudomonas, Enterbacter*: indwelling catheter

Dx:
1. UA
   - Leukocyte esterase *indicates white blood cells in urine (pyuria)
   - Nitrite (positive for gram-negative bacteria). *Negative nitrite does not exclude cystitis.*

Tx/Mgmt:
- Uncomplicated: Treat only if symptomatic.
  a. Oral TMP/SMX
  b. Nitrofurantoin or fosfomycin or fluoroquinolones
- Complicated: Treat regardless of symptoms.
  a. Known structural abnormalities
  b. Male sex (longer antibiotic course, consider further workup)
  c. Diabetes
  d. Renal failure

  e. Pregnancy (longer antibiotic course, avoid fluoroquinolones)
  f. Pyelonephritis within the past year
  g. Going to have urologic surgery
  h. Indwelling catheter, stent, or nephrostomy tube
  i. Antibiotic-resistant organism
  j. Immunocompromised
  k. Going to have urologic surgery
  l. Obstructive symptoms
  m. Multiple recurrences

Chlamydial Urethritis

Buzz Words: Above 24 years of age + sexually active + purulent discharge + dysuria

Clinical Presentation:

- Men: dysuria, purulent discharge, scrotal swelling, fever
- Women: often asymptomatic, purulent discharge, abnormal bleeding, dysuria

PPx: Condom usage. Screen sexually active nonpregnant women age 24 and younger and nonpregnant women age 24 and older who engage in risky sexual behavior.

MoD: Intracellular pathogen

Dx: Nucleic acid amplification testing (NAAT)

Tx/Mgmt: Azithromycin or doxycycline

STIs are covered in Chapter 9, so they are not repeated in this chapter. Instead, here is a quick overview of infections of the male genitourinary system:

Balanitis refers to inflammation of the glans penis. It is usually secondary to poor hygiene of the foreskin and can lead to *phimosis*, which is the inability to retract the foreskin. These conditions can lead to meatal obstruction. Know that balanitis is not a result of STIs, but these must be ruled out.

Prostatitis, on the other hand, can arise either secondary to STIs or from coliform bacteria. In a young child or elderly man with prostatitis, the most common pathogen is *E. coli*, whereas a young adult might have prostatitis secondary to an STI. Patients with acute prostatitis will present with fever and chills, pain on urination (dysuria), urinary frequency and urgency, and low back pain. On digital rectal exam, one will feel a "boggy, tender prostate" and UA/UCx will be abnormal. Treat with TMP/SMX or ciprofloxacin. Acute prostatitis *may* lead to slight elevations in prostate-specific antigen (PSA), so do not be fooled into thinking a patient has prostate cancer if he does not fit the clinical picture. Chronic prostatitis may be asymptomatic, and diagnosis is made when WBCs are found in prostatic secretions. Chronic prostatitis must be treated with long-term ciprofloxacin or another fluoroquinolone.

Epididymitis refers to infection or inflammation of the epididymis. Clinically this presents similarly to testicular torsion, but the patient will also have fever, pyuria, and an exquisitely tender spermatic cord. Although epididymitis does not threaten the testicle, testicular torsion must be ruled out emergently. Therefore a diagnostic ultrasound must be obtained immediately. Once torsion has been excluded, diagnostic tests for epididymitis may be run. Gonococcal and chlamydial infections are most common in young men, while *E. coli* is common in children and the elderly. Tuberculosis can also cause epididymitis, but usually after generalized spread from the lung.

Orchitis refers to infection of the testicle. It is most commonly tested in the setting of a mumps infection. Understand that this is preventable with appropriate vaccination and can accompany a parotitis. In children, mumps orchitis can lead to infertility, while in adults this is an uncommon outcome. Bacterial infections are less likely to lead to an orchitis.

Inflammatory Processes

Interstitial Cystitis/Hemorrhagic Cystitis

Buzz Words: Gross hematuria + dysuria in a patient with chronic infection, radiation exposure, or malignancy

Clinical Presentation: A patient on cyclophosphamide for leukemia treatment presents with painful, bloody urination.

PPx: Adequate hydration and sodium 2-mercaptoethane sulfonate (Mesna).

Dx:
1. CBC
2. UCx
3. Kidney ultrasound
4. Cystogram
5. Radio-opaque vesicoureterogram
6. Cystoscopy

Tx/Mgmt:
1. Empiric antibiotics
2. Clot evacuation
3. Hydration

Hemorrhagic Cystitis Workup

Neoplasms of the Lower Urinary Tract

Bladder Cancer

When a patient presents with painless hematuria, especially a middle- or older-aged smoker, immediately think of bladder cancer. Bladder cancer is the most common cancer of the genitourinary tract. Of all bladder cancers, transitional cell carcinomas are *by far* the most common type. Squamous cell carcinoma and adenocarcinoma are less common.

The primary risk factor for transitional cell bladder cancer is smoking. Incidentally, this is also the number one risk factor for renal cancer. Other risk factors for transitional cell bladder cancer including aniline dyes, painkillers, and cyclophosphamide.

Recall that cyclophosphamide causes interstitial cystitis. While rarely seen in the United States (test questions will often feature foreign patients), squamous cell carcinoma of the bladder will be seen in a patient with a history of *Schistosoma haematobium* infection. Diagnosis is done with an IV pyelogram and cystoscopy with biopsy. This is the definitive test; however, other causes of dysuria and hematuria should also be ruled out, including infection. A CT scan and chest x-ray are also necessary for staging, although you are not responsible for knowing the various stages. Know that recurrence is common, and that the most common route of spread is through local extension to surrounding tissues. Screening is never indicated for bladder cancer.

Prostate Cancer

Buzz Words: Urinary obstruction + bony metastasis

Clinical Presentation: Prostate cancer is the second most common cancer in men. The primary risk factor is age; other risk factors include African American ethnicity, a high-fat diet, and exposure to pesticides. Early-stage cancers may be asymptomatic and cause urinary obstruction as they enlarge. Prostate cancers often metastasize to the bones, primarily the vertebral bodies.

PPx:
- Transrectal ultrasounds for abnormal rectal exams
- PSA levels
  <4.0, digital rectal examination (DRE) normal→annual follow up
  >10, DRE normal→biopsy

MoD: Adenocarcinomas (90%) develop in the periphery and move centrally.

QUICK TIPS

Think of the mnemonic Pee SAC—pain killer abuse, smoking, aniline dyes, and cyclophosphamide.

QUICK TIPS

Benign prostatic hyperplasia occurs due to central proliferation of the prostate and thus leads to urinary obstruction.

Dx:
1. Transrectal ultrasound
2. Plain radiographs of pelvis and spine
3. CT pelvis

Tx/Mgmt:
- **Localized:** watchful waiting, prostatectomy (complications include erectile dysfunction and urinary incontinence)
- **Locally invasive:** radiation therapy, antiandrogens (flutamide)
- **Metastatic:** orchiectomy, flutamide, luteinizing hormone releasing hormone (LHRH) agonists (leuprolide), GnRH antagonists (abarelix, cetrorelix). Goal is to reduce testosterone
- Treat urinary obstruction with 5-alpha reductase inhibitors (finasteride, decreases libido and may cause erectile dysfunction) or alpha blockers (prazosin, may cause orthostatic hypotension)

Testicular Cancer

Buzz Words: Opaque testicular mass (painless) + gynecomastia (nonseminomatous) + cryptorchidism + Klinefelter

Clinical Presentation: A male 20–25 years old with a history of cryptorchidism presents with a firm, painless testicular mass and gynecomastia.

PPx: Surgical repair of cryptorchidism

MoD:
- Germ cell tumors (95%): malignant
  a. Seminoma is most common
  b. Choriocarcinoma has highest metastatic potential
- Non-germ cell tumor (5%): usually benign

Dx:
1. Physical exam (nontesticular masses within scrotum are generally benign)
2. Testicular ultrasound (r/o spermatocele, etc.)
3. Tumor markers (B-HCG, alfa fetoprotein [AFP])
4. CT chest
5. DO NOT BIOPSY THE MASS

Tx/Mgmt:
All men with a firm, painless testicular mass need an orchiectomy to confirm diagnosis and to prevent scrotal seeding.
- If seminoma: add radiation therapy
- If nonseminoma: retroperitoneal lymph node dissection

Penile Cancer
Buzz Words:
Human papillomavirus (HPV) 16, 18
Clinical Presentation:
Exophytic mass on penis of a sexually active male
PPx:
1. Circumcision
2. HPV vaccination
MoD: HPV 16, 18 causing squamous cell carcinoma
Dx: Biopsy
Tx/Mgmt: Local excision

Development of the Genitourinary and Male Reproductive System and Its Pathologies

The urogenital system arises from intermediate mesoderm that forms on either side of the aorta. The urogenital ridge that forms develops into three sets of tubular nephric structures: the pronephros, mesonephros, and metanephros. During the course of development, the pronephros mostly regresses. The mesonephros develops into mesonephric tubules and the mesonephric (wolffian) duct. Initially, the tubules carry out primitive kidney functions, but these too mostly regress. The Wolffian duct, however, will persist and will open as the cloaca, and the mesonephros will contribute to the development of the male reproductive system. The metanephros gives rise to the definitive adult kidney and comes from the metanephric blastema within the ureteric bud. A mesenchymal-to-epithelial transformation must take place during this time.

Renal agenesis occurs when the ureteric bud fails to form. If both kidneys fail to form, a patient is diagnosed with Potter syndrome. This pathology is found in strictly neonatal populations, as the resulting oligohydramnios (secondary to anuria) leads to fetal compression, limb and facial deformities, and a pulmonary hypoplasia that is usually fatal. Retinoic acid plays a significant role in the development of the kidney. Any signaling interruption throughout the renal organogenesis, especially those involving perturbations in retinoic acid, may thus lead to renal abnormalities, including renal hypoplasia and agenesis. Vesicoureteral reflux, in a similar but unrelated etiology, may arise from defects in the mesothelial-to-epithelial transformation process. This is also high-yield for the Pediatrics Shelf.

Double Collecting System, Double Ureter, Bifid Ureter

Buzz Words: Hydronephrosis + vesicoureteral reflux

Clinical Presentation: A patient with Fanconi anemia presents with hydronephrosis.

PPx: N/A

MoD: Premature division of the ureteric bud prior to penetration of the metanephros. This disorder presents on a spectrum ranging from double ureter to complete duplication.

Dx: CT.

Tx/Mgmt:

- Manage associated conditions (vesicoureteral reflux, recurrent UTIs, hydronephrosis).
- Vesicoureteral reflux is often congenital and can be due to obstructive lesions at the bladder neck, including posterior ureteral valves. It predisposes to interstitial nephritis and recurrent UTIs and may lead to an obstructive uropathy. Diagnose with voiding cystourethrography. This is the same test used to diagnose a urethral diverticulum in men and children.

Horseshoe Kidney

Buzz Words: Inferior mesenteric artery + Turner syndrome + pyelonephritis + kidney stones

Clinical Presentation: A 6-year-old girl with Turner syndrome frequently suffers from pyelonephritis and kidney stones.

PPx: N/A

MoD: Kidneys initially form near the tail of the embryo. The growth of the embryo in a caudal-rostral direction leads to renal "ascension." Horseshoe kidney arises during ventral fusion, with subsequent entrapment below the inferior mesenteric artery.

Dx: In utero ultrasound or CT

Tx/Mgmt: Manage associated conditions.

As mentioned previously, the mesonephric (wolffian) ducts ultimately give rise to the male genital ducts. The development of the male reproductive system is discussed here and the female reproductive system is largely reviewed elsewhere; however, a brief review of the difference between the two is necessary. Differentiation is determined by the presence of the *SRY* gene on the Y chromosome. The *SRY* gene will induce the primitive gonad to develop into the testis, which is composed of spermatogonia, Leydig cells, and Sertoli cells. Leydig cells produce testosterone. Sertoli cells produce

gg AR

Horseshoe kidney radiographs

anti-Müllerian hormone, which leads to the regression of the paramesonephric duct (female reproductive system). Both Sertoli cells and Leydig cells function improperly in Klinefelter syndrome, the commonly tested pathology.

Klinefelter Syndrome

Buzz Words: Female hair distribution + atrophic testis + azoospermia + long extremities + testicular neoplasm + XXY karyotype

Clinical Presentation: A 24-year-old man presents with infertility. On exam, he has long extremities, female hair distribution, gynecomastia, azoospermia, and testicular atrophy. He had developmental difficulties as a child. A sperm count reveals no sperm in his ejaculate.

PPx: N/A

MoD:

47 XXY from nondisjunction or translocation

- Loss of Sertoli cells and lack of seminiferous tubules
  - No Sertoli cells to produce inhibin → no inhibin to inhibit FSH → increased FSH → increased aromatase → convert testosterone to estrogen
- Leydig cell dysfunction
  - No Leydig cells to produce testosterone → loss of negative feedback → elevated luteinizing hormone (LH) and low testosterone

Dx: Chromosomal analysis

Tx/Mgmt: Look out for testicular neoplasms!

Normally, the testes arise in the lumbar region and descend through the inguinal canal to their final location within the scrotum. This descent is due to the anterior attachment of the gubernaculum. Thus, inappropriate attachment of the gubernaculum may lead to an undescended testicle.

The external genitalia arise from proliferation of mesoderm and ectoderm around a primordial cloacal membrane. This produces the primordial external genital tissues of both sexes: the genital tubercle, genital folds, and genital swellings. Abnormal development of the urogenital folds around the urogenital sinus potentially leads to a high-yield pathology: hypospadias.

Hypospadias/Epispadias

Buzz Words:

- **Hypospadias:** urethral opening on ventral penis
- **Epispadias:** urethral opening on dorsal penis

Clinical Presentation: Neonate with urethral opening

PPx: N/A

MoD: Improper formation of the penile raphe due to incomplete fusion of the urogenital fold around the urogenital sinus

Dx: Clinical presentation

Tx/Mgmt:

- These patients should NOT be circumcised, as urology may use the foreskin to repair the defect.
- Circumcision should also be avoided in patients with a spiral raphe.
- Manage increased risk of UTI.

Genitourinary Trauma and Mechanical Disorders

Kidney, Bladder, or Urethral Trauma

Buzz Words:

- **Kidney** = flank pain + CVA tenderness + upper quadrant mass + blunt trauma
- **Bladder**
- Extraperitoneal rupture: pelvic instability, suprapubic tenderness and mass
- Intraperitoneal rupture: acute abdomen
- Urethra = high-riding prostate + hematuria + penile/scrotal swelling + blood at meatus

Clinical Presentation: Most commonly from blunt trauma with a high association with pelvic fractures

PPx: N/A

MoD:

Most frequently traumatic

- Urethra
- **Posterior**: most commonly at junction of membranous and prostatic portion due to shearing forces at this fixed location
- **Anterior**: straddle injury leads to crushing of bulbar urethra against pubic ramus

Dx:

- Pelvis: radiograph with anteroposterior (AP) views
- Kidney: IVP, CT
- Bladder: UA, urethrogram, retrograde cystoscopy, and cystogram
- Urethra: retrograde urethrogram

Tx/Mgmt:

- Kidney
- Minor hematoma or laceration = conservative management
- High-grade injury = surgical repair
- Bladder

- Minor injury to extraperitoneal portion = Foley catheter
- Major injury to extraperitoneal portion = surgical repair
- Intraperitoneal = the abdomen must be drained and the bladder repaired surgically.
- Urethra
- DO NOT PLACE A FOLEY
- Posterior injury = suprapubic cystostomy and surgical repair
- Anterior injury = conservative management. If void-limiting, suprapubic cystostomy may be performed.

Penile Fracture

Buzz Words: "Eggplant penis" + acute pain + erection

Clinical Presentation: A male presents with acute onset of penile pain following trauma to his erect penis during sexual intercourse.

PPx: N/A

MoD: Fracture of the tunica albuginea surrounding the corpus cavernosa

Dx:

1. Clinical presentation
2. Diagnostic cavernography or MRI

Tx/Mgmt: Surgical repair of tunica albuginea. Complications include erectile dysfunction and urethral injury.)

Testicular Rupture/Avulsion/Hematocele

Buzz Words: Scrotal mass + testicular pain + trauma

Clinical Presentation: A male playing sports presents with testicular pain and a scrotal mass following a traumatic collision with another player. He is nauseous and vomiting and the right testicle is elevated.

PPx: N/A

MoD:

- **Hematocele:** hematoma within the tunica vaginalis
- **Rupture:** disruption of the tunica albuginea

Dx: Ultrasound

Tx/Mgmt: Ruptures always require surgical repair.

Peyronie Disease

Buzz Words: Penile curvature + infertility + pain + Dupuytren contracture

Clinical Presentation: A male with a connective tissue disorder and Dupuytren contractures on both hands presents with infertility and penile pain. On exam, his penis is unusually curved.

PPx: N/A

MoD: Fibrosis of the tunica albuginea, which surrounds the corpus cavernosa.

Dx:

1. Clinical presentation
2. Ultrasound (fibrous penile plaques)

Tx/Mgmt:

1. Observation if stable
2. Potassium aminobenzoate or vitamin E
3. Nesbit surgery for refractory cases

Sexual Dysfunction

There are many types of sexual dysfunctions, including those due to impotence, premature ejaculation, dyspareunia (pain), and arousal disorders.

Impotence/Erectile Dysfunction

Buzz Words: *Persistent* inability to maintain erection

Clinical Presentation: A 47-year-old man with a history of diabetes, dyslipidemia, coronary artery disease, and anxiety presents with a consistent and persistent inability to maintain an erection during both sexual intercourse and masturbation.

PPx: Diabetic and lipid control

MoD: If organic, then a vascular pathology is usually at play. The same atherosclerotic process that leads to peripheral vascular disease also affects the hypogastric artery. If a patient is younger and/or able to maintain in erection nocturnally or during masturbation, the etiology is likely psychological.

Dx: Clinical presentation

Tx/Mgmt:

- Psychological = psychotherapy
- Organic = Phosphodiesterase 5 (PDE5) inhibitors (sildenafil)

Premature Ejaculation

Clinical Presentation: A male (any age) with a history of anxiety presents with persistent ejaculation prior to or immediately upon penetration.

PPx: N/A

MoD: Usually secondary to anxiety

Dx: Clinical presentation

Tx/Mgmt:

1. "Stop and squeeze" technique
2. Psychotherapy
3. Selective serotonin reuptake inhibitors (SSRIs)

QUICK TIPS

ALWAYS ASK ABOUT THE ABILITY TO OBTAIN NIGHTTIME ERECTIONS.

Dyspareunia

Buzz Words: Painful intercourse + fear of intercourse + sexual abuse + history of STIs

Clinical Presentation: Broadly, *dyspareunia* refers to pain associated with sexual intercourse. This may be physiologic or psychologically induced pain that localizes in the external genitalia (<50 years old) or deep within the pelvis (>50 years old). Postmenopausal women may experience the pain because of vaginal atrophy.

Dyspareunia is often chronic and can be associated with interstitial cystitis, *Candida* (excoriations caused by itching), hypoestrogenic states such as menopause, urethral diverticula, and endometriosis.

PPx: N/A

MoD: Be on the lookout for past trauma or abuse.

Dx: Rule out all medical causes of pain.

Tx/Mgmt: Psychotherapy if no medical causes found.

Arousal Disorder

Buzz Words: None

Clinical Presentation:

Absence of three of the following for 6 months *leading to distress* (very important)
- Interest in sexual activity
- Sexual/erotic thoughts
- Initiation/reception of sexual activity
- Excitement and pleasure with sexual activity
- Sexual arousal in response to both internal and external stimuli
- Genital and nongenital sensations

PPx: N/A

MoD: Multifactorial psychosocial disorder

Dx: History and physical

Tx/Mgmt: Psychotherapy

Adverse Effects of Drugs on the Renal, Urinary, and Male Reproductive System

(Table 10.1)

GUNNER PRACTICE

1. A 42-year-old African American male presents to your office for a routine physical examination. On arrival, his blood pressure is elevated to 153/92. He has no significant past medical history, but family history is significant for hypertension and coronary artery

TABLE 10.1 The Adverse Effects of Selective Drugs on the Genitourinary System

Drug	Genitourinary Side Effects	Minimizing Toxicity	Contraindications
ACE inhibitors	• Acute renal failure • Hyperkalemia	—	• Renal insufficiency • Bilateral renal artery stenosis • Pregnancy
Aminoglycosides	• Acute tubular necrosis	—	—
Amphotericin B	• Hypokalemia • Hypomagnesemia • Amphotericin toxicity → "shake and bake"	—	—
Cisplatin	• Acute tubular necrosis	—	—
Furosemide	• Hypokalemia • Metabolic alkalosis • Hypomagnesemia • Ototoxicity is exacerbated in those with renal insufficiency • Hyperuricemia: increased urate absorption caused my increased proximal Na + reabsorption	—	• Sulfa allergy—use ethacrynic acid in those with sulfa allergy
Gadolinium	• Nephrogenic systemic fibrosis	—	• GFR <30 mL/min
Heroin	• Focal segmental glomerulosclerosis	—	—
Iodinated contrast dye	• Contrast induced nephropathy	• Hydration • N-Acetyl-cysteine • Bicarbonate • Statins	• Chronic kidney disease
Lithium	• Nephrogenic diabetes insipidus	—	• Pregnancy • Volume depletion • Renal disease
NSAIDs	• Renal insufficiency→Na retention, HTN, CHF exacerbation • Interstitial nephritis • Papillary necrosis	—	—
Penicillins	• Interstitial nephritis (nafcillin)	—	—
Sulfa drugs	—	—	—
Tenofovir	• Nephrotoxic to proximal convoluted tubule	• Probenecid	—
Alcohol	• Testicular atrophy • Gynecomastia	—	—
Androgens	• Acne • Gynecomastia • Testicular atrophy • Azoospermia • Prostatic hypertrophy • Aggression	—	—

TABLE 10.1 The Adverse Effects of Selective Drugs on the Genitourinary System—cont'd

Drug	Genitourinary Side Effects	Minimizing Toxicity	Contraindications
Antipsychotics	• Galactorrhea • Sexual dysfunction	—	—
Antidepressants (SSRIs)	• Sexual dysfunction • Decreased libido	—	—
Beta Blockers	• Impotence • Decreased libido	—	—
Diuretics (thiazide)	• Sexual dysfunction • Decreased libido • Delayed ejaculation	—	—
Trazadone	• Priapism	—	—
Finasteride, Dutasteride	• Decreased libido • Erectile dysfunction	—	—
Sildenafil	• Priapism	—	—
Marijuana	• Sexual dysfunction	—	—

ACE, Angiotensin-converting enzyme; *NSAIDs*, nonsteroidal anti-inflammatory drugs; *SSRIs*, selective serotonin reuptake inhibitors.

disease. He was hospitalized once as in his 20s after developing a desquamating rash while being treated with TMP/SMX for a skin infection. He has since been advised to avoid sulfa-containing drugs. Which of the following antihypertensive medications should be used in this man?

A. Chlorthalidone

B. Furosemide

C. Ethacrynic acid

D. Esmolol

2. A 53-year old homeless male was admitted to the hospital 3 days ago after he vomited blood. His past medical history includes cirrhosis, peripheral artery disease, hypertension, and chronic kidney disease. On admission, his INR was 1.7; BUN, 22; and Cr, 2.2. Physical exam revealed abdominal tenderness with a significant fluid wave, and the patient was taken to interventional radiology (IR) for draining of his abdominal ascites on hospital day 2. Since returning from the IR suite, he has been oliguric. The patient's BUN has increased to 34 and his Cr is now 3.5. He received a fluid bolus of 1000 mL lactated Ringer (LR) overnight but his urine output has failed to improve. Which of the following is the likely diagnosis?

A. Traumatic ureteral disruption during abdominal tap

B. Prerenal azotemia

C. Hepatorenal syndrome

D. Acute tubular necrosis

E. Focal sclerosing glomerulonephritis

3. Which of the following is the leading cause of death among patients with chronic kidney disease?

A. Cardiovascular disease

B. Infection

C. Cerebrovascular disease

D. Cancer

Notes

ANSWERS: What Would Gunner Jess/Jim Do?

1. WWGJD? A 42-year-old African American male presents to your office for a routine physical examination. On arrival, his blood pressure is elevated to 153/92. He has no significant past medical history, but family history is significant for hypertension and coronary artery disease. He was hospitalized once as in his 20s after developing a desquamating rash while being treated with sulfamethoxazole-trimethoprim for a skin infection. He has since been advised to avoid sulfa-containing drugs. Which of the following anti-hypertensive medications should be used in this man?

Answer: C. Ethacrynic acid

> Explanation: Ethacrynic acid should be used in hypertensive patients with severe sulfa allergies.
>
> A. Incorrect → Although the thiazide diuretic class is first line treatment in African Americans with hypertension, this patient's severe allergy precludes him from taking chlorthalidone or furosemide.
>
> B. Incorrect → Furosemide is a sulfa-containing drug.
>
> C. Incorrect → Esmolol is a cardioselective beta blocker that can be dosed only IV and would not be used in the treatment of outpatient hypertension.

2. WWGJD? A 53-year old homeless male was admitted to the hospital 3 days ago after he was found vomiting blood. His past medical history includes cirrhosis, peripheral artery disease, hypertension, and chronic kidney disease. On admission, his INR was 1.7, BUN was 22, and Cr was 2.2. Physical exam revealed abdominal tenderness with a significant fluid wave, and the patient was taken to IR for draining of his abdominal ascites on hospital day 2. Since returning from the IR suite, he has been oliguric. The patient's BUN has increased to 34 and his Cr is now 3.5. He received a fluid bolus of 1000 mL LR overnight but his urine output has failed to improve. Which of the following is the likely diagnosis?

Answer: C. Hepatorenal syndrome

> **Explanation:** Hepatorenal syndrome represents the most advanced stage of cirrhotic liver failure. The pathophysiology is incompletely understood but is thought to arise from a combination of peripheral arterial vasodilation and subsequent renal vasoconstriction, stimulation of the renal sympathetic nervous system, renal hypoperfusion, and an increase in vasoactive cytokines circulating within the renal vascular bed. Sudden fluid shifts may send a

cirrhotic patient into complete kidney failure that is refractory to fluids. The only definitive treatment is a liver transplant.

A. Incorrect → Traumatic ureteral disruption during abdominal tap. The ureter is located very posteriorly and is unlikely to be damaged.

B. Incorrect → Prerenal azotemia has a BUN:Cr ratio of >20:1 and may have responded to the 1L LR bolus.

D. Incorrect → Acute tubular necrosis. Given a history of cirrhosis and signs of severe disease such as esophageal varices (vomiting blood), hepatorenal syndrome is more likely.

E. Incorrect → Focal sclerosing glomerulonephritis. See earlier.

3. WWGJD? Which of the following is the leading cause of death among patients with chronic kidney disease?

Answer: A. Cardiovascular disease

Explanation:The leading cause of death among patients with chronic kidney disease remains cardiovascular disease. Therefore interventions aimed at minimizing the risk of CAD are extremely important in these patients. Aspirin is almost always indicated in patients over 50 years old, and dialysis patients are no exception.

Disorders of the Skin and Subcutaneous Tissues

Jacob Charny, Hao-Hua Wu, Leo Wang, Rebecca Gao, and Temitayo Ogunleye

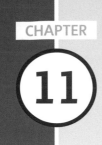

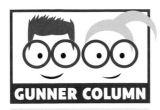

GUNNER COLUMN

Introduction

Diseases of the skin and subcutaneous tissues are esoteric and therefore often presented classically on exams. The skin is the largest organ in the body, consisting of the epidermis, dermis, and subcutaneous tissue. It serves as a physical and immunologic barrier to the outside world. It is also important for sensation, thermoregulation, and fluid regulation. Skin dysfunction can lead to disfigurement, dehydration, infection, pain or anesthesia, immune dysfunction, sepsis, and death.

This chapter includes a wide array of the most common disease of the skin and subcutaneous tissues grouped into infectious, inflammatory and immunologic, neoplasms, and other. Infections are the highest yield and therefore take up almost half of the chapter. The inflammatory and immunologic conditions are less intuitive, but tend to have classical presentations that show up on exams. Skin cancer is the most prevalent cancer in the United States. Neoplasms should come to mind for any chronic painless skin lesion. The last part of the chapter consists of other disorders known to show up on subject exams.

Only about 5%–10% of the NBME Medicine Subject Test will focus on disease of the skin and subcutaneous tissues. While this is a small percentage, these questions are often obscure or make use of slightly ambiguous visual aids. Questions almost always relate to other organ systems. While the emphasis in this chapter is on particular skin diseases, connections to other organ systems are presented. When approaching a tough question about a patient with a skin disease, determine a focused differential before choosing a next step.

Diseases
Infections and Infestations
Bacterial
Cellulitis
Buzz Words: Pain + redness + warmth + swelling

Clinical Presentation: A tender, erythematous, warm, and swollen area of skin with or without fever in a patient of any age. Predisposing factors include venous or lymphatic insufficiency and local skin breakage due to superficial inflammation or trauma.

PPx: N/A

MoD: Inflammation of dermis and subcutaneous fat in response to a bacterial pathogen, which gains access via breaks in the epidermis. Most common pathogens are Group A Streptococci or *Staphylococcus aureus* (including MRSA). Can be due to gram-negative rods, especially in diabetic patients.

Dx:

1. Clinical presentation
2. Wound cultures

Tx/Mgmt:

1. First generation cephalosporin or antistaphylococcal penicillin for streptococcus and MSSA, TMP-SMX, clindamycin, doxycycline for MRSA in the outpatient setting
2. IV vancomycin for MRSA in inpatients or those with systemic symptoms

Erysipelas

Buzz Words: Well-demarcated + history of lymphatic obstruction

Clinical Presentation: A sharply demarcated, red, painful, raised lesion on the extremity or face. Predisposing factors are the same as for cellulitis. Can be complicated by fever, sepsis, and necrotizing fasciitis.

PPx: N/A

MoD: Inflammation localized to the dermis and dermal lymphatic vessels. Most likely due to Group A Strep.

Dx: Clinical presentation

Tx/Mgmt:

1. For mild infections, give oral penicillin or erythromycin.
2. For infections with systemic symptoms, give intravenous ceftriaxone.

Impetigo

Buzz Words: Honey-colored crusting (Fig. 11.1)

Clinical Presentation: Areas of erythema and erosion with overlying golden or honey-colored crusting. Generally located on the face or upper extremities in children or adults without systemic symptoms. There is also a bullous variant that presents with large erosions bordered by scale, as bullae are too flaccid to remain intact.

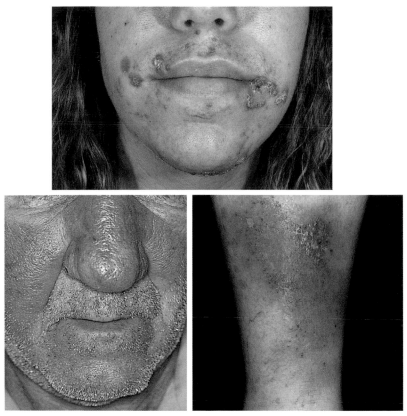

FIG. 11.1 Impetigo, cellulitis, and erysipelas. (From Netter Images. https://www.netterimages.com/impetigo-cellulitis-and-erysipelas-unlabeled-pathology-60693.html. ©2017 Elsevier, Inc.)

Poststreptococcal glomerulonephritis or rheumatic fever can result after impetigo resolves.

PPx: Contact precautions in healthcare settings.

MoD: Superficial infection with *S. aureus* or, less likely, Group A Streptococci via breaches in the skin. Staphylococcal exfoliative toxin A cleaves desmoglein 1 to cause superficial skin blisters in bullous impetigo.

Dx: Clinical. Gram stain and culture of lesions will guide treatment by determining if the infection is due to Strep or Staph.

Tx/Mgmt:
1. For limited infections, topical mupirocin ointment.
2. For extensive infections, empiric oral antibiotics (cephalexin, dicloxacillin, doxycycline).
3. If MRSA is suspected or confirmed, choose clindamycin.

Skin Abscesses, Furuncles, and Carbuncles

Buzz Words: Fluctuance + pus

Clinical Presentation: A pink, painful, tender, fluctuant nodule often surrounded by swelling and erythema. Spontaneous draining of pus can occur. Systemic symptoms are rare unless abscess is secondary to seeding of the subcutaneous tissue in a septic patient.

PPx: Contact precautions in healthcare settings

MoD: Abscesses are collections of pus within the subcutaneous tissues that result from bacterial entry via skin barrier breakdown, trauma, or septic seeding of the area. Abscesses of the hair follicle and surrounding tissue are called a furuncle or boil. A group of inflamed hair follicles with pus collecting is known as a carbuncle. *S. aureus* is the major pathogen.

Dx: Clinical presentation. Can consider ultrasound for confirmation of deep pus collection.

Tx/Mgmt: Incision and drainage with pus sent for bacterial culture. Patients at risk for infective endocarditis should receive vancomycin prior to incision and drainage. Further antibiotic treatment depends on culture results and is only necessary if there are multiple lesions, lesions greater than 2 cm, ineffective incision and drainage, extensive surrounding cellulitis, immunosuppression, systemic infection, presence of indwelling medical device, or high risk of transmission to others.

Folliculitis

Buzz Words: Rash after shaving or hot tub use

Clinical Presentation: Pustules and papules centered on hair follicles. Patients may report a history of recent hot tub or heated pool use, shaving against the grain, or prolonged use of corticosteroids.

PPx:

- Avoid tight occlusive clothing, shaving against the grain, use of hot tubs or heated pools.
- Decolonization with mupirocin or clindamycin ointment or chlorhexidine wash to prevent recurrences.

MoD: Inflammation of the hair follicle due most commonly to *S. aureus* or *Pseudomonas aeruginosa.* Staphylococcal folliculitis often occurs in scalp or face. Pseudomonal folliculitis presents more acutely and is often linked to contaminated water such as hot tubs or heated pools.

Dx: Clinical presentation

Tx/Mgmt: Not always indicated
- For staphylococcal cases, can give topical mupirocin.
- If refractory or extensive, give oral dicloxacillin and cephalexin (for MSSA) or either TMP-SMX or doxycycline (for suspected MRSA).
- For pseudomonal cases, give ciprofloxacin only if patient is immunocompromised.

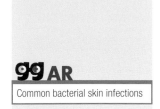

Pilonidal Disease

Buzz Words: Recurrent draining mass in intergluteal cleft + waxing and waning course

Clinical Presentation: Presents as a pore or pit in the inter-gluteal cleft that can be asymptomatic or acutely or chronically inflamed with palpable mass and purulent malodorous discharge. Patients may be overweight and/or have a family history.

PPx: N/A

MoD: Predisposition to the creation of pores or pits in hair follicles leading to sinus tracts that can become infected and inflamed. Exact etiology is unclear.

Dx: Clinical presentation.

Tx/Mgmt:
1. Incision and drainage for abscesses
2. Antibiotics for cellulitis are indicated
3. Definitive treatment is surgical excision of all sinus tracts. Asymptomatic patients do not need definitive treatment

Cutaneous Anthrax Infection

Buzz Words: Bioterrorism or outbreak + black eschar on exposed skin

Clinical Presentation: Presents 5–7 days after exposure as a painless pink bump on exposed skin (face, neck, upper extremities) that blisters and erodes into a necrotic lesion with extensive surrounding erythema and lymphadenopathy. Systemic symptoms include fever and headache and can progress to organ dysfunction and death if left untreated. Can be seen in IV drug users, people who work with animals or animal products, or victims of bioterrorism.

PPx: Airborne precautions in healthcare settings. For postexposure prophylaxis, give a 60-day course of antimicrobial therapy and three-dose anthrax vaccine.

MoD: Cutaneous anthrax results when spores of *Bacillus anthracis* are introduced into the subcutaneous tissues via breaks in the skin. Spores multiply and spread locally releasing toxins that cause tissue edema and necrosis.

Dx:
1. Gram stain, culture, and polymerase chain reaction (PCR)
2. Full-thickness punch biopsy

Tx/Mgmt:
1. Ciprofloxacin or doxycycline PO
2. For systemic infections, give IV ciprofloxacin, clindamycin, and antitoxin for 2 weeks before switching to oral regimen

Cutaneous Mycobacterial Infection

Buzz Words:
- Armadillos contact for *Mycobacterium leprae*
- Recent aquarium or tide pool exposure for *Mycobacterium marinum*

Clinical Presentation: Varies. Mycobacteria tend to cause polymorphic skin lesions that range from plaques to nodules to ulcerations with lymphangitis. *M. marinum* can also demonstrate sporotrichoid spread (linear distribution of nodules starting distally and progressing proximally, usually on upper limb). *M. leprae* in particular causes characteristic hypopigmented and anesthetic plaques associated with neuropathy and nonspecific ophthalmic symptoms.

PPx: Rifampin prophylaxis for close contacts of patients with leprosy

MoD: Infection of the skin with one of multiple species of mycobacteria. *M. leprae* shows a predilection for invading neural tissues. For skin, be sure to know *M. leprae* and *M. marinum* in particular. *M. avium* complex and *M. tuberculosis* are very important clinically, but rarely have cutaneous manifestations unless via hematogenous spread.

Dx: Skin biopsy with acid-fast bacteria culture. PCR is available for *M. leprae*.

Tx/Mgmt:
- For *M. leprae*: dapsone and rifampin
- For *M. marium*: depends on susceptibility of the isolate

Viral

Herpes Simplex Virus Types 1 and 2

Buzz Words: Cold sores + fever blisters + "punched out" painful erosions + recurrences (Fig. 11.2)

Clinical Presentation: Classically, marked by grouped vesicles on an erythematous base occurring in the perioral (type 1) or genital area (type 2). Risk factors for genital

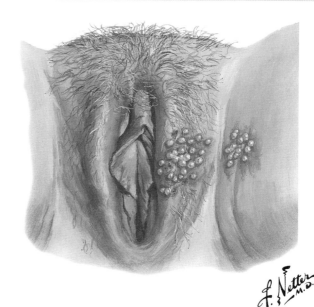

FIG. 11.2 Herpes genitalis. (From Netter Images. https://www.netteri
mages.com/herpes-genitalis-unlabeled-dermatology-frank-h-netter-
47664.html ©2017 Elsevier, Inc.)

lesions include multiple sexual partners, men who
have sex with men, low socioeconomic level, being
black or Hispanic, and having HIV infection. Primary
herpes simplex virus (HSV) infection tends to be more
severe than recurrences.

- Herpetic whitlow presents with herpes lesions on
  distal digits classically in a healthcare worker.
- Herpetic gingivostomatitis presents with fever,
  bleeding painful gums, and oral pain. Primary
  genital herpes presents with headache, fever, and
  dysuria in addition to genital lesions.
- Herpes keratoconjunctivitis presents with eye pain,
  eyelid edema, and photophobia.
- Eczema herpeticum presents with painful erosion
  and crusting of eczema in an atopic patient.
- Disseminated infection can occur and affect
  lungs, liver, and central nervous system (CNS).
  Complications include temporal hemorrhagic
  encephalitis, Bell palsy, erythema multiforme, and
  bacterial superinfection.

PPx: Oral valacyclovir or acyclovir to prevent recurrence in
patients with history of HSV infection. Oral acyclovir to
prevent reactivation in immunocompromised patients
(chemotherapy, organ-transplant, HIV). Contact precautions for healthcare workers.

MoD: Viral shedding transmitted via saliva and bodily fluids. Establishes lifelong latency in dorsal root ganglia. Classically, HSV type 1 infects trigeminal root ganglia causing perioral lesions and HSV type 2 infects sacral root ganglia causing genital lesions, although both types can infect either area. HSV infection of eye, distal digits, and active eczema leads to keratoconjunctivitis, herpetic whitlow, and eczema herpeticum, respectively.

Dx:

1. Clinical presentation
2. Confirmatory studies include Tzanck smear looking for multinucleated giant cells, viral culture, or HSV DNA PCR of infected epithelial cells

Tx/Mgmt:

1. Supportive care and antiviral therapy (oral acyclovir, valacyclovir, or famciclovir)
2. IV antiviral therapy for severe disseminated infections

Herpes: Merck Manuals

Varicella-Zoster Virus

Buzz Words: Chickenpox + shingles + "dewdrop on a rose petal" + rash in a unilateral dermatomal distribution (Fig. 11.3)

Clinical Presentation: Varicella-zoster virus (VZV) causes two distinct syndromes: chickenpox and herpes zoster. Chickenpox is seen in unvaccinated children and adults as diffuse painful or itchy discreet vesicles on an erythematous base with individual lesions in different stages of evolution. Systemic symptoms include fever, myalgia, and headache. Lesions tend to crust over and heal within a few weeks.

Shingles is the reactivation of VZV in dorsal root ganglia of a given nerve. It seen in adults, immunocompromised patients, and the elderly as an intensely painful vesicular eruption on a base of erythema confined to one or a few dermatomes. Ramsay-Hunt syndrome is the reactivation of VZV in the vestibulocochlear nerve. Postherpetic neuralgia is residual pain in the affected dermatome after resolution of skin findings. Disseminated infection can occur in immunocompromised patients and can affect the liver, lungs, and CNS, leading to organ failure, bacterial superinfection, and death.

PPx: Two-dose varicella vaccine at 12–15 months and 4–6 years. Postexposure prophylaxis with varicella vaccine within 72 hours of exposure. One-dose shingles vaccine Food and Drug Administration (FDA) approved for age 50+ and recommended by the Centers for Disease

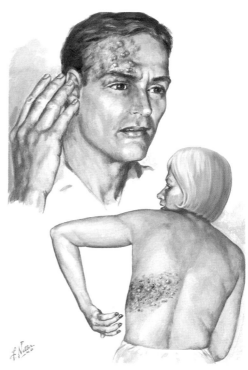

FIG. 11.3 Herpes zoster. (From Netter Images. https://www.netterim ages.com/herpes-zoster-unlabeled-neuroanatomy-frank-h-netter-68113.html ©2017 Elsevier, Inc.)

Control and Prevention (CDC) for age 60+. Both vaccines are live vaccines and should be avoided in pregnant and immunocompromised patients. Airborne precautions for healthcare workers.

MoD: Respiratory droplet or direct contact transmission of the VZV, a member of the *Herpesviridae* family. Incubation period is about 14 days and rash appears within a few days of systemic symptoms. Herpes zoster presents due to reactivation of VZV from dorsal root ganglia of a peripheral or cranial nerve, leading to dermatomal distribution of lesions.

Dx:
1. Clinical presentation
2. PCR
3. Direct fluorescent antibody (DFA) test and Tzanck smear are less common

Tx/Mgmt: For chickenpox, supportive care with antiviral therapy (acyclovir) reserved for severe infections. For herpes zoster, early antiviral (acyclovir) and analgesic (amitriptyline, nonsteroidal antiinflammatory drugs [NSAIDs], gabapentin) therapy. For postherpetic neuralgia, tricyclic

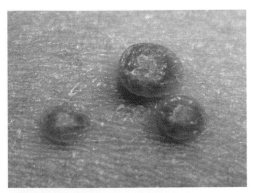

FIG. 11.4 Molluscum contagiosum, or water wart. (From Wikimedia Commons: https://commons.wikimedia.org/wiki/File:Molluscaklein. jpg. Licensed under the Creative Commons Attribution-Share Alike 3.0 Unported. Created by Evanherk, 7/7/2005.)

antidepressants, gabapentin, opioids, topical lidocaine, or topical capsaicin.

Molluscum Contagiosum

Buzz Words: Umbilicated papules in a child or immunocompromised patient + sexually transmitted infection (STI) in young adults (Fig. 11.4)

Clinical Presentation: Itchy or asymptomatic flesh colored dome shaped papules. Some may be umbilicated with central core of viral material. Some may be larger and more inflamed than others. Often occur in areas of dry or eczematous skin. In adults, lesions tend to occur in genital area as often transmitted through sexual contact. Chronic course, lasting up to 2 years. Large amount of lesions may be seen in immunocompromised patients.

PPx: Contact precautions in healthcare settings. Avoid direct contact and sharing baths, pools, or towels with affected people. Avoid manipulation of lesions to prevent spread.

MoD: Direct contact causes transmission of molluscum contagiosum, a member of the *Poxviridae* family. Virus forms core in the epidermis, where it is relatively protected from the immune system.

Dx:
1. Clinical presentation
2. Biopsy examination under light microscopy can show molluscum bodies (Henderson-Patterson bodies)
3. Skin biopsy indicated in immunocompromised patients to rule out opportunistic infections

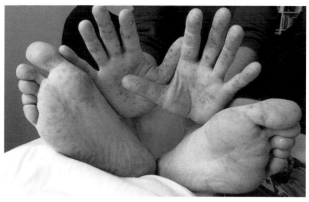

FIG. 11.5 Lesions caused by the hand, foot, and mouth virus on a 36-year-old male. (From Wikimedia Commons: https://upload.wiki media.org/wikipedia/commons/5/5f/Hand_Foot_Mouth_Disease_ Adult_36Years.jpg. By KlatschmohnAcker (Own work) [CC BY-SA 3.0 (http://creativecommons.org/licenses/by-sa/3.0)].)

Tx/Mgmt: Self-limited infection. May treat cryotherapy with liquid nitrogen, physical removal of lesions via curettage, or topical cantharidin solution.

Hand-Foot-and-Mouth Disease

Buzz Words: Football shaped vesicles + rash on hands, feet, and mouth (and perianal area; Fig. 11.5)

Clinical Presentation: Development of erythematous macules in oropharynx and extremities, including palmar and plantar surfaces. Macules evolve into painful football shaped vesicles on an erythematous base that can ulcerate. Although rare, certain strains may be associated with diarrhea, encephalitis, pneumonia, and myocarditis.

PPx: Hand hygiene and surface disinfection prevent spread to close contacts.

MoD: Transmission of virus via contact with nasal, oral, and fecal secretions. Most commonly caused by one of the *coxsackievirus* A serotypes of the *enterovirus* genus. Certain strains such as *enterovirus* A71 and *coxsackievirus* A6 and are associated with more severe infections and systemic symptoms. Infections are highly contagious and tend to occur in outbreaks, especially in groups such as day cares, military camps, and dormitories.

Dx: Clinical presentation

Tx/Mgmt: Supportive; infection is self-limited.

Parvovirus B19

Buzz Words: "Slapped-cheek" rash (Fig. 11.6)

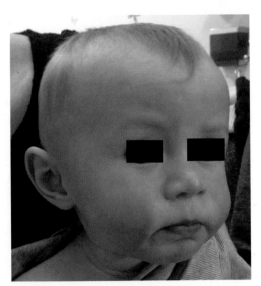

FIG. 11.6 Erythema infectiosum or fifth disease, due to an infection by parvovirus B19. The disease is also referred to as "slapped cheek syndrome." (From Wikimedia Commons: https://commons .wikimedia.org/wiki/File%3AErythema_infectiosum.jpg. By Gzzz (Own work) [CC BY-SA 4.0 (http://creativecommons.org/licenses/ by-sa/4.0)].)

Clinical Presentation: Nonspecific prodromal symptoms followed by erythematous patches on cheeks and reticulated pink rash on limbs and trunk. Infection in adults may also present as symmetric arthropathy of small joints of limbs, which typically resolves within 6 weeks. Transient aplastic crisis may occur in patients with pre-existing hematologic diseases. Chronic red cell aplasia may occur in immunocompromised patients. Fetal infection can lead to hydrops fetalis and death.

PPx: Droplet precautions in healthcare settings for immunocompromised and transient aplastic crisis patients. Immunocompetent patients are not contagious once symptoms present.

MoD: Respiratory droplet transmission of the parvovirus B19, which infects erythroid progenitor cells. Can also be transmitted vertically or hematogenously.

Dx:

- For immunocompetent patients, presence of antiparvovirus B19 IgM in serum indicates acute infection.
- For immunocompromised patients, parvovirus B19 PCR or nucleic acid amplification test (NAAT) can indicate acute infection.
- Bone marrow biopsy in parvovirus B19 induced red cell aplasia shows giant pronormoblasts.

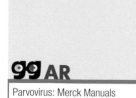

Tx/Mgmt:
- For immunocompetent patients, supportive care is sufficient as this infection is self-limited. Those with symptomatic anemia require blood transfusions until the bone marrow recovers.
- Immunocompromised patients require intravenous immunoglobulin (IVIG) in addition to blood transfusions if infection is persistent or severe.

Rubella

Buzz Words: Pinpoint petechiae on soft palate + unvaccinated patient (Fig. 11.7)

Clinical Presentation: Prodrome of fever, lymphadenopathy, and malaise followed by eruption of pinpoint pink macules on the face after a few days. Rash becomes coalescent within a day and spreads caudally to the trunk and extremities. Often accompanied by arthralgia and arthritis in adults. Pinpoint petechiae on the soft palate called Forchheimer spots are evident during prodromal phase. Rarely complicated by encephalitis.

PPx: Two-dose measles, mumps, rubella (MMR) vaccine at 12–15 months and 4–6 years. MMR is alive, attenuated

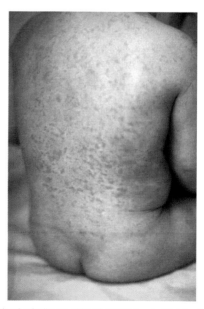

FIG. 11.7 Rash of rubella on skin of child's back. Distribution is similar to that of measles but the lesions are less intensely red. (This image is a work of the Centers for Disease Control and Prevention, part of the United States Department of Health and Human Services, taken or made as part of an employee's official duties. As a work of the US federal government, the image is in the public domain.)

vaccine that should be avoided in pregnant and immunocompromised patients. Droplet precautions in healthcare workers.

MoD: Respiratory droplet transmission of the rubella virus, a member of the *Togaviridae* family. Incubation takes about 14 days and rash appears up to 1 week after prodromal symptoms.

Dx: Clinical presentation. Enzyme immunoassay is available to detect rubella specific IgM, but usually used only for confirming congenital rubella.

Tx/Mgmt: Supportive. Infection is self-limited.

Rubeola

Buzz Words: Measles + fever and rash in unvaccinated + triad of cough, coryza, and conjunctivitis

Clinical Presentation: Prodrome of high fevers, cough, coryza, conjunctivitis for 3–4 days before emergence of diffuse red confluent maculopapular rash. Small blue-white oral lesions known as Koplik spots can form on oral mucosa a few days before rash. Pneumonia and ear infections are common. Subacute sclerosing panencephalitis can be a late complication and presents as altered mental status, seizures, coma, and death.

PPx: Two-dose measles, mumps, rubella (MMR) vaccine at 12–15 months and 4–6 years. Postexposure prophylaxis with MMR vaccine within 72 hours of exposure. MMR is live attenuated vaccine that should be avoided in pregnant and immunocompromised patients. Airborne precautions in healthcare workers.

MoD: Respiratory droplet transmission of the measles virus, a member of the *Paramyxoviridae* family. Incubation in respiratory epithelium takes about 10 days, and rash appears about 14 days after exposure.

Dx: Clinical presentation. Confirmatory testing with nasopharyngeal swab (measles RNA PCR) or serology (anti-measles IgM).

Tx: Vitamin A has been shown to reduce morbidity and mortality.

CDC Information on Measles

Verrucae Vulgaris

Buzz Words: Wart, irregular and rough lesions, extensive in immunosuppression

Clinical Presentation: One or multiple painless flesh colored papules with rough and irregular surface texture. More likely on the extremities but can be on mucosal surfaces.

PPx: Verruca vulgaris is used for warts on the body, and condyloma acuminata is used for genital warts.

MoD: Infection of skin and mucosal epithelial cells with human papilloma virus (HPV). Immunosuppression in HIV and organ-transplant patients can unmask latent infection leading to extensive wart formation.

Diagnosis

Clinical presentation

Tx/Mgmt: Most resolve spontaneously. Over the counter topical salicylic acid or cryotherapy with liquid nitrogen is first line treatment.

Fungal

Candidiasis

Buzz Words: Yeast + oral thrush (Fig. 11.8)

Clinical Presentation: Candidal intertrigo presents as macerated pink plaques with satellite papules and pustules in skin folds such as groin, axilla, inframammary creases, and web spaces of digits. Other localized cutaneous candida infections include folliculitis, balanitis, paronychia, onychomycosis, diaper rash, and cheilitis. Oral thrush presents as white furry plaques on the tongue or oropharyngeal mucosa that can be easily scraped off with an instrument. Oral thrush, candidal esophagitis, fungemia, and disseminated infection (liver, spleen, heart valves, skin, etc.) are all important clinical presentations in immunocompromised patients. Candidal

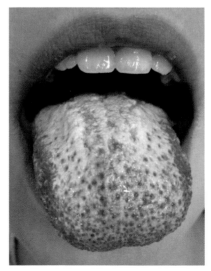

FIG. 11.8 Thrush in a child who had taken antibiotics. (From Wikimedia Commons: https://commons.wikimedia.org/wiki/File%3AHuman_tongue_infected_with_oral_candidiasis.jpg. By James Heilman, MD [Own work] [CC BY-SA 3.0 (http://creativecommons.org/licenses/by-sa/3.0) or GFDL (http://www.gnu.org/copyleft/fdl.html)].)

vulvovaginitis presents with itching, burning, dysuria, and a curd-like vaginal discharge.

PPx: Avoid occlusive clothing. Topical drying agents (not talc!) applied to intertriginous areas after infection can help prevent recurrence. Treating predisposing factors such as diabetes and obesity to reduce risk of infection. Antifungal prophylaxis is only indicated for the highest risk immunocompromised patients and is not routinely used.

MoD: Infection with the budding yeast, Candida albicans. Often occurs in areas of moisture such as intertriginous areas and mucosa. Associated with an imbalance of normal mucocutaneous flora. For example, patients using inhaled corticosteroids or systemic antibiotics are at higher risk of developing oral thrush and vulvovaginal candidiasis, respectively.

Dx:

1. Clinical presentation
2. Skin or mucosa scraping stained with 10% KOH will reveal budding yeast with pseudohyphae
3. Fungal culture of skin swab
4. Blood culture may be useful in fungemic patients but is often negative

Tx/Mgmt:

1. Topical nystatin for localized infections
2. Swish-and-spit or swish-and-swallow nystatin medication for oral or esophageal thrush
3. Intravaginal antifungals or oral fluconazole for candidal vulvovaginitis
4. IV antifungals for systemic infections

Tinea (Pedis, Cruris, Corporis, Capitis) and Onychomycosis

Buzz Words: Ringworm + athlete with localized lesion + jock itch (Fig. 11.9)

Clinical Presentation: Annular itchy erythematous scaly plaques with central clearing and advancing borders. Pedis (feet and toes), cruris (groin), corporis (body), and capitis (scalp) refer to the corresponding area affected on the body. Scalp involvement can cause a local area of hair loss leaving behind black dots as affect hair follicles break, leaving roots behind. Nail involvement, or onychomycosis, causes nail dystrophy, thickening, discoloration, and odor that is notoriously difficult to treat.

PPx: Good hygiene is the hallmark of prevention including thorough bathing and drying, wearing socks when wearing closed toes shoes, not showering barefoot in

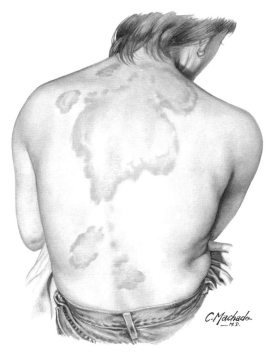

FIG. 11.9 Tinea corporis. (From Netter Images. https://www.netterima ges.com/tinea-corporis-unlabeled-dermatology-carlos-a-g-machado-2556.html ©2017 Elsevier, Inc.)

public showers, not sharing clothing, avoiding skin-to-skin contact with affected individuals.

MoD: Localized infection of skin and nails with dermatophyte fungi, a group consisting of many species that can cause tinea.

Dx: Scraping of scaly border of lesions or under nails stained with 10% KOH will show branching fungal hyphae. Fungal culture is useful for speciation but takes too long to be clinically relevant.

Tx/Mgmt:
1. Topical over-the-counter or prescription antifungals for localized infection. Choose an -azole, terbinafine, or griseofulvin.
2. Systemic treatment for onychomycosis and tinea capitis. Watch out for antifungal-induced liver failure.
3. Terbinafine is the first line for nail involvement.

Tinea Versicolor

Buzz Words: Teenager with skin color changes + hot environment + "spaghetti and meatballs" (Fig. 11.10)

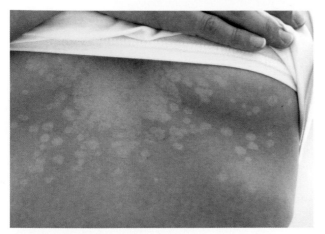

FIG. 11.10 Tinea versicolor. (From Wikimedia Commons: https://comm ons.wikimedia.org/wiki/File%3ATinea_versicolor1.jpg. By Sarahrosenau on Flickr.com [Flickr.com] [CC BY-SA 2.0 (http://creativecommons.org/ licenses/by-sa/2.0)].)

Clinical Presentation: Hypo- or hyperpigmented macules and patches with fine scale on chest, back, and shoulders. Generally asymptomatic. Seen in teenagers, pregnancy, oily skin, excessive sweating, and corticosteroid use.

PPx: Not contagious or related to poor hygiene. Prevent recurrence with topical antifungal to affected areas.

MoD: Infection of skin due to overgrowth of *Malassezia furfur* or other *Malassezia* spp., which is part of normal skin flora. Thought to be promoted by oily, warm, high hormonal conditions.

Dx:

1. Clinical presentation
2. Skin scraping stained with 10% KOH show spores and hyphae that look like "spaghetti and meatballs."

Tx/Mgmt: Topical ketoconazole or selenium sulfide

Sporotrichosis

Buzz Words: Rose thorn injury, landscaper, florist (Fig. 11.11)

Clinical Presentation: Initial inflamed papule or nodule progressing over weeks via ascending lymphatics. Linear distribution of nodules starting distally and progressing proximally, usually on upper limb. Nodular lesions may ulcerate and are associated with lymphangitis and lymphadenopathy. Systemic symptoms usually absent.

PPx: Wear gloves while gardening.

MoD: Traumatic inoculation and subsequent infection with dimorphic fungus, *Sporothrix schenckii.* Fungus infects subcutaneous tissues and invades lymphatic vessels over the course of weeks.

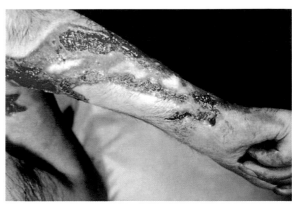

FIG. 11.11 This patient's arm shows the effects of the fungal disease sporotrichosis, caused by the fungus Sporothrix schenckii. The first symptom is usually a small painless bump that is red, pink, or purple. This is followed by one or more additional bumps/nodules that open and may resemble boils. Eventually lesions look like open sores, or ulcerations, and heal slowly. (From the CDC/Dr. Lucille K. Georg 1964, https://phil.cdc.gov/phil_images/20030610/25/PHIL_3940_lores.jpg.)

Dx: Not a very specific presentation. Skin biopsy with fluorescent-labeled antibodies and special fungal stains (Periodic Acid-Schiff [PAS] and GMS) for speciation. Fungal and bacterial culture. Acid-fast bacterial culture to rule out mycobacterium.

Tx/Mgmt: Systemic itraconazole or potassium iodide

Parasitic

Cutaneous Larva Migrans

Buzz Words: Creeping itch + barefoot on sand or soil (Fig. 11.12)

Clinical Presentation: Itchy raised serpiginous or curved eruption on legs or feet with a history of skin exposure to soil or sand weeks or months previously. Systemic symptoms are absent.

PPx: Wear shoes outdoors.

MoD: Parasitic infestation with hookworm, *Ancylostoma braziliense.* Hookworms endemic to southern United States and Caribbean. Larvae move through tissues overtime leading to the evolving nature of the eruption.

Dx: Clinical presentation

Tx/Mgmt: Oral albendazole or ivermectin

Cutaneous Leishmaniasis

Buzz Words: International traveler or immigrant with ulcerative skin lesions

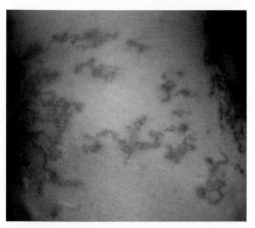

FIG. 11.12 Heavy attack of Larva Migrans Cutanea. (From Wikimedia Commons: https://commons.wikimedia.org/wiki/File%3ALarva_Migrans_Cutanea.jpg By WeisSagung [Own work] [Public domain].)

Clinical Presentation: Presents with a slowly evolving smooth red papule or nodule that ulcerates. Ulcerative plaques can be up to 10 cm large and have heaped inflamed borders. Lymphadenopathy and lymphangitis common, but systemic symptoms are rare.

PPx: N/A

MoD: Cutaneous infection with obligate intracellular protozoa of *Leishmania* genus. Vector is the sand fly. Various *Leishmania* spp. are implicated and vary based on geography.

Dx: Tissue biopsy with evidence of amastigotes (stages of protozoa life cycle) in macrophages with Giemsa stain. Parasite DNA PCR.

Tx/Mgmt:
1. IV Sodium stibogluconate
2. Infectious disease consult. Monitor at regular intervals for resolution and relapse.

Infestations and Bites

Scabies

Buzz Words: Visible burrows, intense itching, afflicted close contacts

Clinical Presentation: Intensely pruritic pinpoint pink papules and serpiginous burrows in web spaces, areola, genitals, flexor surfaces, and axilla. Secondary lesions may be larger and more nodular with hemorrhagic scale from excoriation.

PPx: Treat close contacts of affected individuals. Wash all linens and clothes with hot water and high heat drying. Contact precautions in healthcare settings.

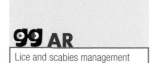

Lice and scabies management

MoD: Infestation with *Sarcoptes scabiei* mite. The mite burrows into the epidermis and lays eggs, causing intense itching. Extremely contagious.

Dx: Scraping and mineral oil prep with visualization of mite, ova, or feces under light microscopy.

Tx/Mgmt:
1. Permethrin cream vs. two doses of oral ivermectin 2 weeks apart.
2. For pregnant patients: ivermectin.
3. Antihistamines and topical steroids for itch as lesions make take up to 2 weeks to clear after treatment.

Lice
Buzz Words: Nits, crabs + homelessness or sex workers

Clinical Presentation: Three distinct clinical manifestations. Head lice usually manifests in school-aged children with intensely pruritic hair and visible nits in hair or on combs. Body lice infest clothes and lead to intensely pruritic rash. Can transmit typhus, relapsing fever, or trench fever. Pubic lice are sexually transmitting and infest pubic hair and eyelashes.

PPx: Contact precautions in healthcare settings. For body lice, wash all clothing and linens in hot water and dry with high heat.

MoD: Infestation with one of three species of louse. Head lice, *Pediculous humanus capitis.* Body lice, *Pediculus humanus corporis.* Public lice, *Phthirus pubis.* All three forms are extremely contagious as the human is the natural host.

Dx: Visualization of lice and nits in hair, eyelashes, pubic hair, on the body, or in clothes.

Tx: Permethrin cream applied and then washed off. Manual removal of nits with a fine-toothed comb.

Arthropod Bites and Bed Bugs
Buzz Words: "Breakfast, lunch, and dinner" lesions + history of bug bite

Clinical Presentation: A variety of arthropod bites can cause various clinical presentation. Insect bites typically result in pink pruritic or painful wheals at the location of the bite. Bed bugs bites form lesions in straight lines called a "breakfast, lunch, and dinner" pattern. Stings tend to be pink or white with central punctum where stinger entered the skin. Swelling is variable in bites and stings. Anaphylaxis, especially with bee stings, is the most feared complication and presents with swelling, difficulty breathing due to airway edema, tachycardia, and hypotension.

PPx: Bug spray, mosquito nets, citronella. Use of professional exterminators for infestations.
MoD: Localized inflammatory response from bite or sting
Dx: Clinical presentation
Tx:

1. Antihistamines and topical corticosteroids
2. IM epinephrine for anaphylactic reaction

Inflammatory and Immunologic Disorders

Psoriasis

Buzz Words: Silvery scaly plaques on extensor surfaces
Clinical Presentation: Chronic presentation, well-demarcated pink plaques on scalp and extensor surfaces, knees, and elbows, with overlying, thick silver scale. Auspitz sign refers to the pinpoint bleeding that occurs if scale is picked off. Nail pitting is common. Can be associated with arthritis in up to 30% of patients. A more acute form known as guttate psoriasis can occur after upper respiratory or streptococcal infections. Important to be aware of increased incidence of depression, metabolic syndrome, and risk for cardiovascular disease in patients with psoriasis.
PPx: N/A
MoD: Unknown, thought to be related to T-cell and keratinocyte dysfunction.
Dx:

1. Clinical presentation
2. Punch biopsy helpful if diagnosis is unclear
3. KOH preparation of scale can rule out fungal infection

Tx/Mgmt:

1. Topical steroids or topical vitamin D for isolated lesions
2. Narrowband UV-B light, three times a week
3. Systemic therapy: immunomodulation with methotrexate, mycophenolate mofetil, cyclosporine, tacrolimus, or injectable antitumor necrosis factor (TNF)α such as etanercept or adalimumab and IV infliximab.

99 AR

Psoriasis

Lichenoid Disorders

Lichen Planus

Buzz Words: The 5Ps: purple, planar, polygonal, pruritic papules
Clinical Presentation: Often located on wrists and flexor surfaces but can be diffuse including mucous membranes. Can be associated with nonspecific nail changes. Can be associated with hepatitis B and C infections.

PPx: N/A

MoD: Keratinocytes targeted by autoreactive T cells

Dx:

1. Clinical presentation
2. Punch biopsy helpful if diagnosis is unclear
3. Hepatitis B and C serologies in at-risk populations

Tx/Mgmt: Topical corticosteroids. Adjunctive antihistamines and phototherapy for pruritus.

Lichen Sclerosis

Buzz Words: Cigarette paper skin, anogenital skin lesion (Fig. 11.13)

Clinical Presentation: Atrophic or sclerotic white plaques with surrounding pink border, mostly on anogenital skin. Can be itchy or asymptomatic. Ulceration or erosion can occur. There is an increased risk of squamous cell carcinoma in these lesions.

PPx: N/A

MoD: Unknown

Dx: Skin biopsy

Tx/Mgmt: Topical corticosteroids or immunomodulators such as tacrolimus ointment

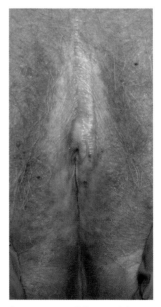

FIG. 11.13 Lichen sclerosus on an 82-year-old woman, showing an ivory white coloring in the vulva, also stretching downward to the perineum. (From Wikimedia Commons: https://commons.wikimedia .org/wiki/File%3ALichen_sclerosus.jpg. By Mikael Häggström 2014 [Own work] [CC0] [Public domain].)

Lichen Simplex Chronicus

Buzz Words: Lichenified patches, history of atopic dermatitis

Clinical Presentation: Well-demarcated itchy patches of thickened lichenified skin often with associated hypo- or hyperpigmentation. Lesions are self-induced and often on scalp, neck, limbs, or anogenital area.

PPx: Control underlying urge to scratch.

MoD: Self-induced via scratching or rubbing

Dx: Clinical presentation. Punch biopsy may be necessary if diagnosis is unclear.

Tx/Mgmt: Topical corticosteroids. Adjunctive antihistamines for pruritus.

Pityriasis Rosea

Buzz Words: Herald patch + Christmas tree distribution (Fig. 11.14)

Clinical Presentation: Salmon colored pruritic patch or plaque with subsequent eruption of smaller circular or oval pink patches, plaques, or papules with or without scale. Eruption usually spreads across trunk in a Christmas tree distribution. A prodromal flu-like illness may occur prior to eruption.

PPx: N/A

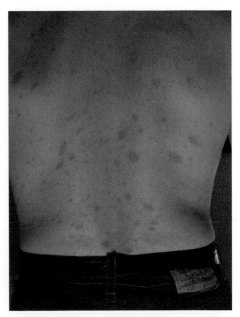

FIG. 11.14 Pityriasis rosea. (From Wikimedia Commons: https://commons.wikimedia.org/wiki/File%3APityriasis_rosea-4.jpg. By Aceofhearts1968 [Own work] [Public domain].)

MoD: Thought to be mediated by infection with HHV-6 and/or HHV-7

Dx: Clinical. KOH preparation to rule out fungal infection if there is significant scaling.

Tx/Mgmt: Self-limiting in 4–6 weeks

Dermatitis

Atopic Dermatitis (Eczema)

Buzz Words: Pruritic pink patches + flexural surfaces

Clinical Presentation: Chronic pruritic pink patches located in flexural areas or on face in children. Can become super-infected with HSV, streptococci, or staphylococci, as barrier function of skin is compromised from repeated scratching. Can give rise to patches of lichen simplex chronicus. Associated with other atopic disorders such as asthma, allergic rhinitis, and food allergies. Can be diffuse and severe, especially in children and young adults.

PPx: Frequent moisturization, sensitive skin care, avoiding triggers such as excessive bathing and irritation

MoD: Unknown

Dx: Clinical presentation. Cultures for bacteria or viral PCR helpful in diagnosing infection. Low threshold to test for allergies or asthma.

Tx/Mgmt: Topical corticosteroids intermittently. Extensive disease may require systemic immunomodulation. Adjunctive antihistamines for pruritus. Antibiotic or antiviral therapy as needed for infection.

Allergic and Irritant Contact Dermatitis

Buzz Words: Nickel + dermatitis near belt buckle + chemical worker + poison ivy + new exposures

Clinical Presentation: Weepy pink eruption. Morphology can be vesicular, papular, plaque-like or bullous. Occurs in the location of exposure such as earlobes for nickel allergy or ankles for poison ivy contact. A history of exposure to some irritant or chemical such as fragrances or dyes is typical.

PPx: Determination and avoidance of the irritant or allergen

MoD: Type IV hypersensitivity reaction (cell mediated)

Dx: Clinical presentation. Careful history and physical to determine irritant or allergen. Punch biopsy will show dermatitis, nonspecific. Patch testing can elucidate allergen or irritant if trigger is unknown.

Tx/Mgmt: Avoidance of trigger. Topical corticosteroids. Adjunctive antihistamines for pruritus.

Urticaria

Buzz Words: Hives + wheals + rash after exposure to allergen

Clinical Presentation: Acute onset of pink plaques or papules with surrounding erythema. Lesions are itchy and swollen and individual lesions do not last more than 24 hours. Can be diffuse or localized. Can be associated with angioedema and symptoms of anaphylaxis.

PPx: Determination and avoidance of allergen

MoD: Type I hypersensitivity reaction mediated by mast cell degranulation

Dx: Clinical presentation. Biopsy useful if individual lesions last more than 24 hours.

Tx/Mgmt: Avoidance of triggers. Nonsedating antihistamines (loratadine or fexofenadine) or sedating antihistamines (diphenhydramine or hydroxyzine). If anaphylaxis is occurring, epinephrine IM.

Erythema Multiforme

Buzz Words: Dusky targetoid lesions + rash in patient with previous HSV eruption

Clinical Presentation: Well-defined circular targetoid macules and papules with three distinct zones of color. Central zone may be bullous or crusted. Occurs on face, hands, limbs, and trunk. Mucous membrane involvement is common, especially the lips. Patients may have HSV, mycoplasma, salmonella, or histoplasma infections. Typically resolves within 2 weeks, but can recur.

PPx: N/A

MoD: Unknown but thought to stem from cutaneous immune system response to infection exposure. Formerly part of a continuum with Stevens-Johnson syndrome (SJS) and toxic epidermal necrolysis (TEN) but now thought to be its own disease entity.

Dx:
1. Clinical presentation
2. Viral culture or HSV PCR of associated grouped vesicles

Tx/Mgmt:
1. Discontinue possible causative drugs
2. Treat any underlying infection
3. Analgesia with NSAIDs
4. Adjunctive antihistamines or topical corticosteroids for pruritus

Stevens-Johnson Syndrome and Toxic Epidermal Necrolysis

Buzz Words: Dermatologic emergency + skin and mucous membrane detachment + new drug

Clinical Presentation: Both disease entities lie on a continuum with SJS involving less than 10% body surface area and TEN involving greater than 30% body surface area. Often begins as dusky macules, patches, or targetoid lesions that coalesce and blister. Bullae are flaccid and slough off leading to large erosions and ulcerations with hemorrhagic crust. Systemic symptoms such as fever are often present in SJS and always present in TEN. There is mucous membrane involvement in both entities. Widespread breakdown of the skin leads to fluid loss, temperature dysregulation, and death secondary to sepsis, adult respiratory distress syndrome, gastrointestinal bleeding, or pulmonary emboli.

PPx: Avoidance of triggering agent

MoD: Unknown. Most cases involve recent exposure to prescription medication. Culprit drugs include anticonvulsants, antibiotics, and NSAIDs.

Dx: Skin biopsy

Tx:
1. Admit to intensive care unit or burn unit. Careful management of vitals, fluids, nutrition, electrolytes. Wound care, pain management, and infection prevention are paramount
2. Identify and discontinue culprit drug
3. Urology or gynecology consult for genital involvement
4. Ophthalmology consultation for eye involvement
5. Consider IVIG and plasmapheresis

99 AR

Steven Johnson Syndrome

Dermatitis Herpetiformis

Buzz Words: Rash with celiac disease

Clinical Presentation: Clustered pruritic vesicles symmetrically on extensor surfaces such as elbows, knees, shoulders, and buttocks. Vesicles can be excoriated with hemorrhagic crust. 90% of patients with dermatitis herpetiformis have gluten sensitivity.

PPx: Gluten-free diet

MoD: In the papillary dermis, IgA immune complexes are deposited leading to small areas of inflammation that form vesicles. Associated with HLA DQ2.

Dx: Skin biopsy. Antigliadin or antiendomysial antibody serology.

Tx/Mgmt: Strict, gluten-free diet. Dapsone.

Pyoderma Gangrenosum

Buzz Words: Ulcerative skin lesions in a patient with inflammatory bowel disease

Clinical Presentation: One or few large shaggy ulcerated lesions with dusky purple borders and surrounding erythema. Ulcers progress to develop purulence and odor. Most commonly on the limbs. Some patients have an underlying systemic disease such as inflammatory bowel disease, arthritis, myeloma, or leukemia.

PPx: N/A

MoD: Unknown. While they can become superinfected, they are not infectious in nature.

Dx:

1. Skin biopsy with culture
2. Complete blood count (CBC), blood smear, comprehensive metabolic panel, urinalysis, serum/urine protein electrophoresis, and autoantibody panel may be useful

Tx/Mgmt:

1. Determination and treatment of the underlying condition
2. Wound care and systemic corticosteroids
3. Intralesional or topical corticosteroids can be used for mild disease
4. TNF-α inhibitors, dapsone, or tacrolimus can be used if systemic corticosteroids fail

Erythema Nodosum

Buzz Words: Nodules on shin in a patient with sarcoid or inflammatory bowel disease

Clinical Presentation: Tender pink to purple-brown nodules on the bilateral anterior shin or other areas of limbs and buttocks. Flu-life symptoms may accompany the rash. Triggers include recent streptococcal infection, sarcoidosis, inflammatory bowel disease, and prescription medications such as oral contraceptive pills. Lasts up to 6 weeks.

PPx: Avoid known trigger drugs.

MoD: Inflammation of the subcutaneous fat

Dx: Skin biopsy. More specialized testing depending on suspected trigger.

Tx/Mgmt:

1. Determination and treatment of underlying condition. Avoidance of triggering medications
2. Best rest, limb elevation and compression, and analgesia with NSAIDs or colchicine

Pemphigus Vulgaris, Foliaceus, and Bullous Pemphigoid

Buzz Words: Basal cell "tombstones" on H&E for pemphigus vulgaris; tense bullae for bullous pemphigoid

Clinical Presentation: These are three flavors of autoimmune blistering diseases. Pemphigus vulgaris is marked by flaccid bullae and erosions with mucous membrane involvement leading to increased risk for infection and sepsis. Pemphigus foliaceus is marked by very superficial flaccid bullae formation leading to widespread scaling and erythema involving the scalp and face, especially. Bullous pemphigoid is marked by tense bullae formation with sparing of the mucous membranes.

PPx: N/A

MoD: IgG autoantibodies to desmoglein-1 desmoglein-3 (pemphigus vulgaris), desmoglein-1 only (pemphigus foliaceus), and hemi-desmosome (bullous pemphigoid).

Dx: Skin biopsy with direct immunofluorescence. ELISA for antidesmoglein 1.

Tx/Mgmt:
1. Systemic corticosteroids are first line for all three blistering disorders
2. Immunosuppressive agents such as dapsone, mycophenolate mofetil, or rituximab for severe cases

Merck Manuals: Pemphigus Vulgaris

Vitiligo

Buzz Words: White patches + fluorescence under UV light

Clinical Presentation: Painless asymptomatic sharply demarcated depigmented patches that fluoresce under UV light (Wood lamp test). No surface changes to the skin. Can be associated with other autoimmune diseases such as hypothyroidism or diabetes mellitus type 1.

PPx: N/A

MoD: Unknown. Thought to be mediated by autoantibodies or autoreactive T cells against melanocytes.

Dx:
1. Wood lamp test
2. Screen for other autoimmune disorders with ANA, CBC, thyroid-stimulating hormone (TSH), and fasting blood glucose.

Tx/Mgmt:
1. Sun protection
2. Topical or oral corticosteroids depending on extent of disease and psychosocial burden on the patient. Phototherapy or depigmentation options

Neoplasms

Benign Neoplasms

Actinic Keratosis

Buzz Words: Solar keratosis + rough patches on sun-exposed area

Clinical Presentation: Subtle. These rough, scaly patches often are easier to feel than see. They present on sun-exposed areas, especially in older, fair-skinned patients. Can be light pink base with white or yellowish scale. More common in immunocompromised patients.

PPx: Sun protection

MoD: Chronic UV damage leading to precancerous proliferation of keratinocytes. These lesions can develop into squamous cell carcinoma.

Dx:
1. Clinical presentation
2. Shave biopsy can be performed to confirm the diagnosis

Tx/Mgmt:
1. Cryotherapy with liquid nitrogen
2. Topical 5-fluorouracil cream for more extensive involvement

Seborrheic Keratosis

Buzz Words: Stuck-on waxy growth (Fig. 11.15)

Clinical Presentation: Rapidly growing waxy papules with a stuck-on appearance. Can be pink to dark brown in color. More common with advancing age. The rapid onset of many seborrheic keratosis, known as the sign of Leser-Trélat, is a paraneoplastic syndrome signaling internal malignancy.

PPx: N/A

MoD: Proliferation of keratinocytes possibly linked to aberrant growth factor receptor signaling

Dx: Clinical presentation. Shave biopsy for suspicious lesions.

Tx/Mgmt: Removal is only necessary for cosmetic reasons or lesions suspicious of malignancy.

Nevus

Buzz Words: Moles

Clinical Presentation: Skin colored, brown, or black macules or papules that occur anywhere on the body. Lesions can be typical or atypical, meaning they can be flat, raised, round, irregular, uniform in color or not. Atypical nevi confer a greater risk for melanoma.

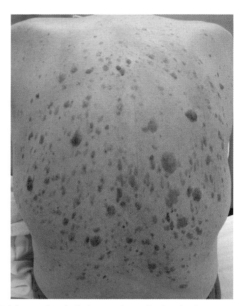

FIG. 11.15 Many seborrheic keratosis on the back of a person with Leser–Trélat sign due to colon cancer. (From Wikimedia Commons: https://commons.wikimedia.org/wiki/File:Seborrheic_keratosis_on _human_back.jpg. By James Heilman, MD [Own work] [CC BY-SA 3.0 (http://creativecommons.org/licenses/by-sa/3.0) or GFDL (http:/ /www.gnu.org/copyleft/fdl.html)].)

PPx: Sun protection

MoD: Benign proliferation of melanocytes

Dx: Clinical. Suspicious lesions can be biopsied to rule out melanoma. Remember the ABCDE of melanoma: asymmetry, borders, color, diameter, evolution.

Tx/Mgmt: None necessary. Can be removed for cosmetic reasons.

Epidermoid Cyst

Buzz Words: Thick, cheesy material

Clinical Presentation: A dome-shaped, firm nodule located anywhere on the body, but especially the face and neck. Can become inflamed or extrude cheesy, foul-smelling material from a punctum. Congenital occurrence of multiple epidermoid cysts is indicative of Gardner syndrome, a GI neoplastic syndrome.

PPx: N/A

MoD: May be secondary to iatrogenic implantation of epidermis into deeper layers of skin, causing subcutaneous proliferation of keratinocytes and sebaceous material

Dx:

1. Clinical presentation
2. Punch biopsy can confirm diagnosis

Tx/Mgmt: None necessary. Symptomatic lesions can be excised.

Lipoma
Buzz Words: Soft, mobile, subcutaneous mass
Clinical Presentation: Most common soft tissue tumor. Soft, mobile, subcutaneous mass. Occurs on back, legs, arms, or neck preferentially.
PPx: N/A
MoD: Benign proliferation of mature adipocytes
Dx: Clinical presentation
Tx/Mgmt: None necessary. Excision can be performed for cosmetics.

Xanthoma
Buzz Words: Yellow, waxy, firm mass
Clinical Presentation: Can be inflammatory or not. Rapidly presenting yellowish waxy papules or plaques. Located mostly on extensor surfaces, tendons, palms, or around the eye. Can be one or several hundred lesions at a time, depending on the type of xanthoma. Different types: tuberous, eruptive, palmar, etc. Associated with hypercholesterolemia syndromes, hypertriglyceridemia, or primary biliary cirrhosis.
PPx: Lipid lowering therapy, diet control
MoD: Accumulation of lipid-laden macrophages, often in patients with extremely high blood cholesterol or triglyceride levels
Dx: Fasting serum lipid panel. Skin biopsy.
Tx/Mgmt: Statins, fibrates, and/or niacin

Malignant Neoplasms
Basal Cell Carcinoma
Buzz Words: Pearly pink papule in elderly (Fig. 11.16)
Clinical Presentation: Most common skin cancer. Slowly growing pearly pink papule with raised edges. Sometimes telangiectatic blood vessels are visible. Occurs in sun-exposed areas and does not tend to metastasize.
PPx: Sun protection
MoD: Malignant proliferation of basal keratinocytes
Dx: Biopsy
Tx/Mgmt: Surgical removal

Squamous Cell Carcinoma
Buzz Words: Nonhealing ulcer
Clinical Presentation: A scaly erythematous papule that grows slowly on chronic sun-exposed areas. Lesions grow

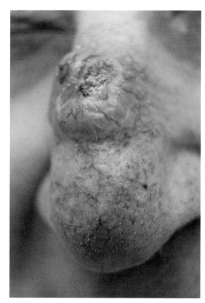

FIG. 11.16 Basal-cell carcinoma. (From Wikimedia Commons: https:/
/commons.wikimedia.org/wiki/File%3ABasaliom_am_Nasenr%C3%
BCcken_5.JPG. By Bin im Garten [Own work] [CC BY-SA 3.0 (http:/
/creativecommons.org/licenses/by-sa/3.0)].)

locally and ulcerate. Can occur in areas of chronic ulceration, scars, or burns. Has a low potential to metastasize. Common cancer in immunosuppressed patients.

PPx: Sun protection

MoD: Malignant proliferation of squamous keratinocytes

Dx: Biopsy

Tx:

1. Mohs surgery or excision
2. Topical imiquimod and 5-fluorouracil

Melanoma

Buzz Words: Changing mole

Clinical Presentation: Most deadly skin cancer, highest
metastatic potential. Various clinical presentations.
Superficial spreading melanoma can be raised or flat,
asymmetric, irregularly shaped, black, brown, or skin
colored, and changing over time. Nodular melanoma
can be a rapidly growing black nodule that ulcerates
and bleeds. Lentigo maligna melanoma is a brown or
black patch that spreads irregularly. Acral lentiginous
melanoma presents as a brown or black macule on
palms, soles, or under fingernails often in African American patients. Can metastasize to lungs, liver, brain, and
heart.

PPx: Sun protection
MoD: Malignant proliferation of melanocytes
Dx: Full-thickness biopsy. Clinical suspicion using the ABCDEs of melanoma.
Tx/Mgmt:

1. Surgical excision. Margins depend on the depth of the lesion ranging from 0.5 cm for melanoma in situ to 2 cm for melanoma invading greater than 4 mm. Sentinel lymph node sampling for staging for select patients based on depth, pathologic findings such as mitoses or ulceration, patient age.
2. Adjuvant chemotherapy required for metastatic disease. Vemurafenib is a biologic drug that targets BRAF and is approved for melanoma treatment.
3. Regular surveillance.

99 AR

Melanoma and Nevi

Kaposi Sarcoma

Buzz Words: AIDS patient with purple skin growth
Clinical Presentation: Dark red or purple plaques on skin or mucous membranes. Can be AIDS or non-AIDS associated. Non-AIDS associated Kaposi sarcoma is classically seen in older men of Mediterranean or Eastern European descent and located on lower extremities.
Prophylaxis
HIV prevention via safe sexual practices and avoidance of IV drug use
MoD: Human herpes virus 8 mediated proliferation of vascular endothelial cells
Dx: Skin biopsy
Tx/Mgmt: Treat underlying AIDS. Radiation, cryosurgery, or excision of isolated lesions is helpful in non-AIDS associated Kaposi sarcoma.

99 AR

Cutaneous manifestations of HIV infection

Cutaneous T-cell Lymphoma

Buzz Words: T cells with cerebriform nuclei; erythroderma with constitutional symptoms
Clinical Presentation: Multiple subtypes. Often begins as one or multiple patches, nodules, or tumors with ulceration. Mycosis fungoides and Sézary syndrome are the most tested. Mycosis fungoides is the most common presentation, presenting as erythematous patches or plaques with possible itching and ulceration. Sézary syndrome is rare but severe, presenting as erythroderma and lymphadenopathy. Constitutional symptoms are common.
PPx: N/A
MoD: Malignant proliferation of T cells localized to the skin. Mycosis fungoides malignant cells are CD3+, CD4+,

and thought to be related to abnormal CD8+ stimulation. Sézary syndrome cause is unknown but is marked by a very high CD4:CD8 ratio and Sézary cells (T cells with cerebriform nuclei).

Dx: Punch biopsy. Referral to a specialist. CBC, CMP, peripheral smear. Cytology and immunophenotyping may be helpful. Biopsy of lymph nodes if lymphadenopathy. PET-CT scan and/or bone marrow biopsy is helpful for staging.

Tx/Mgmt: Phototherapy, topical corticosteroids. Systemic treatment with interferon-alpha, methotrexate, or more specialized chemotherapy for advanced stage mycosis fungoides and Sézary syndrome.

Other Disorders

Disorders of the Hair

Alopecia

Buzz Words: Patchy hair loss

Clinical Presentation: Multiple different types of alopecia. Alopecia areata is the most common. Presents as smooth nonscarring oval or circular patches of hair loss. Can be limited to the scalp or involve the eyebrows, eyelashes, and other body hair. Hair can spontaneously regrow or never return. Associated with autoimmune diseases such as Hashimoto thyroiditis, vitiligo, pernicious anemia, and lupus. Often fingernail pitting can be seen.

PPx: N/A

MoD: Autoimmune T-cell mediated damage to hair follicles.

Dx:

1. Clinical. Look for exclamation point hairs and a positive peripheral hair pull test.
2. Scalp biopsy when diagnosis is unknown.
3. Helpful labs include CBC, ANA, TSH, and vitamin D.

Tx/Mgmt: Not very effective. Intralesional or topical corticosteroids. Methotrexate for severe disease.

Seborrheic Dermatitis

Buzz Words: Greasy, scaly rash, dandruff

Clinical Presentation: Inflammatory, greasy-appearing, scaly rash often on the nasolabial folds, around the eyebrows, skin folds, and scalp. Can be widespread in immunocompromised patients.

PPx: N/A

MoD: Unknown

Dx:
1. Clinical presentation
2. Skin scraping with KOH stain is helpful for ruling out tinea
3. HIV test in widespread or severe cases

Tx/Mgmt:
1. Ketoconazole 2% shampoo, facial cleanser, or cream
2. Mild topical corticosteroids

Disorders of the Nails

Paronychia

Buzz Words: Nail infection

Clinical Presentation: Swelling, tenderness, and redness around the nail. Pus formation is common. More likely in patients with diabetes or immunocompromised patients.

PPx: N/A

MoD: Infection of the nail bed with bacterial or yeast

Dx: Bacterial and fungal culture

Tx/Mgmt:
1. Incision and drainage if abscess is present
2. Warm soaks and topical antibiotics or antifungals
3. For severe infections, systemic antibiotics

Ingrown Nail

Buzz Words: Improper trimming of the toe nails

Clinical Presentation: Swelling and inflammation of the nail bed, especially the distal digit of toe nails. Most commonly the great toe.

PPx: Properly fitting shoes and avoiding improper toe nail trimming

MoD: Trimming nail too short and/or wearing tight athletic shoes leads to abnormal nail growth leading to pain and inflammation

Dx: Clinical presentation

Tx/Mgmt: Debridement and nail softening with urea

Disorders of Sweat and Sebaceous Glands

Acne Vulgaris

Buzz Words: Adolescent with facial eruption, whiteheads/blackheads

Clinical Presentation: Inflammatory papules and pustules, open and closed comedones, cystic lesions. Located on face, chest, and back. More prevalent in adolescence. Women's acne tends to flare during menstruation. Can be a result of hyperandrogenism secondary to polycystic ovarian syndrome or Cushing syndrome.

PPx: Avoid touching or picking skin and overcleansing.

MoD: Increased sebum production, proliferation of *Propionibacterium acnes* bacteria, plugging of follicles, and subsequent inflammation

Dx:
1. Clinical presentation.
2. Check testosterone level in women with acne and hirsutism.
3. AM cortisol level in suspected Cushing syndrome or adrenal hyperplasia.

Tx/Mgmt:
- **Mild acne:** Topical regimen of benzoyl peroxide, retinoids, or clindamycin
- **Moderate acne:** Topical + systemic antibiotics such as tetracycline, doxycycline, or minocycline
- **Severe or cystic acne:** Isotretinoin. Side effects of isotretinoin include elevated liver enzymes, depression, and teratogenicity.
- Spironolactone can be effective for women.

Rosacea

Buzz Words: Red face, nasal hypertrophy

Clinical Presentation: Erythema and swelling of the central face, especially the nose. Often with associated papules and telangiectasia. More common in light-skinned patients and can be exacerbated by various nonspecific triggers.

PPx: N/A

MoD: Unknown

Dx:
1. Clinical presentation.
2. A urine 5-HIAA can be done to rule out carcinoid syndrome, which causes flushing that may mimic rosacea.

Tx/Mgmt:
1. Avoiding triggers such as sunlight and spicy or extremely hot foods.
2. Topical metronidazole, azelaic acid, or clindamycin for mild disease.
3. Oral tetracycline for moderate disease.

Hidradenitis Suppurativa

Buzz Words: Groin and axillary cysts + obese female patient + boils

Clinical Presentation: Painful nodules and cysts in axilla, groin, inframammary folds, and gluteal cleft. Lesions form draining sinus tracts and scar when healed. Noninfectious and tends to affect obese and/or African American women preferentially. Cigarette smoking is associated.

PPx: N/A

MoD: Occlusion of follicles leading to rupture and deep inflammation

Dx: Clinical presentation

Tx/Mgmt:

1. Smoking cessation and weight loss.
2. Benzoyl peroxide wash and oral tetracycline.
3. TNF alpha inhibitors.

Hyperhidrosis

Buzz Words: Too much sweating

Clinical Presentation: Perspiration, often in the hands or axilla, in excessive amounts. Secondary hyperhidrosis seen in hyperthyroidism, malignancy, or tuberculosis.

PPx: N/A

MoD: Unknown

Dx: Clinical presentation. TSH, PPD, CBC, CMP.

Tx/Mgmt:

1. Topical antiperspirants
2. Twenty percent aluminum chloride solution, botulinum toxin, glycopyrrolate, oxybutynin

Ichthyosis Vulgaris

Buzz Words: Fish-scale skin

Clinical Presentation: Dry skin with fish-scale-like appearance. Mostly on the limbs, palms, and soles.

PPx: N/A

MoD: Autosomal dominant mutation in profilaggrin expression.

Dx:

1. Clinical presentation
2. Skin biopsy can give definitive diagnosis

Tx/Mgmt:

1. Moisturizing creams
2. Topical vitamin D, urea, or salicylic acid can help with descaling

Oral Disease

Aphthous Ulcers

Buzz Words: Canker sore

Clinical Presentation: Painful erosion of the oral mucosa, red border, and covered with a white pseudomembrane.

Not on the hard palate or gingiva. Seen in nutritional deficiencies, lupus, HIV, inflammatory bowel disease, and Behçet syndrome.

PPx: N/A

MoD: Unknown

Dx: Clinical presentation

Tx/Mgmt:

1. Topical anesthesia or analgesia
2. Topical corticosteroids or cautery
3. Prednisone for multiple lesions

Leukoplakia

Buzz Words: White plaque on the tongue

Clinical Presentation: White plaque on the tongue can be hairy in appearance. Not able to be scraped off. Sometimes with an erythematous base. Often in patients who use tobacco. Precursor of squamous cell carcinoma.

PPx: Cessation of tobacco use

MoD: Dysplastic proliferation of squamous cells of oral mucosa

Dx: Biopsy

Tx: Excision

Disorders of Pigmentation

Albinism

Buzz Words: Lack of pigment on skin and eyes

Clinical Presentation: Whole body and ocular depigmentation or hypopigmentation. Hair is white or blonde.

PPx: N/A

MoD: Autosomal recessive mutation in tyrosinase, leading to an absence of melanin

Dx: Clinical presentation

Tx/Mgmt:

- None
- Sun protection/avoidance
- Eye protection

Lentigo

Buzz Words: Sun spots

Clinical Presentation: Tan or light brown macule on sun-exposed skin. Can coalesce into patches or develop into lentigo maligna.

PPx: Sun protection

MoD: Unknown

Dx: Clinical presentation. Biopsy to rule out lentigo maligna if lesions change or grow.

Tx/Mgmt: Cryotherapy, lasers, or topical retinoid.

Traumatic, Mechanical, and Latrogenic Disorders

Animal Bites

Buzz Words: History of animal exposure

Clinical Presentation: Cellulitis or purulent drainage at the site of the bite, lymphadenopathy, or fever can occur.

PPx: N/A

MoD: Traumatic inoculation of bacteria into patient causing localized and possible systemic infection

Dx:

1. Clinical presentation
2. Bacterial culture and gram stain

Tx/Mgmt:

1. Wound care and debridement as needed.
2. Radiographs for retained teeth or nails in the wound.
3. Prophylactic antibiotics for deep wounds or those near bones. Amoxicillin-clavulanic acid is first line treatment for infections from dog and cat bites.

Burns

Buzz Words: History of fire, chemical, or electrical exposure

Clinical Presentation: First-degree burns are superficial and present as painful erythema with no blisters. Second-degree burns are partial thickness and present as pink, painful patches with blistering. Third-degree burns are full thickness and present as white, painless patches with areas of eschar. Sunburns are typically first degree, but blistering can occur.

PPx: Proper precautions around fire, chemicals, and electrical equipment. Sun protection.

MoD: Tissue damage from chemicals, heat, UV light, or electricity

Dx: Clinical presentation

- For severe burns, consider CBC, CMP, coagulation panel, carboxyhemoglobin, type and screen, urine analysis.
- Electrocardiogram (EKG) for electrical burns
- Peripheral neurovascular exam important to monitor for compartment syndrome in circumferential burns
- Biopsy nonhealing burns to monitor for squamous cell carcinoma

Tx/Mgmt:

1. Airway, breathing, circulation.
2. IV fluids for severe burns.
3. Wound care. Debridement of necrotic tissue.
4. Skin grafting can help facilitate wound healing.
5. Patients with electrical burns require cardiac monitoring.

Management of Burn Injuries of Various Depths

Pernio and Frostbite

Buzz Words: History of exposure to cold

Clinical Presentation: Perniosis presents as painful pink or purple papules on the hands and feet that present about a day after cold exposure and last for a few weeks. Frostbite begins as painful erythema on distal toes, fingers, ears, or nose, and progresses to anesthesia, discoloration, necrosis, and gangrene.

PPx: Proper protection from cold

MoD: Tissue damage and necrosis form cold exposure

Dx: Clinical presentation

Tx/Mgmt:

1. Frostbitten areas must be rapidly rewarmed via soaking in cold water that is warmed gradually.
2. Necrotic areas should be debrided.

Pressure Ulcers

Buzz Words: Decubitus ulcers + bedsores + elderly immobile patients

Clinical Presentation: Ulcer on sacrum, heels, occiput, or other areas of chronic pressure. Especially seen in elderly and immobile patients, diabetes can develop pressure ulcers on feet secondary to impaired sensation. Stage I through IV based on depth.

PPx: Changing position of immobile patients every 2 hours, maintain hygiene and nutrition in immobile patients. Special mattresses and pillows can be used to reduce pressure on body.

MoD: Chronic pressure on a specific area leading to ischemia and eventual skin breakdown.

Dx: Clinical presentation. Wound culture to rule out infection.

Tx/Mgmt: Wound care. Débridement of necrotic tissue and treatment of infection as necessary.

Keloids and Hypertrophic Scars

Buzz Words: Growth on a scar especially after ear piercing or surgery

Clinical Presentation: Both keloids and hypertrophic scars appear as smooth, shiny growths on an area of scar tissue. Keloids extend beyond the borders of the original scar, while hypertrophic scars do not. These areas are firm, painless, and do not resolve on their own. Keloids can uncommonly arise in areas without prior trauma and can cause discomfort. They are more common in African Americans.

PPx: Avoid unnecessary procedures and traumatic skin breakage such as ear piercing as much as possible.

MoD: Benign proliferation of scar tissue

Dx: Clinical presentation. Biopsy if diagnosis is unclear.

Tx/Mgmt: Extremely difficult

1. Topical silicon sheeting
2. Intralesional corticosteroid injections, intralesional bleomycin, excision, radiation

Keloids and Hypertrophic Scarring

Drug and Vaccine Eruptions

Buzz Words: Rash after drug or vaccine

Clinical Presentation: Fixed drug eruption presents as a painful well-circumscribed dark red to purple patch that recurs with repeated exposure to the drug. Morbilliform eruptions begin as macules or papules that coalesce into patches and plaques and spread diffusely. Urticaria and anaphylaxis are possible reactions if there is an allergy to an ingredient in a drug or vaccine. Localized swelling or cellulitis at injection site is common. Drug eruptions may also be vesicular or pustular. Systemic symptoms such as fever can occur and signal a more serious reaction.

PPx: Avoid the offending agent.

MoD: Unknown. Common culprit drugs include NSAIDs, antibiotics, sulfa drugs, angiotensin converting enzyme (ACE) inhibitors, angiotensin receptor blockers, anticonvulsants, diuretics, and allopurinol.

Dx: Clinical presentation

Tx/Mgmt:

1. Determine the culprit drug and stop usage immediately.
2. IM epinephrine for anaphylaxis.
3. Antihistamines, prednisone, or topical steroids help in urticarial eruptions.

GUNNER PRACTICE

1. A 40-year-old female with a history of hypertension, asthma, and depression presents to the emergency room with difficulty breathing for the past 30 minutes. Her husband explains that they were out to dinner when she began to complain of difficult breathing. She currently takes amlodipine, albuterol, and sertraline. She is allergic to shellfish. Her vitals are: HR 110, BP 90/65, RR 30. She is afebrile. She appears anxious but is able to speak. Her lips are swollen. The patient is covered in pink papules and plaques with surrounding erythema. The remainder of the physical exam is normal. What is the next best step in management?

A. Albuterol nebulizer
B. Intramuscular epinephrine
C. Intubation and mechanical ventilation
D. Establish IV access and deliver 2L of normal saline
E. Oral diphenhydramine

2. A 24-year-old African American man with G6PD deficiency presents to clinic with a painful skin lesion on his chest. He noticed the area began feeling tender and swollen over the past few days. He has tried to lance the lesion on his own, but the area has since become more inflamed and painful. The patient has a temperature of 39°C, HR 100, BP 118/75, RR 18. On exam, there is a 2 cm fluctuant nodule on the anterior chest draining green pus from a small opening. There is surrounding erythema, edema, and tenderness. The remainder of the physical exam is normal. Gram stain shows gram-positive cocci in clusters. Wound cultures grow many colonies of *S. aureus* that are resistant to methicillin. What is the treatment for this patient?
A. Incision and drainage
B. Oral trimethoprim-sulfamethoxazole
C. IV vancomycin
D. Oral doxycycline
E. Surgical debridement

3. A 72-year-old retired construction worker with history of osteoarthritis, hypertension, hyperlipidemia, and chronic kidney disease status post kidney transplantation presents for a full skin exam. He is currently taking metoprolol, atorvastatin, tacrolimus, and azathioprine. He has no complaints. Skin exam shows several small slightly scaly pink lesions over his hands and face, several small round light brown macules of various sizes scattered diffusely, and a well-healed surgical scar on his lower abdomen. The findings on exam put this patient at greatest risk for developing which of the following diseases?
A. Basal cell carcinoma
B. Squamous cell carcinoma
C. Melanoma
D. Kaposi sarcoma
E. Cutaneous T-cell lymphoma

Notes

ANSWERS: What Would Gunner Jess/Jim Do?

1. WWGJD? A 40-year-old female with a history of hypertension, asthma, and depression presents to the emergency room with difficulty breathing for the past 30 minutes. Her husband explains that they were out to dinner when she began to complain of difficult breathing. She currently takes amlodipine, albuterol, and sertraline. She is allergic to shellfish. Her vitals are: HR 110, BP 90/65, RR 30. She is afebrile. She appears anxious but is able to speak. Her lips are swollen. The patient is covered in pink papules and plaques with surrounding erythema. The remainder of the physical exam is normal. What is the next best step in management?

Answer: B, Intramuscular epinephrine

Explanation: This patient is having an anaphylactic reaction to something she ate while out to dinner. She has a known food allergy and could certainly have been exposed at the restaurant. The patient is tachycardic, hypotensive, and tachypneic, with urticarial and angioedema on exam. This is a classic presentation of anaphylaxis. The patient is speaking in sentences, a sign that her airway is intact.

A. Albuterol nebulizer → Incorrect. An albuterol treatment is indicated for an asthma exacerbation, which does not present like this.

C. Intubation and mechanical ventilation → Incorrect. While there should be a low threshold to intubate this patient given the potential for her condition to worsen rapidly, epinephrine should be given first as it may quickly improve her ability to breath.

D. Establish IV access and deliver 2 L of normal saline → Incorrect. Establishing IV access is important in hypotensive patients, but this patient needs intramuscular epinephrine and reassessment before large amounts of fluids are given.

E. Oral diphenhydramine → Incorrect. Oral diphenhydramine can help relieve the itching of her urticaria, but it will not treat anaphylaxis and the patient will have difficulty swallowing pills at this time.

2. **WWGJD?** A 24-year-old African American man with G6PD deficiency presents to clinic with a painful skin lesion on his chest. He noticed the area began feeling tender and swollen over the past few days. He has tried to lance the lesion on his own, but the area has since become more inflamed and painful. The patient has a temperature of 39°C, HR 100, BP 118/75, RR 18. On exam, there is a **2 cm fluctuant nodule on the anterior chest draining green pus from a small opening. There is surrounding erythema, edema, and tenderness.** The remainder of the physical exam is normal. Gram stain shows gram-positive cocci in clusters. Wound cultures grow many colonies of *S. aureus* that are resistant to methicillin. What is the treatment for this patient?

Answer: D, Oral doxycycline

Explanation: This patient has an abscess with wound infection and surrounding cellulitis after nonsterile incision and drainage was performed. The wound cultures grow MRSA, meaning doxycycline or trimethoprim-sulfamethoxazole is the first line choice.

A. Incision and drainage → Incorrect. Incision and drainage is inappropriate as the abscess is already draining.

B. Oral trimethoprim-sulfamethoxazole → Incorrect. Because of his G6PD deficiency, this patient cannot receive trimethoprim-sulfamethoxazole.

C. IV vancomycin → Incorrect. IV vancomycin is often used for MRSA infections, but is not necessary in this case, given that the patient is generally well-appearing and has a limited infection.

E. Surgical debridement → Incorrect. Surgical débridement is often used in burns and necrotizing fasciitis. It would only be necessary if this patient's wound became necrotic.

3. **WWGJD?** A 72-year-old retired construction worker with history of osteoarthritis, hypertension, hyperlipidemia, and chronic kidney disease status post **kidney transplantation** presents for a full skin exam. He is currently taking metoprolol, atorvastatin, tacrolimus, and azathioprine. He has no complaints. Skin exam shows several small slightly scaly pink lesions over his hands and face, several small round light brown macules of

various sizes scattered diffusely, and a well-healed surgical scar on his lower abdomen. The findings on exam put this patient at greatest risk for developing which of the following diseases?

Answer: B. Squamous cell carcinoma

Explanation: This patient has a long history of sun exposure as a construction worker, is currently immunosuppressed due to his recent kidney transplant, and has multiple actinic keratoses on exam. All of these factors predispose him to squamous cell carcinoma. An actinic keratosis is a dysplastic growth that is a precursor to squamous cell carcinoma. They are often treated with cryotherapy to prevent further dysplastic growth.

A. Basal cell carcinoma → Incorrect. There is no equivalent lesion for basal cell carcinoma, although his history of sun exposure and immunosuppression do put him at a greater risk for this type of skin cancer as well. There are also several benign nevi on exam.

C. Melanoma → Incorrect. Benign nevi are nondysplastic and have a low likelihood of harboring melanoma.

D. Kaposi sarcoma → Incorrect. Kaposi sarcoma is not likely in this patient based on the skin exam.

E. Cutaneous T-cell lymphoma → Incorrect. Cutaneous T-cell lymphoma is not likely in this patient based on the skin exam.

Diseases of the Musculoskeletal System and Connective Tissue

George Hung, Hao-Hua Wu, Leo Wang, Rebecca Gao, and Nadia Bennett

Introduction

This chapter covers the disease processes one can expect to see on the medicine shelf pertaining to the musculoskeletal system and connective tissue.

This chapter is split into 10 sections: (1) infectious disorders; (2) immunologic disorders; (3) benign MSK neoplasms; (4) malignant MSK neoplasms; (5) degenerative and metabolic disorders of bone/tendon/cartilage; (6) degenerative/metabolic disorders of joints; (7) degenerative/metabolic disorders of muscles, ligaments, fascia; (8) traumatic and mechanical disorders; (9) congenital disorders; and (10) adverse effects of drugs on the MSK system.

When perusing this chapter, realize that there are many diseases that sound alike (osteoarthritis, osteomalacia, osteoporosis, osteonecrosis, etc.), so remember to be able to differentiate between them. Also remember that knowing the pathognomonic or unique features to each disorder, as highlighted in the Buzz Words, will help you quickly come to a diagnosis.

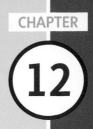

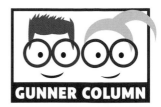

GUNNER COLUMN

Infectious Disorders

Gangrene

Buzz Words:

- **Dry gangrene**: clinical evidence of vascular obstruction, such as pale/blue/gray/purple coloration, numbness, decreased perfusion; common on ends of fingers and toes
- **Wet gangrene**: bullae, ecchymosis, crepitation of gas, cutaneous anesthesia
- **Gas gangrene (clostridial myonecrosis)**: crepitation with palpation, bronze skin discoloration, tense bullae, serosanguineous or dark fluid, and necrotic areas

Clinical Presentation:

An elderly man with a history of diabetes, peripheral vascular disease, recent CABG, and frequent episodes of cellulitis and skin abscesses presents with pain and violaceous discoloration of the left lower extremity. Capillary refill is prolonged.

AR

Gangrene tutorial

PPx: Prevention of risk factors, especially diabetes, peripheral vascular disease, and trauma

MoD:
- Dry gangrene: insufficient blood supply
- Wet gangrene: necrotizing bacterial infection
- Gas gangrene: *Clostridium perfringens* infection of tissue releases alpha toxin, a lecithinase (phospholipase) that degrades tissue and cell membranes → gas bubble formation → gas gangrene (myonecrosis)

Dx:
Clinical diagnosis
- Dry gangrene: peripheral vascular disease workup: reduced ABI (<0.4), absence of vascular flow on ultrasound
- Gas gangrene: gram-positive or gram-variable stain, few polys, bacteremia in 15%, gas dissecting into muscle on radiographs

Tx/Mgmt:
1. Revascularization
2. Antibiotics and wound debridement (surgical removal of dead tissue)
3. Hyperbaric oxygen or maggot debridement therapy
4. Amputation

Discitis (Vertebral Osteomyelitis)

Lower back physical exam

Buzz Words: Back or neck pain exacerbated by physical activity or percussion

Clinical Presentation: A 60-year-old male with a history of intravenous (IV) drug use, endocarditis, diabetes, and HIV presents with lower back pain and lower extremity paresthesias. (May also present with features of epidural abscess: focal severe back pain, radiculopathy, motor weakness and sensory change, eventual paralysis, ± fever.)

PPx: N/A

MoD: Hematogenous spread of a systemic infection, most commonly urinary tract infection (UTI), pneumonia, and soft-tissue infections into the vertebrae. *Staphylococcus aureus*, *Escherichia coli*, and Proteus are most common. Rarely, the infection may spread via direct inoculation from trauma or surgery or by contiguous spread from adjacent tissue.

Dx:
1. Neurologic exam
2. X-ray of corresponding spinal segment (i.e., cervical, thoracic, lumbar)

3. Positive culture from computed tomography (CT)-guided biopsy of involved disc or vertebrae, although suggestive clinical and radiographic findings are enough for diagnosis

Tx/Mgmt:
1. Six weeks of antimicrobial therapy
2. Surgery for inadequate response to antimicrobials or if presence of focal neurologic deficits or epidural or paravertebral abscess

Infective Myositis

Buzz Words: Proximal muscle weakness + no rash + no papules on knuckles

Clinical Presentation: Proximal muscle weakness can manifest as deficits of the deltoid (difficulty carrying heavy objects above shoulder level) or gluteus maximus (difficulty getting out of a chair without hand support).

PPx: Avoid risk factors: *S. aureus* infection, trauma, overseas travel, poorly cooked pork, tick bites, immunocompromised states.

MoD: Inflammation of the muscle 2/2 infection. Viruses (HIV, HTLV-1, influenza, coxsackievirus, echovirus), bacteria (most commonly *S. aureus*, but also Borrelia burgdorferi), fungi, parasites *(Trypanosoma cruzi, Taenia solium).*

Dx:
1. Elevation of muscle serum enzymes (CK, aldolase, aminotransferase)
2. Autoantibodies (e.g., ANA, anti-Jo-1, anti-Mi-2) to rule out (r/o) autoimmune (e.g., dermato- or polymyositis) etiology
3. Test for infection
4. Muscle biopsy to r/o autoimmune etiology

Tx/Mgmt: Treat underlying cause

Necrotizing Fasciitis

Buzz Words: Cellulitic skin + intense disproportionate pain + SIRS (acutely ill)

Clinical Presentation: A homeless patient with a history of IV drug use, diabetes, peripheral vascular disease, cirrhosis 2/2 alcohol abuse, and recent hernia surgery presents with sudden intense pain in the right lower extremity. The leg was initially hyperesthetic and became anesthetic over the past few hours. On exam, there are bullae and darkening of skin to bluish-gray. XR shows gas bubbles within the soft tissue.

PPx: Appropriate hygiene

AR
Discitis imaging

QUICK TIPS
Unlike dermatomyositis, infective myositis does not present with heliotropic rash or Gottron papules.

QUICK TIPS
Fournier's gangrene: necrotizing fasciitis of the male or female genitalia

AR
Necrotizing Fasciitis overview

LRINEC Criteria for necrotizing fasciitis

99 AR

Necrotizing subcutaneous infection seen on XR

99 AR

Osteomyelitis imaging

99 AR

Joint aspirates

MoD: Tissue ischemia 2/2 occlusion of small subcutaneous vessels → skin infarction and necrosis → infection of deep soft tissues that rapidly tracks along fascial planes → sepsis, shock, and death. Often due to Group A Streptococci or *C. perfringens.*

Dx:
1. Clinical presentation
2. Complete blood count (CBC; high WBC)
3. XR of affected area can show gas bubbles

Tx/Mgmt:
1. Broad-spectrum IV antimicrobials
2. Emergency surgical exploration and excision of devitalized tissue

Osteomyelitis

Buzz Words: Focal bone pain ± fever, malaise, and night sweats

Clinical Presentation: For osteomyelitis, the key is to figure out the etiology of the infection. For instance, osteomyelitis in sickle cell patients on the shelf is most frequently due to salmonella. Patients present with focal bone pain with possible fever, malaise, and night sweats.

PPx: Avoid risk factors: prosthetic joints, animal bites, IV drug use.

MoD: Hematogenous or direct spread.

Dx:
1. XRP, ESR
2. XR
3. Surgical culture or needle biopsy, NOT ulcer swab or fistulae drainage
4. Magnetic resonance imaging (MRI) most sensitive

Tx/Mgmt:
1. Four to eight weeks of antibiotics
2. Surgery for severe or chronic disease

Septic Arthritis

Buzz Words: Swollen, warm, and painful joint + limited active and passive range of motion + palpable effusion + fevers/chills/malaise

Clinical Presentation: Patients with septic arthritis, or infection of a joint, have extreme pain with even small movements of the affected joint. The joint may be erythematous and swollen. If only one joint is affected (e.g., left knee), while the other joint is normal, it should increase your suspicion of infection rather than an autoimmune process.

PPx: Prevention of risk factors: immunocompromised states, systemic lupus erythematosus (SLE), elderly, damaged joints (RA, OA, gout, trauma, surgery, prosthetic joint).

MoD: Hematogenous or contiguous spread of microorganisms or trauma to joint space.

Dx:
1. Aspiration of the joint with synovial fluid findings of: WBC > 50K, greater than 90% polys, Gram stain positive in ¾ of staph and ½ of GNR, culture positive
2. BCx positive in more than ½ of cases

Tx/Mgmt:
1. Empiric antibiotics
2. If elderly or immunosuppressed, add antipseudomonal agent

Immunologic Disorders

Adhesive Capsulitis (Frozen Shoulder Syndrome)

Buzz Words: Gradual onset of limited and painful shoulder range of motion + no other apparent pathology

Clinical Presentation: Adhesive capsulitis is the diagnosis given to shoulders with idiopathic capsular thickening and fibrosis, leading to pain and limitation of range of motion. Thus, in order to make this diagnosis on the shelf, all other diseases on the differential (such as rotator cuff tear) must be ruled out. A typical patient is a middle-aged female with a history of diabetes, hypothyroidism, and previous trauma/surgery to the shoulder presenting with a gradual onset of limited range of motion of her shoulder.

PPx: N/A

MoD: Chronic inflammation of capsule subsynovial layer produces capsular thickening, fibrosis, and adherence.

Dx: Global limitation of glenohumeral motion with normal x-ray, no specific underlying cause

Tx/Mgmt:
1. Physical therapy
2. Nonsteroidal anti-inflammatory drugs (NSAIDs)
3. Intraarticular corticosteroid injections
4. Operative manipulation or capsular release

Ankylosing Spondylitis

Buzz Words: Low back pain that improves with activity and worsens with rest + morning stiffness + bamboo spine + HLA-B27 + enthesitis + uveitis + aortic regurgitation

Clinical Presentation: Ankylosing spondylitis is a seronegative spondyloarthropathy characterized by chronic back pain from inflammation of the joints of the spine. Key associations include HLA-B27, chronic back pain, progressive loss of motion of the spine, morning stiffness, and achiness over the sacroiliac joint bilaterally and lumbar spine,

QUICK TIPS

The presence of crystals on aspiration does NOT rule out septic arthritis.

QUICK TIPS

The most common joint affect is the knee, but patients with immunosuppression or connective tissue disease may have polyarticular arthritis.

99 AR

Shoulder anatomy

QUICK TIPS

Back or joint pain that is worse in the mornings and improves with activity is more likely to be autoimmune. Pain that gets worse as the day progresses is more likely to be caused by "wear-and-tear."

QUICK TIPS

Other commonly tested seronegative spondyloarthropathies: reactive arthritis, psoriatic arthritis, and juvenile spondyloarthritis

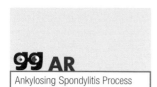

Ankylosing Spondylitis Process

which can lead to ankylosis (joint fusion). Patient can also present with limitation of chest wall expansion. Patients with advanced disease can have brittle "bamboo spine" that predisposes to vertebral fractures. A typical patient is a 20- to 40-year-old male with a history of an inflammatory autoimmune condition presenting with chronic back pain.

PPx: Avoid risk factors: Klebsiella synovitis, pulmonary fibrosis, renal amyloidosis, history of total joint replacement.

MoD: Unknown but likely 2/2 autoimmune reaction to environmental antigen

Dx:
1. Rheumatoid factor negative (hence seronegative).
2. Imaging via plain film, MRI, or CT showing sacroiliitis (sclerotic changes in the sacroiliac area). Advanced disease will show bamboo spine (vertebral fusion) on imaging.
3. Elevated ESR in 75% of patients.

Tx/Mgmt:
1. NSAIDs (indomethacin)
2. Physical therapy
3. Anti-TNF-alpha agents (etanercept, adalimumab, certolizumab, infliximab)
4. Surgery for cases of spinal deformity

Bursitis

AR
Knee anatomy

Buzz Words: Painful swelling at the knee, shoulder or elbow + no other constitutional symptoms

Clinical Presentation: Bursitis is the swelling of bursa, which are small fluid-filled sacs positioned near joints that act as cushions for muscles, tendons, and bones. Any bursa can lead to bursitis; the key is to be able to differentiate the swelling of a bursa with other more emergent diseases, such as septic arthritis. Bursitis can be diagnosed examining relevant anatomic landmarks (e.g., tenderness to palpation of greater trochanteric bursa) and ruling out other systemic causes on the differential. A typical patient has a history of diabetes, gout, RA, or other recurrent, noninfectious inflammation, and presents with swelling at the knee or elbow.

PPx: N/A

MoD:
- Direct trauma, percutaneous inoculation, or contiguous spread of *S. aureus* (most common).
- Commonly affected bursa as seen on the shelf are the subacromial (shoulder), olecranon (elbow), or prepatellar (knee).

Dx: Physical exam shows discrete bursal swelling, erythema, preserved joint range of motion, and maximal tenderness at center of bursa.

Tx/Mgmt:

1. Antibiotics for 1–4 weeks
2. Serial aspirations every 1–3 days until sterile or no reaccumulation of fluid
3. Surgery if refractory, presence of foreign body, or necrosis.

Osteochondritis Dissecans

Buzz Words: Child or adolescent + knee pain, swelling + precipitated by physical activity + catching or locking

Clinical Presentation: Osteochondritis dissecans (OD) is a disorder of the joint in which defects form in the subchondral bone (e.g., bone directly beneath the surface of the cartilage) and the cartilage itself. The affected joint can be painful, swollen, and range-limited. Advanced cases may cause joint catching or locking. A typical patient is a child or adolescent complaining of painful swelling in knee, elbow, or shoulder worsened by physical activity with no history of trauma.

PPx: N/A

MoD: Repetitive use results in necrotic bone and degenerative changes in the overlying cartilage. The bone/cartilage piece may separate from the underlying bone, causing pain, catching, and popping.

Dx:

1. Physical exam
2. X-ray
3. CT/MRI

Tx/Mgmt:

1. Joint rest
2. Physical therapy
3. Arthroscopic surgery

Tendinitis

Buzz Words:

Finkelstein test

- **Supraspinatus tendinitis**—pain subacromially and on the lateral aspect of the shoulder with arm abduction. Pain may be referred to lateral arm.
- **Lateral epicondylitis** ("tennis elbow")—excessive supination/pronation results in inflammation/degeneration of extensor tendons of the forearm
- **Medial epicondylitis**—pain distal to medial epicondyle (origin of flexor muscles of forearm), exacerbated by wrist flexion, caused by overuse of flexor pronator muscle.

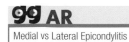

Medial vs Lateral Epicondylitis

- De Quervain tenosynovitis—pain at radial aspect of the wrist with pinch gripping with radiation of pain into elbow or thumb. Due to inflammation of abductor pollicis longus and extensor pollicis brevis. Positive Finkelstein test (grasping the thumb and ulnar deviating the hand sharply causes sharp pain on distal radius).

Clinical Presentation: Tendinitis (or tendinopathy) is an overuse disorder that leads to tendon thickening, and chronic, localized tendon pain. Although tendinitis is clinically manifested by pain with tendon loading and pain with palpation of the tendon, it is important to recognize the specific tendinitis syndromes listed previously. For these types of questions, knowledge of the neuromuscular anatomy will enable you to determine the specific tendinitis in question.

PPx: N/A

MoD: Overuse of tendon

Dx: Physical exam

Tx/Mgmt:

1. Physical therapy
2. Steroid injection
3. Surgery for refractory cases

Temporomandibular Joint Disorders

Buzz Words: Facial pain, ear discomfort or dysfunction, headache that is triggered by jaw movement

Clinical Presentation: Temporomandibular joint (TMJ) disorders have a complex, not very well understood pathophysiology. However, they usually present with acute or chronic facial pain triggered by jaw movement. On the shelf, TMJ disorders will usually come up as a differential diagnosis question, so be able to distinguish between the various etiologies for facial, ear, and jaw pain.

PPx: N/A

MoD: Structural, biologic, behavioral, environment, cognitive factors all contribute to pathophysiology

Dx: Physical exam

Tx/Mgmt:

1. Supportive therapy
2. Ten–fourteen days of NSAIDs
3. NSAID + muscle relaxant (cyclobenzaprine)
4. Tricyclic antidepressants
5. Surgery

Autoimmune Myositis Polymyositis/ Dermatomyositis

Buzz Words: Elevated CK, +ANA, +anti-Jo-1, +anti-SRP, +anti-Mi-2

- Both: gradual onset symmetric proximal muscle weakness (neck, shoulder, and pelvic girdle)
- Dermatomyositis (DM): also features malar rash, Gottron papules (popular, erythematous, scaly lesions over MCP, PIP, DIP), heliotrope (erythematous periorbital) rash, "shawl and face" rash (V and Shawl sign), "mechanic's hands"

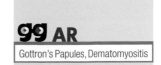

Gottron's Papules, Dermatomyositis

Dermatomyositis vs Polymyositis

Clinical Presentation: DM and PM are multisystem disorders, as is common with autoimmune diseases. The most notable clinical presentation finding is proximal muscle weakness. On the shelf and in clinic, it will be important to realize that the clinical finding of weakness does not always signify a neurologic issue. A classic patient is a 40-year-old female with history of arthralgias and interstitial lung disease presenting with muscle weakness causing difficulty rising from a chair and lifting her arms above her head.

PPx: N/A

MoD:

- PM: CD8+ T-cell mediated endomysial inflammation.
- DM: CD4+ T-cell mediated perimysial and perivascular inflammation and atrophy. May be associated with underlying cancer.

Dx:

Need at least two out of four criteria:

- Symmetric proximal muscle weakness
- Elevated CK
- EMG findings of myopathy
- Biopsy evidence of myositis

Tx/Mgmt:

1. Steroids
2. Immunosuppressants (methotrexate)
3. Physical therapy

Benign Neoplasms

Osteochondroma

Buzz Words: Localized pain, swelling, deformity, or pathologic fracture near metaphysis of distal femur

Clinical Presentation: Osteochondromas are the most common benign tumors of the bones, particularly in childhood or adolescence. They take the form of a cartilage-capped bony spur arising on the external surface of a bone, with the cartilaginous cap as the source of growth. On the shelf, be able to distinguish between various etiologies of musculoskeletal growths based on radiographic features. Classic patients are males less than 25 with joint or bone pain.

PPx: N/A

Bone Neoplasms

99 AR

Osteochondroma images, pathology

QUICK TIPS

Do not confuse Giant cell tumor with Giant cell tumor of the tendon sheath, which is a different entity that is more closely to pigmented villonodular synovitis (PVNS)

99 AR

Giant cell images, pathology

MoD: Aberrant growth plate cartilage

Dx: XR showing outgrowth of bone (exostosis) capped by benign cartilage near metaphysis of distal femur

Tx/Mgmt:

1. Serial exams and radiographs
2. Biopsy and removal of tumor for lesions with a cap greater than 2 cm thick

Giant Cell Tumor

Buzz Words: Soap bubble appearance on XR, pain, swelling, and limited ROM at epiphyseal end of distal femur or proximal tibia

Clinical Presentation: A benign tumor of the bone that has a histologic presentation of many giant cells. Very rarely tested in the shelf exam, and if it is tested, will likely only be the diagnosis of the disease (e.g., soap bubble appearance) in a 20–40-year-old patient.

PPx: N/A

MoD: Unknown

Dx:

1. Physical exam
2. "Soap bubble" appearance on XR
3. Giant cells seen in histologic specimen

Tx/Mgmt:

1. Bisphosphonates
2. Denosumab
3. Wide surgical resection

Malignant Neoplasms

Osteosarcoma

Buzz Words: Localized pain and/or soft tissue mass at metaphysis of long bones (especially knee)

Clinical Presentation: Osteosarcoma is a malignant primary bone-forming tumor that often presents with metaphyseal soft-tissue extension. Patients are more commonly male with a bimodal age distribution of 10–20 and more than 65. Things to look out for on the history include Paget disease of bone, bone infarct, radiation, familial retinoblastoma, and Li-Fraumeni syndrome.

PPx: N/A

MoD: Inherited or sporadic mutations

Dx:

1. Increased alkaline phosphatase
2. "Sunburst" or "Hair on end" lesion on XR
3. Biopsy for definitive diagnosis

Tx/Mgmt: Surgical excision and chemotherapy

Ewing Sarcoma

Buzz Words: Pediatric patient + onion skin appearance on periosteum of bone + localized pain or swelling at pelvic girdle, or diaphysis/metaphysis of proximal femur or rib + constitutional symptoms (fever, anemia, leukocytosis, elevated ESR)

Clinical Presentation: Ewing sarcoma is a small round blue cell tumor possibly related to primitive neuroectodermal cells. The tumor is typically diaphyseal and often associated with a soft-tissue mass. The classic patient is a male less than 15 years old with a chief complaint of boney pain, fevers, and fatigue.

PPx: N/A

MoD: t(11;22) translocation

Dx:

1. XR ("onion skin" periosteal reaction)
2. Biopsy for definitive diagnosis

Tx/Mgmt: Surgery and chemotherapy

Cancer Metastases to Bone

Buzz Words: Bone pain + Constitutional weight loss + BLT KP primary cancer

Clinical Presentation: Mets to the bone are the most common cause of bone cancer seen in the elderly. Any oncology patient you encounter with bone pain should always lead to high suspicion for metastasis. Common primary neoplasms include: breast, lung, prostate, kidney, thyroid, and melanoma (rare).

PPx: N/A

MoD: N/A

Dx: Imaging

Tx/Mgmt: Variable depending on the cancer staging. Likely will not be asked a question about treatment given the complexity of algorithms.

Degenerative and Metabolic Disorders of Bone, Tendon, and Cartilage

Chondromalacia Patellae (Patellofemoral Pain Syndrome)

Buzz Words: Knee pain worsening with squatting, running, prolonged sitting, or using stairs + positive patellofemoral compression test

Clinical Presentation: Chondromalacia patellae is the softening or degeneration of the cartilage on the undersurface of the patellofemoral joint, which presents clinically as pain near the knee cap. Sometimes referred to as

99 AR
Osteosarcoma

99 AR
Ewing sarcoma images, pathology

MNEMONIC
Mnemonic of cancers that metastasize to bone = BLT with a Kosher Pickle (Breast, Lung, Thyroid, Kidney, Prostate)

99 AR
Patellofemoral Compression Test

"runner's knee," patellofemoral pain syndrome is common with sports that involve running or jumping. Pain is often worse with running, stair use, or use after sitting for long periods of time. Be able to distinguish this from other causes of knee pain, such as pes anserinus, bursitis, etc., as this will likely appear as an answer choice among multiple knee pain etiologies.

PPx: Avoid overuse or trauma to knee

MoD: Unknown

Dx: Clinical presentation

Tx/Mgmt:

1. Short-term NSAIDs
2. Physical therapy
3. Surgical evaluation for refractory cases

Herniated Disc

Buzz Words:

- **Lumbar Herniated Disc:** Positive straight leg test + pain shooting down leg from back + paresthesias and weakness of lower extremity + unilateral (Table 12.1)

TABLE 12.1 Disc Herniation: Cervical and Lumbar Radiculopathy

Disc	Root	Pain/Paresthesias	Sensory Loss	Motor Loss	Reflex Loss
C4–5	C5	Neck, shoulder, upper arm	Shoulder	Deltoid, biceps, infraspinatus	Biceps
C5–6	C6	Neck, shoulder, lat. Arm, radial forearm, thumb and index finger	Lat. arm, radial forearm, thumb and index finger	Biceps, brachioradialis	Biceps, brachio-radialis, supinator
C6–7	C7	Neck, lat. arm, ring & index finger	Radial forearm, index and middle fingers	Triceps, extensor carpi ulnaris	Triceps, supinator
C7–T1	C8	Ulnar forearm and hand	Ulnar half of ring finger, little finger	Intrinsic hand muscles, wrist extensors, flexor dig profundus	Finger flexion
L3–4	L4	Anterior thigh, inner shin	Anteromedial thigh and shin, inner foot	Quadriceps	Patella
L4–5	L5	Lat. thigh and calf, dorsum of foot, great toe	Lat. calf and great toe	Extensor hallucis longus, foot dorsiflexion, inversion and eversion	None
L5–S1	S1	Back of thigh, lateral posterior calf, lat. foot	Posterolat. calf, lat. and sole of foot, smaller toes	Gastrocnemius, foot eversion	Achilles

- **Cervical Herniated Disc:** Positive Spurling test + pain shooting down arm + paresthesias and weakness of upper extremity + unilateral
- **L3–L4 disc:** weakness of knee extension, decreased patellar reflex
- **L4–L5 disc:** weakness of dorsiflexion, difficulty in heel-walking
- **L5–S1 disc:** weakness of plantarflexion, difficulty in toe-walking, decreased Achilles reflex

Clinical Presentation: A herniated disc, also referred to as a ruptured disc, or slipped disc. This can lead to irritation or compression of nearby nerves, causing numbness, tingling, paresthesias, and/or motor changes. Patients most commonly present with back pain and pain shooting down their legs.

PPx: N/A

MoD: Posterolateral disc herniation most commonly at L4–L5 and L5–S1.

Dx:
1. Clinical presentation and specific tests like Spurling test and straight leg test
2. XR
3. MRI

Tx/Mgmt:
1. NSAIDs
2. Physical therapy
3. Epidural steroid injections
4. Surgery

Legg-Calve-Perthes Disease

Buzz Words: Four–eight years old + painless/painful limp + XR of dense, contracted femoral capital epiphysis

Clinical Presentation: Perthes disease is avascular necrosis of the proximal femoral epiphysis in children. Its etiology is unknown and often presents in an otherwise healthy 4–8-year-old child (M > F). Patient can have bilateral painless limp and groin pain. Patient can also have gait abnormalities and limited ROM due to synovitis, as well as pain and limp worsened by activity. Over time, may have muscle atrophy and limb shortening from contractures and/or from femoral head collapse.

PPx: N/A

MoD: Etiology is unknown; unknown insult leads to loss of vascularity to femoral head.

Dx: Serial antero-posterior and frog-leg lateral x-rays are necessary and sufficient.

99 AR
Vertebrae 3d model

99 AR
Dermatomes

99 AR
Spurling test used for cervical radiculopathy

99 AR
Straight leg test is only positive if there is pain **shooting down leg** replicated when raising leg off the ground

Legg-Calve-Perthes X-ray

Hip anatomy

Tx/Mgmt:
1. Activity restriction; crutches, bracing, casting
2. Periodic radiographs
3. Physical therapy
4. NSAIDs
5. Surgery

Osgood-Schlatter Disease

Buzz Words:
- Child + anterior knee pain worse with activity or trauma + bony prominence over insertion of patellar tendon onto tibial tubercle + relieved by rest
- Tenderness and prominence of the tibial tubercle with an otherwise normal exam

Clinical Presentation: Osgood-Schlatter disease is a common cause of knee pain in growing adolescents, manifest by inflammation and pain near the tibial tubercle. This most commonly presents following a growth spurt, when structures are changing rapidly or following physical activity. Be able to diagnose this based on history and location of pain. A classic presentation is a 9–14-year-old male that is very active in sports and recently had a growth spurt.

PPx: N/A

MoD: Overuse—repetitive strain and chronic avulsion of secondary ossification center of tibial tubercle

Dx: Clinical presentation

Tx/Mgmt:
1. Ice after activity
2. Analgesics or NSAIDs
3. Physical therapy
4. Hyperosmolar dextrose injection

Osteodystrophy

Buzz Words: CKD + osteitis fibrosa cystica (cystic bone spaces filled with "brown tumor" consisting of osteoclasts and deposited hemosiderin from hemorrhages)

Clinical Presentation: Osteodystrophy is a general term for dystrophic growth of the bone, most commonly due to renal disease or disturbances in calcium and phosphorus metabolism. It is manifested by (1) osteomalacia (decreased mineralization of bone due to decreased calcium and $1,25\text{-}(OH)_2D$) and (2) osteitis fibrosa cystica (due to increased PTH). The patient may have chronic kidney disease or secondary hyperparathyroidism.

PPx: N/A

MoD:
- Renal failure → decreased vitamin D → decreased mineralization of bone → osteomalacia
- Renal failure → increased PTH → osteitis fibrosa cystica

Dx:
1. CMP (hypocalcemia, hyperphosphatemia)
2. Decreased vitamin D, increased parathyroid hormone
3. Increased alkaline phosphatase
4. Bone biopsy

Tx/Mgmt:
1. Vitamin D and/or calcium supplementation
2. Treat chronic kidney disease

Osteomalacia/Rickets

Buzz Words: Waddling gait + difficulty walking + soft, bending bones + vitamin D deficiency + bone pain and muscle weakness

Clinical Presentation: Osteomalacia refers to a softening of the bones, most commonly caused by vitamin D deficiency. Rickets = soft bone in children 2/2 vitamin D deficiency. Osteomalacia = vitamin D induced bone softening in adults, 2/2 to chronic kidney disease or hypocalcemia.

PPx: Vitamin D and calcium supplementation.

MoD: Defective mineralization of osteoid growth plates.

Dx:
1. X-rays show osteopenia and "Looser zones" (pseudofractures)
Decreased serum calcium and phosphate; increased ALP and PTH

Tx/Mgmt: Vitamin D supplementation

Avascular Necrosis of Femoral Head

Buzz Words: Trauma + corticosteroids + excessive alcohol intake + recent total hip replacement + crescent sign (subchondral radiolucency)

Clinical Presentation: Avascular necrosis is due to death of bone tissue due to a lack of blood supply, resulting in arthritis. Risk factors include sickle cell disease, recent total hip replacement, SLE, trauma, and corticosteroid use. On the shelf, remember the risk factors, and be able to identify its appearance on radiograph.

PPx: N/A

MoD: Compromise of bone vasculature 2/2 multiple predisposing etiologies

Dx:
1. Clinical presentation

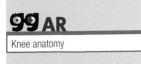

99 AR
Knee anatomy

99 AR
Rickets and global health

99 AR
Looser zones

XR of avascular necrosis of femoral head.

Femoral Head (vasculature)

99 AR

Osteoporosis screening guidelines

2. MRI for early detection due to high sensitivity
3. Anterior-posterior and frog-leg lateral films showing mild density changes, or pathognomonic crescent sign (subchondral radiolucency) in later phases

Tx/Mgmt:
1. Supportive therapy
2. Core decompression surgery
3. If refractory, then total hip replacement

Osteopenia/Osteoporosis

Buzz Words: Vertebral body compression fractures + Colles fracture (distal radius fracture) + hip fractures + long bone fractures

Clinical Presentation: Osteopenia and osteoporosis fall on a spectrum of decreased bone mineral density, where osteopenia can sometimes be considered a precursor to osteoporosis. Osteopenia is a sign of normal aging, while osteoporosis is pathologic. It is important to also realize that osteoporosis in question stems may refer to secondary osteoporosis, caused by excess steroids, Cushing syndrome, hyperthyroidism, long-term heparin, hypogonadism, or vitamin D deficiency. Classic patients are postmenopausal women or elderly men.

PPx: Calcium, vitamin D, weight-bearing exercise, smoking cessation

MoD: Rate of bone resorption exceeds rate of bone formation after peak bone mass is attained

Dx:
- Osteopenia: DEXA Bone Mineral Density T-score between −1.0 and −2.5
- Osteoporosis: DEXA Bone Mineral Density T-score < −2.5

Tx/Mgmt:
1. Nonpharmacologic—adequate calorie, calcium, and vitamin D, weight-bearing exercise, smoking cessation, reduce EtOH intake
2. For established osteoporosis or high-risk osteopenia, bisphosphonates
3. PTH therapy for 24 months

Osteitis Deformans (Paget Disease of Bone)

Buzz Words: Increased hat size + hearing loss + pathologic fractures + osteogenic sarcoma + heart failure due to arteriovenous malformations (AVMs) in vascular bone

Clinical Presentation: Paget disease of bone is common in aging bone, and the majority of patients are asymptomatic. In patients that are symptomatic, it is important to remember pathognomonic clues such as increased hat size, in combination with hearing loss or pathologic fractures in an older patient. Sometimes, the only abnormality in workup will be increased ALP.

PPx: N/A

MoD: Increased osteoclastic activity followed by increased osteoblastic activity, forming poor-quality bone in the pelvis, skull, and femur.

Dx:

1. Normal serum calcium, phosphorus, and PTH
2. Increased ALP
3. Radiographs show thickened bone with shaggy areas of radiolucency
4. Bone scans show "hot spots"

Tx/Mgmt: Bisphosphonates and calcitonin

Spondylolisthesis

Buzz Words: Radiographic Scotty dog sign + low back pain during lumbar extension + minimal tenderness

Clinical Presentation: Spondylolisthesis is a common cause of low back pain in athletes, and refers to anterior slippage of one vertebra over another. Its precursor is spondylosis (a vertebral crack or stress fracture); if the spondylosis weakens the bone sufficiently, then vertebral slippage (spondylolisthesis) will occur. A classic presentation is an adolescent athlete (diving, weightlifting, wrestling, gymnastics) with persistent lower back pain.

PPx: Avoid repetitive hyperextension.

MoD: Bilateral pars defects (spondylolysis) leads to slippage forward of an upper vertebral segment on the lower segment, most commonly L5–S1, then L4–L5, then L3–L4.

Dx:

1. Clinical presentation
2. XR showing Scotty dog sign
3. If severe or persistent pain, then technetium bone scan, SPECT, or MRI

Tx/Mgmt:

1. Restriction of aggravating activities
2. Physical therapy
3. NSAIDs
4. Casting or TLSO (thoracic-lumbar-sacral orthosis)

Degenerative and Metabolic Disorders of Joints

Gout

Buzz Words: Negatively birefringent crystals + recent large meal or alcohol consumption + swollen, red, and painful

99 AR

Paget Disease of the bone

99 AR

Scotty Dog Sign

MTP joint of big toe (podagra) + tophus formation on external ear, olecranon bursa, or Achilles tendon.

Clinical Presentation: Gout, also known as monosodium urate crystal deposition disease, is caused by hyperuricemia and is manifested as recurrent attacks of acute inflammatory arthritis, chronic arthropathy, accumulation of urate crystals, uric acid nephrolithiasis. Deposition is classically on the MTP of the big toe, causing redness, pain, and swelling. On the shelf, be able to distinguish this from arthritis and pseudogout.

PPx: Avoid excess red meats, seafood, alcohol, thiazides. Prophylaxis during chemotherapy with allopurinol.

MoD:

Prolonged hyperuricemia → tissue deposition of monosodium urate. Hyperuricemia can result from:

- Underexcretion of uric acid (lead poisoning, alcoholism, excess red meat, seafood, beer, thiazides)
- Overproduction of uric acid (Lesch-Nyhan syndrome, PRPP excess, increased cell turnover from leukemia or psoriasis treatment)

Dx:

1. Hyperuricemia
2. Absolute neutrophilic leukocytosis
3. Must confirm with joint aspiration showing negatively birefringent MSU crystals

Tx/Mgmt:

1. Acute flare: NSAIDs (indomethacin, ibuprofen), glucocorticoids, colchicine
2. Chronic: xanthine oxidase inhibitors such as allopurinol, febuxostat

Pseudogout (Calcium Pyrophosphate Dihydrate Deposition Disease)

Buzz Words: Positively birefringent crystals + acute pain, redness, swelling + limited ROM in joint + chondrocalcinosis

Clinical Presentation: In calcium pyrophosphate dihydrate deposition disease (CPPD), calcium pyrophosphate crystals deposit in joints, leading to inflammation. Deposition is common in elderly patients with degenerative joint disease, and increases with age and OA of the joints. In most cases, the cause of deposition is unknown, but joint trauma, hemochromatosis, hemosiderosis, hyperparathyroidism, and Bartter syndrome are risk factors. On the shelf, it is important to be able to distinguish the crystals of CPPD from gout.

PPx: Colchicine

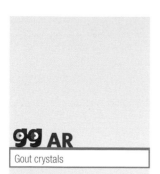
99 AR
Gout crystals

99 AR
Gout vs Pseudogout

MoD: Deposition of calcium pyrophosphate in tissues and cartilage (chondrocalcinosis)

Dx:
1. Chondrocalcinosis on XR
2. Joint aspiration showing rhomboid crystals, weakly birefringent under polarized light

Tx/Mgmt:
1. NSAIDs, colchicine, glucocorticoids
2. Arthroscopic surgery

Osteoarthritis

Buzz Words: Joint crepitus with motion + pain worse with motion + joint stiffness after inactivity + osteophyte enlargement of DIP joints (Heberden nodes) and PIP joints (Bouchard nodes) + joint space narrowing on XR

Clinical Presentation: Osteoarthritis is the most common chronic condition of the joints, and occurs due to non-inflammatory breakdown of articular cartilage. This results in pain, stiffness, and loss of joint mobility, most commonly in hip, knee, back, PIP, and DIP. The pain is worse with use of the joint and improves with rest. Radiographic features include joint space narrowing, subchondral sclerosis, osteophyte formation, and subchondral cysts.

PPx: Maintain healthy weight and engage in physical activity.

MoD: Noninflammatory progressive articular cartilage degeneration at weight bearing joints: femoral head, knee, cervical, and lumbar vertebrae

Dx: XR/imaging

Tx/Mgmt:
1. Heat, decreased weight-bearing, ROM exercises, use of a cane
2. Analgesics
3. Joint replacement

Degenerative and Metabolic Disorders of Muscles, Ligaments, and Fascia

Dupuytren Contracture

Buzz Words: Painless stiffness of fingers + nodules on palmar fascia + palpable cord running longitudinally in subcutaneous tissue which puckers the skin and limits extension

Clinical Presentation: Dupuytren contracture is a contracture of the longitudinal bands of the palmar aponeurosis lying

99 AR

Wrist anatomy

99 AR

Dupuytren contracture

between the skin and flexor tendons in the distal palm and fingers, most commonly in the ring and small fingers. It begins as a nodule and progresses to fibrous bands, with contracture of the fingers and loss of range of motion. Risk factors include: diabetes, cigarettes, alcohol use, repetitive hand use, and a familial history of contractures.

PPx: N/A

MoD: Slowly progressive fibroblastic proliferation and disorderly collagen deposition with fascial thickening

Dx: Clinical presentation

Tx/Mgmt:

1. Glove with padding or modifying casts with cushions
2. Glucocorticoid injection (triamcinolone acetonide and lidocaine)
3. Collagenase injection
4. Surgery (fasciectomy or fasciotomy)

Myositis Ossificans

99 AR
Myositis Ossificans

Buzz Words: Upper or lower extremity mass at site of known blunt trauma

Clinical Presentation: Myositis ossificans is a reactive process of bone formation. It presents as a hard mass that appears after an episode of blunt trauma. This will most likely appear as an answer choice on the shelf, so be able to rule this out based on history.

PPx: Avoid trauma.

MoD: Heterotopic ossification of skeletal muscle following muscular trauma

Dx: XR showing a radiodense white spot "floating" in the muscle

Tx/Mgmt: Symptomatic treatment

Rhabdomyolysis

Buzz Words: Myalgias, weakness + myoglobinuria + AKI + elevated CPK + hyperkalemia + hypocalcemia + hyperuricemia

Clinical Presentation: Rhabdomyolysis is the breakdown of muscle tissue, which leads to release of muscle contents into blood, most notably myoglobin, which is toxic to the kidneys. Causes of muscle breakdown include trauma, crush injuries, prolonged immobility, seizures, snakebites, daptomycin. Patients may present with myalgias, weakness, and red to brown-colored urine.

PPx: N/A

MoD: Skeletal muscle breakdown, release of myoglobin into bloodstream

Dx:
1. Chem 7 (elevated Cr, K)
2. Serum CK > 5× upper limit of normal (usually >5000 IU/L)
3. UA

Tx/Mgmt: IV fluids, mannitol (osmotic diuretic), bicarbonate (drives K back into cells)

Traumatic and Mechanical Disorders

Kyphoscoliosis

Buzz Words: Exercise intolerance + restrictive pulmonary function

Clinical Presentation: Kyphoscoliosis is a combination of kyphosis and scoliosis, and manifests as an abnormal curvature of the spine in both a coronal and sagittal plane. This will likely appear on the shelf as a distractor answer choice, but be able to recall its associations to diseases such as Marfan, neuromuscular disease, neurofibromatosis, etc.

PPx: N/A

MoD: Usually idiopathic, but can be caused by neuromuscular disease (muscular dystrophy, polio, cerebral palsy), vertebral disease (osteoporosis, Pott disease, neurofibromatosis, rickets), connective tissue disorder (Marfan, Ehler-Danlos, Morquio).

Dx: Physical exam, with measurement of Cobb angle

Tx/Mgmt: Supportive care and pulmonary rehab (including noninvasive positive pressure ventilation)

gg AR
Cobb angle of scoliosis

Rotator Cuff Tear

Buzz Words: Weakness/pain with shoulder maneuvers (abduction most common) + difficulty with reaching + painful drop arm test + weakness in external rotation

Clinical Presentation: Rotator cuff tear is a tear of one or more of the tendons of the rotator cuff muscles. It presents with weakness or pain with shoulder abduction or difficulty with reaching in athletes or workers with repetitive shoulder motion. To be best prepared, know your shoulder muscle anatomy and physical exam maneuvers specific or each muscle.

- **Supraspinatus:** abduction
- **Infraspinatus:** external rotation
- **Teres minor:** external rotation
- **Subscapularis:** internal rotation

PPx: N/A

MoD: Multifactorial

gg AR
Rotator Cuff Muscles

gg AR
Shoulder anatomy

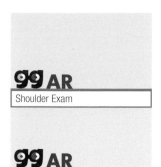

99 AR
Shoulder Exam

99 AR
SCFE

Dx:
1. Physical exam
2. XR
3. MRI

Tx/Mgmt:
1. Rest, analgesics, physical therapy
2. Arthroscopic surgery

Slipped Capital Femoral Epiphysis

Buzz Words: Obese + adolescent + nonradiating, dull, aching hip/groin/thigh/knee pain + altered gait + no trauma

Clinical Presentation: Slipped capital femoral epiphysis (SCFE) presents most commonly with hip or groin pain and altered gait in an obese adolescent, with no history of preceding trauma. It is caused by displacement of the capital femoral epiphysis from the femoral neck.

On the shelf, this will likely appear as an answer choice among multiple etiologies for hip pain (avascular necrosis, Legg-Calve-Perthes, etc.), so be able to distinguish between these etiologies.

PPx: Prevent risk factors such as obesity, endocrinopathy (hypopituitarism, thyroid disease), renal osteodystrophy, growth hormone treatment.

MoD: Displacement of femoral head relative to femoral shaft (slippage of femoral head posterior and inferior to femoral neck); can lead to disruption of the femoral head blood supply 2/2 lesion of the medial femoral circumflex artery.

Dx: Antero-posterior pelvis and frog lateral radiographs.

Tx/Mgmt: Avoid weight-bearing until surgical in situ fixation.

Congenital Disorders

Developmental Dysplasia of the Hip

Buzz Words: Joint laxity/clicking + breech delivery + positive Barlow and Ortolani maneuvers

Clinical Presentation: Developmental dysplasia of the hip (DDH) presents as a spectrum from neonatal instability (subluxation or dislocation) to acetabular dysplasia and is a disease of infancy/early childhood. This will most likely not be directly tested, but appear as an answer choice, so be able to rule this out among etiologies leading to hip pathology. Patients may have a history of breech position birth, oligohydramnios, or torticollis and present with hip joint laxity and "clicking" with movement.

PPx: N/A

MoD: Abnormal development of acetabulum and proximal femur

Dx:
1. Positive Barlow and Ortolani maneuvers
2. Diagnostic imaging (ultrasound in infants, radiographs in older infants) if inconclusive examination findings

Tx/Mgmt:
1. Pavlik harness up to 6 months of age
2. Arthrogram, closed reduction, spica cast
3. Open reduction

Barlow and Ortolani maneuvers

Genu Valgum (Knock-Knee) and Genu Varum (Bow-Leg)

Buzz Words:
- **Physiologic:** Symmetric, normal stature, no thrusts with ambulation, tibiofemoral angle within 2 standard deviations of the mean for age

99 AR
Valgum

- **Pathologic:** Unilateral, short stature, asymmetry, lateral knee-joint protrusion (thrust) with walking, progressive bowing, less than 6 cm between femoral condyles with patella facing forward and medial malleoli together + Blount disease

99 AR
Varum

- **Pathologic:** Unilateral, short stature, asymmetry, medial knee-joint protrusion (thrust) with walking, greater than 8 cm between medial malleoli with patellas facing forward and femoral condyles together, progressive deformity after age 4–5 + mucopolysaccharidosis

Clinical Presentation: Varus and valgus refer to angulation or bowing within the shaft of a bone or at a joint. Varus is the term for inward angulation of the distal segment of a bone or joint, and valgus is the term for outward angulation of the distal segment of a bone or joint.

PPx: N/A

MoD: N/A

Dx: Physical exam

Tx/Mgmt:
- For physiologic varus/valgus: observation and parental reassurance
- For pathologic varus/valgus: imaging, bracing, medical therapy for primary disease if available, and then surgical therapy if refractory

Foot Deformities

Buzz Words: Pes cavus (high arch) + pes planus (flat foot)

Clinical Presentation: A pediatric patient presents with foot pain and has flat feet or a high arch on physical exam.

Tx/Mgmt:
- **Pes planus and pes cavus:** Most are physiologic and asymptomatic. No treatment needed.

MNEMONIC
valGUM = knees sticking together like GUM

QUICK TIPS
Risk factors for both pathologic varus and valgus: trauma, neoplasm, skeletal dysplasia, infection, rickets
    Pathologic varus: Blount disease
    Pathologic valgus: Mucopolysaccharidosis

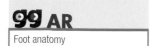

- **Painful flexible pes planus:** Evaluate for ligamentous laxity, tight heel cords, and tibialis posterior tendon dysfunction.
- **Rigid pes planus or pes cavus:** Evaluate for tarsal coalition, neuromuscular disease (Charcot-Marie-Tooth or Friedrich's Ataxia in cases of pes cavus), or talipes equinovarus (residual club foot causing pes cavus).

Osteogenesis Imperfecta ("Brittle Bone Disease")

Buzz Words: Pathologic fractures at birth + blue sclera + deafness + poor dentition + scoliosis + short stature + increased laxity of ligaments and skin

Clinical Presentation: Osteogenesis imperfect is a rare inherited connective tissue disorder with many phenotypic presentations, but be on the lookout in patients with bone fragility and short stature, scoliosis, blue sclera, hearing loss, poor dentition, skin and ligament laxity, and easy bruising. Be able to distinguish this from child abuse, rickets, osteomalacia, and other skeletal syndromes.

PPx: N/A

MoD: Autosomal dominant, defective type I collagen synthesis

Dx: Biochemical/genetic testing

Tx/Mgmt: Bisphosphonates

McArdle Disease (Glycogen Storage Disease V)

Buzz Words: Painful muscle cramps, myoglobinuria with exercise, arrhythmia from electrolyte abnormalities, chronic exercise intolerance with myalgia, fatigue. Muscle biopsy with biochemical testing showing myophosphorylase deficiency, and with periodic acid-Schiff stain showing increased glycogen.

Clinical Presentation: McArdle disease is an autosomal recessive disease caused by mutations in the muscle phosphorylase on chromosome 11, and presents with exercise intolerance, fatigue, myalgia, cramps, myoglobinuria, poor endurance, muscle swelling, and fixed weakness. On the shelf, be able to distinguish this from rhabdomyolysis, weakness, and other causes of fatigue.

PPx: N/A

MoD: Autosomal recessive deficiency of skeletal muscle glycogen phosphorylase (Myophosphorylase) → increased glycogen in muscle, unable to be broken down

Dx:

1. Nonischemic forearm exercise test
2. Genetic testing

Tx/Mgmt:
1. Carbohydrate rich diet
2. Ingestion of sucrose 5 minutes before aerobic exercise and moderation of physical activity

Mitochondrial Myopathies

Buzz Words:
- **Isolated myopathy**: exercise intolerance, fatigue, weakness
- **Chronic progressive external ophthalmoplegia**: gradual EOM paresis, bilateral ptosis
- **Leigh syndrome (subacute necrotizing encephalomyelopathy):** developmental delay, ataxia, dystonia, external ophthalmoplegia, seizures, lactic acidosis, vomiting, weakness
- **MELAS (Mitochondrial Encephalomyopathy with Lactic Acidosis and Stroke-like Episodes):** Hallmark of this syndrome is stroke-like episodes that cause hemiparesis, hemianopia, and cortical blindness. Other features include seizures, headaches, vomiting, short stature, hearing loss, muscle weakness.

Clinical Presentation: Mitochondrial myopathies are rare and variable diseases that typically present with a constellation of symptoms from various organ systems. The shelf likely will not test these directly, but rather a specific mitochondrial myopathy may appear as an answer choice for a clinical scenario relating to fatigue, or weakness. Common mitochondrial myopathies can be ruled out in the absence of multisystem disease.

PPx: N/A

MoD: Mitochondrial DNA mutations

Dx:
1. Genetic testing
2. Muscle biopsy

Tx/Mgmt: Supplementation with coenzyme Q10, creatine, and L-carnitine

Mitochondrial Myopathies

Adverse Defects of Drugs on the MSK System

Drug-induced Myopathy

Buzz Words: Steroids, statins, cocaine, AZT, antimalarials (chloroquine), colchicine, ipecac, chemo, interferon, antipsychotics associated with NMS

MoD: Varied, including direct myotoxicity, immunologically induced, indirect muscle damage

Dx: CK elevation, severe myopathy will show rhabdomyolysis

Tx/Mgmt: Stop offending agent

Malignant Hyperthermia

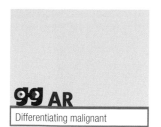

Differentiating malignant

Buzz Words: Anesthesia + hypercapnia + tachycardia, + muscle rigidity + rhabdomyolysis + arrhythmia

Clinical Presentation: A patient with no previous surgeries undergoes anesthesia with succinylcholine and sevoflurane for a hernia repair. Thirty minutes after the surgery begins, the patient becomes tachycardic and hypercapnic. The patient's jaw is clenched tightly. (Hyperthermia is a late sign.)

PPx: Assessment for risk factors during preoperative visit.

MoD: Susceptibility inherited as autosomal dominant with variable penetrance. Mutations in voltage-sensitive ryanodine receptor cause increase calcium release from sarcoplasmic reticulum.

Dx: Clinical presentation

Tx/Mgmt:

1. Dantrolene (ryanodine receptor antagonist)
2. Discontinue inhaled anesthetic; switch to propofol if surgery cannot be halted
3. Add charcoal filters to anesthesia breathing circuit
4. 100% FiO_2
5. Assess for cardiac dysrhythmias
6. Supportive care in ICU for more than 24 hours

GUNNER PRACTICE

1. A 33-year-old man comes to the office because of a 3-month history of low back pain and tightness. His pain is dull and aching, and worsens at night and in the morning. After moving around, the pain improves. He works as a computer programmer, and spends most of his day at a keyboard. He denies any recent trauma. Examination shows T37.0, blood pressure of 131/79, pulse of 72, and respirations of 16/min. His straight leg raise test is negative, and there is no tenderness over the spine or paraspinal areas. Which of the following is the most likely diagnosis?

    A. Idiopathic low back pain
    B. Ankylosing spondylitis
    C. Osteomalacia
    D. Osteoarthritis
    E. Sciatica
    F. Disc herniation

2. A 40-year-old woman comes to the office due to left hip pain for the last 4.5 weeks. The pain is worse when she stands up or walks. The pain is not worse in the morning; there is no history of trauma. She has a history of SLE, which she has treated with medium-dose prednisone and hydroxychloroquine. She denies use of tobacco, or illicit drugs, but does drink 3–4 drinks of alcohol per week. On physical exam, she has full hip range of motion, but pain on hip abduction and internal rotation. A hip plain film radiograph is normal. Which of the following is the best next step in management of this patient?
   A. DEXA scan
   B. MRI of hip
   C. Joint fluid analysis
   D. NSAIDs
   E. Reassurance

3. A 65-year-old man comes to the physician for his annual checkup. He reports feeling fine. His past medical history is significant for asthma, hypertension, hyperlipidemia, and osteoarthritis. His current medications are albuterol, atorvastatin, and amlodipine. His DIP and PIP joints appear to be enlarged. His lab values are as follows:

Na	141
K	4.1
Cl	100
HCO_3	26
BUN	18
Cr	1.0
Calcium	8.9
Serum PSA	1.1
Tbili	1.2
Alk Phos	389
AST	22
ALT	46

ALT, Alanine aminotransferase; *AST*, aspartate aminotransferase.

What is most likely diagnosis?
   A. Alcohol use
   B. Adverse effect of medication
   C. Paget disease of bone
   D. Prostate cancer
   E. Normal healthy individual

ANSWERS: What Would Gunner Jess/Jim Do?

1. WWGJD? A 33-year-old man comes to the office because of a 3-month history of low back pain and tightness. His pain is dull and aching, and worsens at night and in the morning. After moving around, the pain improves. He works as a computer programmer and spends most of his day at a keyboard. He denies any recent trauma. Examination shows T37.0, blood pressure of 131/79, pulse of 72, and respirations of 16/min. His straight leg raise test is negative, and there is no tenderness over the spine or paraspinal areas. Which of the following is the most likely diagnosis?

Answer: B, Ankylosing spondylitis

Explanation: Patient has chronic LBP that is worse at night but improves after physical activity. In a young patient, this pattern suggests an inflammatory spondylarthritis, such as ankylosing spondylitis.

A. Idiopathic low back pain → Incorrect. Patient likely has an autoimmune etiology to his low back pain, and thus, does not have an idiopathic cause to his back pain.

C. Osteomalacia → Incorrect. Osteomalacia can lead to pathologic fractures, but the back pain would be worse with activity.

D. Osteoarthritis → Incorrect. Patient is too young to be suffering from osteoarthritis. In addition, this patient has no joint crepitus with motion, and his pain is better with motion, making osteoarthritis unlikely.

E. Sciatica→ Incorrect. Patient does not have shooting pain down his leg, the classic symptom of sciatica, nor does the patient have a positive straight leg raise test, which is also commonly positive in sciatica.

F. Disc herniation → Incorrect. Patient has a negative straight leg raise test, which decreases the likelihood of disc herniation.

2. WWGJD? A 40-year-old woman comes to the office due to left hip pain for the last 4.5 weeks. The pain is worse when she stands up or walks. The pain is not worse in the morning, and there is no history of trauma. She has a history of systemic lupus erythematosus for the last 10 years, which she has treated with medium-dose prednisone and hydroxychloroquine. She denies use of tobacco, or illicit drugs, but does drink 3–4 drinks of alcohol per week. Her BMI is 25.6 kg/m². On physical exam, she has full hip range of motion, but pain on hip

abduction and internal rotation. A plain film radiograph of the hip is normal. Which of the following is the best next step in management of this patient?

Answer: B, MRI of hip

Explanation: This woman most likely has avascular necrosis. The risk of avascular necrosis is significantly increased with use of glucocorticoids, and with SLE. Pain is also classically worse with weight-bearing, hip abduction, and internal rotation, and there is a lack of erythema, swelling, and point tenderness, all features of which this woman manifests. Since her x-ray was normal, MRI is the next best test because it is the most sensitive diagnostic modality.

A. DEXA scan → Incorrect. Although she has some symptoms and risk factors for osteopenia/osteoporosis, she is too young to manifest with DEXA—she hasn't gone through menopause, and is not in a low-estrogen state.

C. Joint fluid analysis → Incorrect. Joint fluid analysis would be used to evaluate septic or crystal-induced arthritis (gout, CPPD). Her presentation is not typical for these arthritides.

D. NSAIDs → Incorrect. Treatment for avascular necrosis includes core decompression, bone graft, or joint replacement, but not NSAIDs.

E. Reassurance → Incorrect. She likely has avascular necrosis, and needs an MRI to confirm this diagnosis.

3. WWGJD? A 65-year-old man comes to the physician for his annual checkup. He reports **feeling fine.** His past medical history is significant for asthma, hypertension, hyperlipidemia, and osteoarthritis. His current medications are albuterol, atorvastatin, and amlodipine. His DIP and PIP joints appear to be enlarged. His lab values are as follows:

Na: 141
K: 4.1
Cl: 100
HCO3: 26
BUN: 18
Cr: 1.0
Calcium: 8.9
Serum PSA: 1.1
Tbili: 1.2
Alk Phos: 389
AST: 22
ALT: 46

What is most likely diagnosis?

Answer: C, Paget disease of bone

Explanation: The only abnormality in this patient is an elevated alkaline phosphatase level. Alkaline phosphatase is expressed at high levels in bone and hepatobiliary tissues, which makes it a marker for diseases of high bone turnover and cholestatic liver disease. A common presentation of Paget disease in an elderly patient is asymptomatic with isolated elevated alkaline phosphatase.

A. Alcohol use → Incorrect. In alcoholic hepatitis, the AST:ALT ratio is usually >2:1, which is not the case in this patient. In addition, his absolute AST and ALT values are not high enough to warrant the diagnosis of alcoholic hepatitis.

B. Adverse effect of medication → Incorrect. Although the patient's statin use could precipitate elevations in liver associated enzymes, the pattern of LAE elevation is usually hepatocellular rather than cholestatic.

D. Metastases to bone → Incorrect. Metastatic cancer to bone can cause elevated alkaline phosphatase, but would usually also cause other symptoms, including constitutional symptoms, bone pain, hypercalcemia, etc.

E. Normal healthy individual → Incorrect. The patient's elevated alkaline phosphatase is abnormal and warrants further workup.

Endocrine and Metabolic Disorders

Sierra Centkowski, Rebecca Gao, Daniel Gromer, Hao-Hua Wu, Leo Wang, and Eric Goren

CHAPTER

13

Introduction

The endocrine system is described as a collection of different organs that secrete hormones directly into the blood stream. While these organs are physically located all over the body, they are intricately connected through a system of feedback loops within the body. This system is unique because it controls various bodily functions, including metabolism, development, sex, hunger and thirst, sleep, mood, and electrolyte balances.

Simplified, the hypothalamus in the brain connects the nervous system to the endocrine system via the pituitary gland. The hypothalamus secretes specific excitatory (positive) and inhibitory (negative) hormones to the pituitary gland. These "on-off" signals from the hypothalamus tell the pituitary when to secrete its own hormones, including adrenocorticotropic hormone (ACTH), thyroid stimulating hormone (TSH), luteinizing hormone (LH), follicle-stimulating hormone (FSH), prolactin, and growth hormone (GH). Each of these hormones travel through the blood stream to stimulate specific organs (i.e., ACTH stimulates the adrenal glands to secrete cortisol) that regulate the functional mechanisms of the body mentioned earlier.

Initially, it may seem overwhelming to memorize the diseases of each endocrine organ independently. The best approach is to understand the feedback loops, the primary function of each hormone, and key signs and symptoms of common electrolyte abnormalities. For example, a patient who presents with hyperreflexia, involuntary muscle contractions, and QT prolongation should make you think of low serum calcium levels or hypocalcemia. What hormones are involved in calcium level regulation? Parathyroid hormone (PTH) is the major positive regulator of calcium, meaning if there isn't enough PTH, there isn't enough calcium floating around.

This chapter is divided primarily by the endocrine organ or disease, including (1) Diabetes mellitus, (2) Thyroid disorders, (3) Parathyroid disorders, (4) Adrenal disorders, (5) Pituitary disorders, and (6) Practice (application of the material learned). As always, each disease process is put

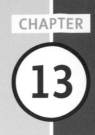

GUNNER COLUMN

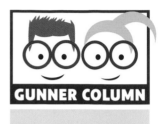

Endocrine System Overview Video

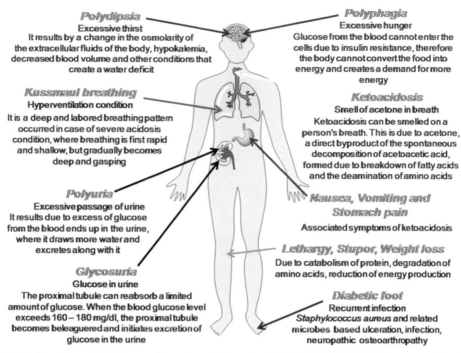

Polydipsia
Excessive thirst
It results by a change in the osmolarity of
the extracellular fluids of the body, hypokalemia,
decreased blood volume and other conditions that
create a water deficit

Kussmaul breathing
Hyperventilation condition
It is a deep and labored breathing pattern
occurred in case of severe acidosis
condition, where breathing is first rapid
and shallow, but gradually becomes
deep and gasping

Polyuria
Excessive passage of urine
It results due to excess of glucose
from the blood ends up in the urine,
where it draws more water and
excretes along with it

Glycosuria
Glucose in urine
The proximal tubule can reabsorb a limited
amount of glucose. When the blood glucose level
exceeds 160 – 180 mg/dl, the proximal tubule
becomes beleaguered and initiates excretion of
glucose in the urine

Polyphagia
Excessive hunger
Glucose from the blood cannot enter the
cells due to insulin resistance, therefore
the body cannot convert the food into
energy and creates a demand for more
energy

Ketoacidosis
Smell of acetone in breath
Ketoacidosis can be smelled on a
person's breath. This is due to acetone,
a direct byproduct of the spontaneous
decomposition of acetoacetic acid,
formed due to breakdown of fatty acids
and the deamination of amino acids

**Nausea, Vomiting and
Stomach pain**
Associated symptoms of ketoacidosis

Lethargy, Stupor, Weight loss
Due to catabolism of protein, degradation of
amino acids, reduction of energy production

Diabetic foot
Recurrent infection
Staphylococcus aureus and related
microbes based ulceration, infection,
neuropathic osteoarthropathy

FIG. 13.1 Symptoms of diabetes mellitus. (From Mahapatra DK, Asati V, Bharti SK: Chalcones and their therapeutic targets for the management of diabetes: structural and pharmacological perspectives. *Eur J Med Chem* 92:839–865, 2015, Figure 1.)

into the four physician tasks that the shelf exam will test you on: (1) Prophylactic management (PPx), (2) Mechanism of Disease (MoD), (3) Buzz words establishing a diagnosis, and (4) Treatment/Management (Tx/Mgmt).

Diabetes and the Endocrine Pancreas

Diabetes

Diabetes Mellitus Type 1

Buzz Words: Young patient + polyuria, polydipsia + abdominal pain + altered mental status + fast, deep breathing (Fig. 13.1).

Clinical Presentation: An 18-year-old presents with abdominal pain, nausea/vomiting, confusion, and tachypnea. The patient complained of increased thirst and urination frequency over the past few weeks.

PPx: N/A

MoD: Diabetes mellitus type 1 is an autoimmune disease (associated with HLA DQ/DR) that involves autoantibodies that destroy beta cells in the pancreas that produce insulin.

Dx: Requires one of the following measurements at two separate visits:
- Fasting glucose greater than 126 mg/dL
- Random plasma glucose greater than 200 mg/dL with symptoms
- Hemoglobin A1c (HbA1c) greater than 6.5% (second measurement taken 3 months later).

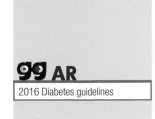
2016 Diabetes guidelines

Tx/Mgmt:
1. Injectable insulin
2. Every 3 months, check HbA1c (goal < 7%)
3. Every year, check urinalysis for urine micro albumin/creatinine ratio (if high, start on angiotensin converting enzyme [ACE] inhibitor or angiotensin receptor blocker [ARB]), serum creatinine (monitor for diabetic nephropathy), eye screening with ophthalmologist (monitor for diabetic retinopathy), podiatry, and cholesterol levels
4. Check blood pressure (if > 130/80, start ACE inhibitor or ARB)

Diabetes Mellitus Type 2

Buzz Words: Obese + poor diet + family history of diabetes

Clinical Presentation: An obese patient with a strong family history of DMT2 presents with increased thirst and urinary frequency.

DMII overview and management

PPx: Modify risk factors for obesity, as it can worsen insulin resistance.

MoD: Patients with poor diet who are obese have high levels of free fatty acids, which both make muscles more resistant to insulin and reduce the beta cells' ability to secrete enough insulin in response to increase the level of circulating free fatty acids. The beta cells become desensitized and, over time, stop secreting as much insulin, resulting in high levels of circulating glucose in the body.

Dx: See DMT1

Tx/Mgmt:
1. Diet and exercise is first line for DMT2.
2. Oral medications, starting with metformin (prevents gluconeogenesis in the liver). Other medications include sulfonylureas (glipizide), pioglitazone, DDP-IV inhibitors (sitagliptin), and GLP-1 receptor agonist (exenatide).
3. Insulin
   - Avoid metformin in renal failure.
   - Metformin can rarely cause lactic acidosis.
   - Sulfonylureas can cause weight gain and hypoglycemia.

- Pioglitazone can cause weight gain and CHF.
- DPP-IV inhibitors are weight neutral and both DPP-IV inhibitors and GLP-1 receptor agonists carry low risk of hypoglycemia but may have dose-limiting gastrointestinal symptoms.

Tx/Mgmt:
- Every three months, check HbA1c (goal <7%).
- Every year, check urinalysis for urine micro albumin/creatinine ratio (if high, start on ACE inhibitor or ARB), serum creatinine (monitor for diabetic nephropathy), eye screening with ophthalmologist (monitor for diabetic retinopathy), podiatry, and cholesterol levels.
- Every visit check blood pressure (if >130/80, start ACE inhibitor or ARB) and feet (for ulcers).
- Note: when diabetic patients are hospitalized, they take insulin sliding scale and stop other medications (metformin is stopped because of increased burden on renal function, especially for patients undergoing imaging studies requiring contrast dye).

Acute Complications of Diabetes Mellitus
Hyperosmolar Coma, or Hyperosmolar Hyperglycemic Nonketotic Syndrome
- Most common in DMT2, especially elderly patients.
- **Symptoms:** severe dehydration (low BP, high HR), nausea/vomiting, abdominal pain, polyuria, polydipsia, seizures, and altered mental status.
- **Lab findings:** high glucose (usually >900 mg/dL), hyperosmolarity (>320 mOsm/L), normal pH, and high BUN (due to dehydration).
- **Treatment:** IV normal saline and low dose insulin.

Hypoglycemic Shock
- Brain is most at risk during hypoglycemia. Causes include too much insulin (high insulin, low C-peptide in blood), insulinoma, ethanol ingestion, etc.
- **Symptoms:** tremor, palpitations, sweating, altered mental status, seizure, and coma in some cases
- **Lab findings:** low glucose (usually <50 mg/dL)
- **Treatment:** IV dextrose (give glucose!)

Ketoacidosis
- Most common in DMT1, but it can occur in both DMT1 and DMT2 patients. It is usually precipitated by stress (illness or trauma) or missed insulin doses.
- **Symptoms:** acute onset nausea/vomiting, abdominal pain, "fruity" breath (cause by high ketones), rapid and

deep breathing, dehydration, polyuria, polydipsia, and altered mental status
- **Lab findings:** high glucose (usually >450 mg/dL), anion gap metabolic acidosis (pH < 7.3 and serum HCO_3 < 15 mEq/L), ketosis, high serum beta-hydroxybutanone
- **Treatment:** IV normal saline, insulin, and potassium supplementation
- **Note:** monitor for anion gap closure as treatment end point.
- Rapid correction of hyperglycemia can cause cerebral edema.

Electrolyte Abnormalities
- Hyperkalemia, but decreased total body potassium; hyponatremia; hypophosphatemia; hypomagnesemia

Chronic Complications of Diabetes Mellitus
These chronic complications of diabetes mellitus are caused by poor glycemic control, which results in damage of the microvasculature and microvasculature.

Gastrointestinal/Gastroparesis
- **Symptoms:** intractable nausea and vomiting, secondary to delayed gastric emptying or esophageal dysmotility
- **Treatment:** pro-kinetic agents, including metoclopramide

Neurologic/Neuropathy
- **Symptoms:** foot ulcers, dry/itchy skin, erectile dysfunction, incontinence, cranial nerve III (oculomotor), and neuropathy (droopy eyelid with "down and out" eye)
- **Treatment:** Gabapentin or tricyclic antidepressants

Ophthalmologic/Retinopathy
- **Symptoms:** vision loss or blindness
- **Funduscopic exam:** small hemorrhages and exudates
- **Treatment:** laser photocoagulation

Peripheral Vascular
- **Symptoms:** poor wound healing

Renal/Diabetic Nephropathy
- **Symptoms:** usually asymptomatic at first
- **Diagnosis:** urine albumin/creatinine ratio
- **Treatment:** ACE inhibitor or ARB

QUICK TIPS

The three most important chronic complications of diabetes mellitus are the "-opathies" = nephropathy, neuropathy, and retinopathy.

Metabolic Syndrome
- **Diagnosis**: weight gain and excess body fat (leading to high blood sugars), high blood pressure, and high cholesterol

Hypoglycemia and Islet Cell Disorders

Hypoglycemia (secondary to insulinoma, surreptitious insulin use, sepsis, liver failure).

Buzz Words: Altered mental status + sweating + tremor + tachycardia + palpitations + headache + seizure or coma.

PPx: Appropriate use of insulin (too much can cause hypoglycemia)

MoD: Most commonly iatrogenic due to inappropriate medication dosing or use of insulin. Insulinomas are benign tumors of the beta cells within the pancreas, which cause over production of insulin. Liver failure can cause hypoglycemia because of decreased glycogen break down. Systemic illness, such as sepsis (widespread infection), can also cause hypoglycemia.

Dx:
- 72-hour fast demonstrates inappropriately elevated insulin levels with low glucose levels.
- Hypoglycemia in diabetic patients is less than 70 mg/dL, but symptoms are usually experienced at a level below that.
- Insulinoma versus surreptitious insulin use? Insulinomas (endogenous insulin source) will cause elevated nightly insulin, pro-insulin, and C-peptide, while surreptitious use of insulin (exogenous insulin source) will have normal C-peptide levels.

Tx/Mgmt:
- Give IV dextrose (glucose) and treat underlying cause (i.e., surgical resection is first line treatment for insulinoma, which is benign). Note: screen patients with insulinomas for MEN 1 syndrome!

Hyperglycemia (Glucagonoma)

Buzz Words: Blistering rash (necrolytic migratory erythema) below the waist + weight loss + diarrhea

PPx: N/A

MoD: Glucagonomas are neuroendocrine tumors of the alpha-cells within the pancreas that secrete glucagon. Glucagon increases the level of glucose in the body, causing hyperglycemia.

Dx: Hyperglycemia with a high glucagon level (>500 pg/mL) Note: normocytic anemia may also be seen.

Tx/Mgmt: Surgical resection of the tumor is first line therapy.

Thyroid Disorders

Thyroid Nodule

Clinical Presentation: These are often noted incidentally and are benign (Table 13.1; Fig. 13.2). However, be aware of suspicious signs. A rapidly growing, fixed, solitary nodule in a patient with prior radiation therapy (specifically to the neck), cervical adenopathy, vocal cord involvement, and a family history of thyroid cancer should make you think malignancy!

Dx:

1 Physical exam and ultrasound
2. TSH
3. Fine-needle aspiration (FNA)
   - If FNA shows malignant cells, surgery is required.
4. Thyroid scan with iodine-123 scintigraphy
   - "Hot" nodule (hyperfunctioning, increased iodine uptake) → treat for hyperthyroidism
   - Cold" nodule (hypofunctioning, decreased iodine uptake) → surgery is required

Tx/Mgmt:

1 Benign nodules require close follow-up and observation.
2. Malignant nodules require surgery.

Euthyroid Sick Syndrome

Clinical Presentation: Abnormal thyroid function tests (TFTs) in the setting of an acute, severe nonthyroidal illness (i.e., acute hepatitis, acute intermittent porphyria, nephrotic syndrome, Cushing syndrome, and psychiatric disturbances).

PPx: N/A

Dx: Usually decreased total T3, decreased free T3, normal T4 and normal/low TSH.

Tx/Mgmt: Usually transient changes in thyroid hormones; do not treat with thyroid hormone replacement therapy.

TABLE 13.1 General Features of Thyroid Disorders

Hyperthyroidism	Hypothyroidism
Anxiety	Depression
Palpitations or atrial fibrillation	Bradycardia
Weight loss	Weight gain
Heat intolerance, sweating	Cold intolerance
Proximal muscle weakness, eye lid lag, tremors, hyper-reflexia	Fatigue, constipation, cognitive slowing, dry skin, hyporeflexia

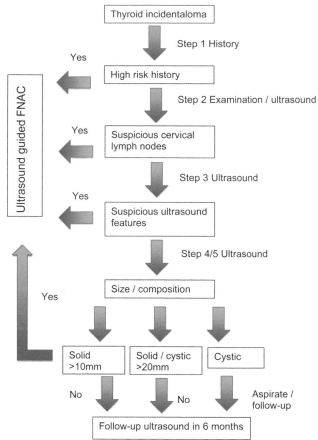

FIG. 13.2 Algorithm for evaluation of a thyroid nodule. (From Aspinall SR, Ong SG, Wilson MS, Lennard TW: How shall we manage the incidentally found thyroid nodule? *Surgeon* 11:96–104, 2013, Figure 8.)

Hypothyroidism

Buzz Words: Cold intolerance, fatigue, weakness, bradycardia, goiter, dry skin; symptoms progress over years.

PPx: N/A

MoD: Depends on etiology.

1 Chronic autoimmune hypothyroidism (Hashimoto's) → presence of thyroid peroxidase (TPO) antibodies mediate destruction of the thyroid (covered in detail in Hashimoto thyroiditis section below)

2. Iodine insufficiency → decreased levels of iodine lead to decreased levels of thyroid hormones produced, resulting in hypothyroidism. Rare in developed countries.

Dx: High TSH, low free T4, possibly increased antimicrosomal antibodies or TPO antibodies (indicating Hashimoto thyroiditis)

Tx/Mgmt: Levothyroxine (T4), daily for life; monitor TSH

Hashimoto Thyroiditis

Buzz Words: Goiter, TPO antibodies, increased thyroglobulin, family history, more common in women

MoD: Autoimmune.

Tx/Mgmt: See above; also, increases risk for lymphoma of thyroid.

Subacute (Viral) Thyroiditis

Buzz Words: Preceded by weeks of flu-like illness + painful thyroid +HLA-B35

MoD: Transient leakage of thyroid hormones from an inflamed thyroid causes depletion of hormones. Transition from hyperthyroid state to euthyroid state to hypothyroid state as damage to thyroid progresses (leakage of hormones to depletion of hormones).

Dx:
1. Low TSH, high T3 and T4, high ESR
2. Low radioiodine (iodine-123) uptake

Tx/Mgmt: Nonsteroidal antiinflammatory drugs (NSAIDs). Steroids for severe symptoms.

Myxedema Coma

Buzz Words: Profound hypothermia + decreased consciousness+ respiratory depression + inciting event like an infection or trauma

MoD: Chronic untreated hypothyroidism (usually undiagnosed) with inciting event

Tx/Mgmt: MEDICAL EMERGENCY! Supportive care to maintain hemodynamic stability (fluids, pressors, mechanical ventilation), IV thyroxine, and IV steroids.

Hyperthyroidism

Buzz Words: Heat intolerance (excessive sweating or "hot flashes"), insomnia, anxiety, weight loss, arrhythmias, proptosis, middle-aged female (Fig. 13.3).

PPx: N/A

Dx:
1. Low TSH, high T4, increased radioactive iodine-123 uptake
2. If both TSH and T4 are increased, consider secondary hyperthyroidism caused by pituitary.
3. Note: order pregnancy test for increased thyroid-binding globulin and low radioactive T3 uptake.

Tx/Mgmt:
1. Beta-blocker (propranolol) for immediate adrenergic symptom management

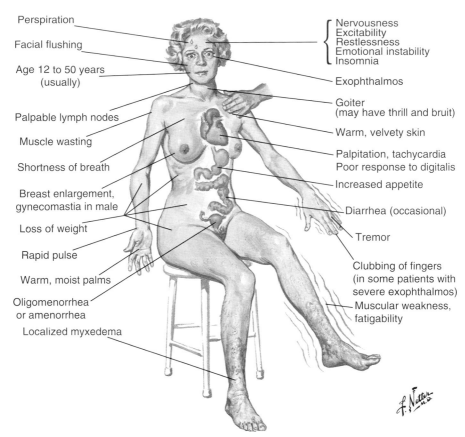

Perspiration

Facial flushing

Age 12 to 50 years
(usually)

Palpable lymph nodes

Muscle wasting

Shortness of breath

Breast enlargement,
gynecomastia in male

Loss of weight

Rapid pulse

Warm, moist palms

Oligomenorrhea
or amenorrhea

Localized myxedema

Nervousness
Excitability
Restlessness
Emotional instability
Insomnia

Exophthalmos

Goiter
(may have thrill and bruit)

Warm, velvety skin

Palpitation, tachycardia
Poor response to digitalis

Increased appetite

Diarrhea (occasional)

Tremor

Clubbing of fingers
(in some patients with
severe exophthalmos)

Muscular weakness,
fatigability

FIG. 13.3 Hyperthyroidism with diffuse goiter (Graves' disease). (From Netter Images. https://www.netterimages.com/hyperthyroidism-with-diffuse-goiter-graves-disease-unlabeled-endocrinology-frank-h-netter-5742.html. ©2017 Elsevier, Inc.)

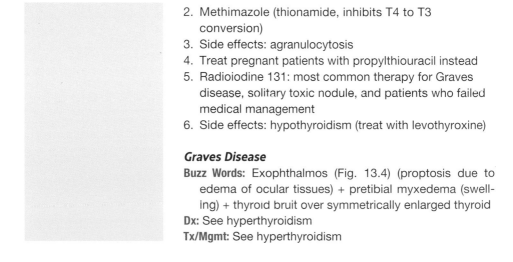

2. Methimazole (thionamide, inhibits T4 to T3 conversion)
3. Side effects: agranulocytosis
4. Treat pregnant patients with propylthiouracil instead
5. Radioiodine 131: most common therapy for Graves disease, solitary toxic nodule, and patients who failed medical management
6. Side effects: hypothyroidism (treat with levothyroxine)

Graves Disease

Buzz Words: Exophthalmos (Fig. 13.4) (proptosis due to edema of ocular tissues) + pretibial myxedema (swelling) + thyroid bruit over symmetrically enlarged thyroid

Dx: See hyperthyroidism

Tx/Mgmt: See hyperthyroidism

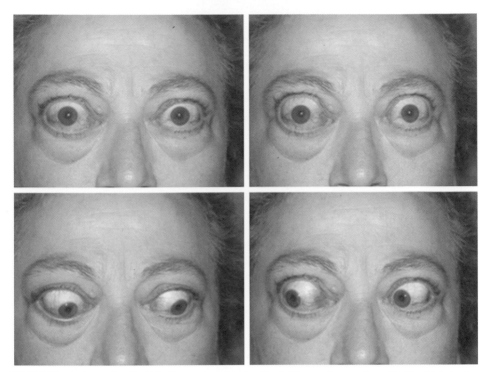

FIG. 13.4 Proptosis, conjunctival injective, and eyelid retraction in Graves disease. (From De Groot LJ, Jameson JL: *Endocrinology: adult and pediatric*, ed 7, Elsevier, 2016, 1437–1464. Chapter 82, Figure 82.5.)

Thyroid Storm

Buzz Words: Recent inciting event (infection, trauma) or contrast study (acute iodine load) + high fever + autonomic instability + CHF + delirium + lid lag + nausea/vomiting/diarrhea + seizures

Tx/Mgmt: Medical Emergency!

1. Beta-blocker (to reduce adrenergic manifestations)
2. PTU (to decrease hormone synthesis/release)
3. Glucocorticoids (to decrease peripheral T4 to T3)
4. Supportive therapy (IV fluids, cooling, etc.)

Thyrotoxicosis

Buzz Words: Symptoms of hyperthyroidism (tachycardia, weight loss, heat intolerance, increased total/free T4, decreased TSH) + *low* radioactive iodine-123 uptake

MoD: Subacute lymphocytic (painless) thyroiditis, subacute (viral) thyroiditis, iodine-induced thyroidtoxicosis, levothyroxine overdose, struma ovarii (ovarian teratoma that produced thyroid hormones)

Dx: Increased total/free T4, decreased TSH, *low* uptake of radioactive iodine-123

Tx/Mgmt: See hyperthyroidism

Neoplasms

Buzz Words: History of radiation therapy to head/neck, solitary thyroid nodule.

PPx: Avoid radiation to head and neck.

MoD:

1 Types of thyroid cancer
   a. **Papillary:** most common type, best prognosis, usually associated with history of radiation exposure, involves epithelial cells, + iodine uptake.
   b. **Follicular:** second most common, worse prognosis due to hematogenous spread and metastasis, associated with iodine deficiency, involves epithelial cells, +++ iodine uptake.
   c. **Medullary:** associated with MEN2, worse prognosis, involves parafollicular C-cells (high calcitonin level).
   d. **Anaplastic:** worst prognosis with high mortality, more common in elderly, involves epithelial cells, and invades adjacent organs and tissue in neck.

Dx: FNA

Tx/Mgmt:

1 Radioactive iodine ablation
2. Total thyroidectomy +/- radical neck lymph node dissection
3. Chemotherapy and radiotherapy directly for anaplastic type

Thyroid Deficiency from Pituitary Disorder (Refer to Pituitary Section)

1 Prolactinoma (common pituitary adenoma) → hypothyroidism
2. Hypopituitarism → low TSH → hypothyroidism

Secondary Hypothyroidism and Hyperthyroidism

1 **Anorexia nervosa:** can cause cold intolerance, thyroid dysfunction
2. **Warfarin:** levothyroxine and thyroid hormones increase warfarin effects, thus increasing bleeding risk.
3. **Amiodarone:** can cause both hypo- and hyperthyroidism

Parathyroid Disorders

Hyperparathyroidism

Buzz Words: Dialysis patient with kidney stones + asymptomatic patient with high calcium on routine labs

Clinical Presentation: A patient may present with a history of kidney stones, hypertension (not well controlled with appropriate medical therapy), and back pain (due to vertebral compression caused by low bone density). Consider familial disorders such as MEN1 syndrome, familial hypocalciuric hypercalcemia (FHH).

PPx: Modify risk factors for chronic kidney disease, maintain healthy vitamin D intake, genetic testing for MEN1 syndrome.

MoD: Primary hyperparathyroidism is caused by a problem at the parathyroid level, with inappropriate release of PTH, no longer responsive to the calcium levels in the blood (remember, high PTH increases plasma calcium levels up to a point, and then a negative feedback mechanism kicks in, where high calcium signals the parathyroid to stop producing PTH). This is almost always caused by a parathyroid adenoma and is very common in younger women.

Secondary hyperparathyroidism is almost always caused by chronic kidney disease that leads to an inability to clear phosphate. This up regulates PTH release to try to clear the phosphate, but that has little effect because the kidney can't clear it. Low levels of vitamin D can also cause secondary hyperparathyroidism or lithium toxicity. Secondary hyperparathyroidism can be distinguished from primary hyperparathyroidism because calcium levels are typically low in secondary hyperparathyroidism. Additionally, in primary hyperparathyroidism, phosphate levels are low, while they are high in secondary hyperparathyroidism.

Hyperparathyroidism due to FHH is caused by an autosomal dominant mutation that results in abnormal calcium-sensing receptors at both the parathyroid cells and renal tubules, so the feedback mechanism of high calcium does not appropriately suppress PTH release (Fig. 13.5).

Dx:
1. **Primary:** normal/high PTH, high serum calcium, and high urine calcium (calciuria)
2. **Secondary:** high PTH, low/normal serum calcium

Tx/Mgmt:
- Surgical resection of one or more of the parathyroid glands is first line.
- If primary hyperparathyroidism is caused by carcinoma, removal of the ipsilateral thyroid and enlarged lymph nodes is recommended.

99 AR
Secondary hyperparathyroidism

Biochemical pathology renal osteodystrophy

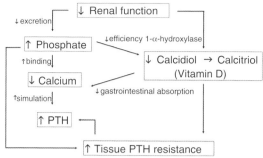

FIG. 13.5 Renal osteodystrophy. (From Lim CY, Ong KO: Various musculoskeletal manifestations of chronic renal insufficiency. *Clin Radiol* 68:e397–e411, 2013, Figure 1, Elsevier.)

- Medical management includes fluids and possibly furosemide if severe hypercalcemia
- For secondary hyperparathyroidism, treat the underlying cause (i.e., give vitamin D or calcitriol and calcium).

Hypoparathyroidism

Buzz Words: History of neck/thyroid surgery + perioral numbness + muscle cramps + hyperreflexia + paresthesias + arrhythmias + prolonged QT interval on EKG

Clinical Presentation: A patient is post-op day two from a total thyroidectomy and is complaining of muscle weakness, perioral numbness, and tingling in the fingers and toes.

PPx: N/A

MoD: The most common cause of hypothyroidism is removal or damage of parathyroid gland tissue during treatment for thyroid disease, which causes low PTH and hypocalcemia. Symptoms are usually from the hypocalcemia.

Dx: Low serum calcium and low PTH with high serum phosphate.

Tx/Mgmt: Calcium and calcitriol supplementation (IV calcium gluconate if severe and in acute hospital setting). Note: calcium supplementation may cause kidney stones.

Metabolic Bone Disease

Buzz Words: Dialysis patient with fractures or bone pain + pain worse when standing

Clinical Presentation: A patient with ESRD on dialysis presents with weakness and back pain that worsens when standing.

PPx: Modify risk for chronic kidney disease (CKD) and subsequent dialysis.

MoD: CKD can stimulate parathyroid glands through feedback loops by altering levels of calcium, vitamin D, and phosphate. CKD patients are frequently on dialysis, which may precipitate symptoms of metabolic bone disease. The main hallmarks that contribute to the secondary hyperparathyroidism seen in metabolic bone disease are high serum phosphate, low free ionized calcium, low vitamin D, and high FGF-23.

Dx: Low serum calcium, low vitamin D, and high PTH.

Tx/Mgmt: Phosphate binders, calcitriol, and calcium supplementation are first line, along with diet modifications.

Adrenal Disorders

Addison Disease

Buzz Words: Hyperpigmentation + hypotension + high potassium + upper lobe cavitary lesion + syncope

Clinical Presentation: A patient from Cambodia with a possible history of TB presents with darkening of the gums, fatigue, and lightheadedness over the past several weeks.

PPx: N/A

MoD: The two most common causes of primary adrenal insufficiency are tuberculosis (worldwide), which causes calcifications within the adrenals, and autoimmune adrenalitis (industrialized countries), which involves immune destruction of the adrenals. Patients on anticoagulants may have hemorrhagic adrenal destruction. Other causes of primary adrenal insufficiency include CMV, fungal infections, and post-partum pituitary infarction (see pituitary apoplexy). Destruction of adrenal gland tissue results in decreased cortisol and aldosterone levels (produced in the adrenals), which causes increased levels of ACTH and renin (attempting to stimulate the adrenals).

Dx: Low AM cortisol and aldosterone, high ACTH and renin; minimal cortisol response to cosyntropin test (synthetic ACTH, which should increase cortisol levels in healthy patients).

Tx/Mgmt: Adrenal crisis is a medical emergency, during which adrenal insufficiency causes severe hypotension, renal failure, and possibly death if untreated. Admit and treat with IV steroids (hydrocortisone) and fluids and identify the underlying cause.

Secondary Adrenal Insufficiency

Buzz Words: Long-term steroid use with abrupt stop

Clinical Presentation: A patient with lupus on chronic steroids is diagnosed with acute appendicitis and receives and appendectomy. On post-op day 1, the patient reports severe weakness and dizziness.

PPx: Steroid tapering or abrupt disruption in the setting of long-term steroid use.

MoD: Secondary adrenal insufficiency is caused by processes outside the adrenal glands that cause decreased levels ACTH, resulting in low cortisol and aldosterone, which include abrupt cessation of long term steroids, high dost progestins, and pituitary process causing hypopituitarism (like prolactinoma, craniopharyngioma, etc.). In the United States, it is most commonly caused by exogenous steroid use.

Dx:
- Low AM cortisol and ACTH
- Normal aldosterone and renin

Tx/Mgmt: Glucocorticoids

Cushing Syndrome

Definition

Cushing syndrome versus Cushing disease (Fig. 13.6):
- Cushing syndrome is a constellation of signs and symptoms caused by high cortisol primarily (other glucocorticoids are increased as well).
- Cushing disease is Cushing syndrome caused specifically by a pituitary adenoma.

Buzz Words: Female patient on steroids + long-term smoker with weight gain (specifically around abdomen) + purple abdominal stretch marks + "buffalo hump" + moon facies with acne + male-pattern facial hair in women

Clinical Presentation: An obese woman with a 50-pack-year smoking history and diabetes presents with weight gain, increased facial hair, irregular periods, muscle weakness, and easy bruising. She also complains of boney hip pain (think avascular necrosis of femoral head).

PPx: Reduce steroid dosages.

MoD: Cushing syndrome is caused by increased levels of cortisol in the body, which may be caused by exogenous steroid use, ectopic ACTH production (most commonly associated with small cell lung cancer), and adrenal tumors. Symptoms include myopathy, high blood pressure, hypokalemia, hypernatremia (with volume overload), and metabolic alkalosis.

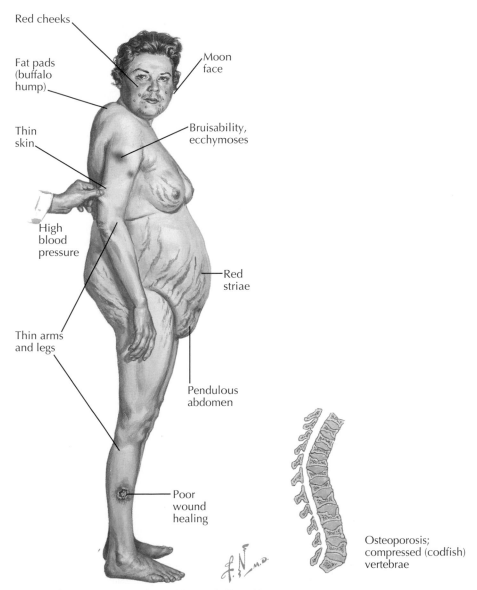

Red cheeks

Fat pads
(buffalo
hump)

Moon
face

Thin
skin

Bruisability,
ecchymoses

High
blood
pressure

Thin arms
and legs

Red
striae

Pendulous
abdomen

Poor
wound
healing

Osteoporosis;
compressed (codfish)
vertebrae

FIG. 13.6 Cushing syndrome (clinical findings). (From Netter Images. https://www.netterimages.com/ cushings-syndrome-clinical-findings-labeled-runge-im-2e-endocrinology-frank-h-netter-19953.html. ©2017 Elsevier, Inc.)

Dx:
- Low dose dexamethasone suppression test fails to suppress cortisol (AM cortisol levels > 5)
- High 24-hour urinary free cortisol level
- High ACTH → pituitary source or ectopic ACTH production; low ACTH → adrenal source

- CRH stimulation test that causes no increase in ACTH or cortisol demonstrates an adrenal or ectopic ACTH source for Cushing syndrome
- Chest CT and abdominal CT to identify mass in lung or on adrenals

Tx/Mgmt: Taper glucocorticoid or treat underlying cause (i.e., surgical excision of tumor in lung)

Cushing Disease

Buzz Words: Hyperpigmentation + features of Cushing syndrome

Clinical Presentation: A female patient presents with weight gain, purple streaks over her belly, amenorrhea, facial hair growth, hyperpigmentation around the neck, headache, and decreased peripheral vision (suggestive of bitemporal hemianopsia). Recently diagnosed with diabetes.

PPx: N/A

MoD: Cushing disease is caused primarily by small pituitary adenomas that increase secretion of ACTH, causing adrenal hyperplasia (from overstimulation), which results in hyperpigmentation, increased cortisol and aldosterone.

Dx:

Cushing diagnostic flowchart

- Low dose dexamethasone suppression test fails to suppress cortisol (AM cortisol levels >5)
- High 24-hour urinary free cortisol level
- High ACTH → pituitary source or ectopic ACTH production
- CRH stimulation test that causes increase in ACTH or cortisol indicates Cushing disease
- Brain magnetic resonance imaging (MRI)

Tx/Mgmt: Surgical resection of pituitary adenoma and bilateral adrenalectomies are first line.

Hyperaldosteronism

Buzz Words: patient with medication resistant hypertension and hypokalemia, without edema

Clinical Presentation: A young, otherwise healthy patient presents with hypertension unresponsive to first, second, or third line anti-hypertensive medications.

PPx: N/A

MoD: Causes of hyperaldosteronism include adrenal adenomas (most common cause, usually unilateral), adrenal hyperplasia (bilateral), and adrenal carcinoma (rare). Elevated aldosterone levels cause hypernatremia, hypokalemia, metabolic alkalosis, high plasma aldosterone/renin ratio (>30).

Dx:

- High plasma aldosterone to renin ratio (> 30)
- Saline infusion does not reduce aldosterone levels
- Adrenal venous sampling, which measures aldosterone in venous blood (bilateral and unilateral to help differentiate etiology—bilateral adrenal hyperplasia or unilateral adenoma)
- Adrenal computed tomography (CT)

Tx/Mgmt:

- Adrenal adenoma—surgical resection is first line therapy.
- Bilateral adrenal hyperplasia—medical management with aldosterone antagonists like spironolactone or eplerenone is indicated.

Pheochromocytoma

Buzz Words: Hypertension + headache + palpitations + anxiety

Clinical Presentation: A 45-year-old patient presents with frequent episodes of severe headaches, sweating, and tachycardia. His BP in your office is 160/100. Consider a family history of MEN2 syndromes, von Hippel-Lindau syndrome and neurofibromatosis type 1 (NF1).

PPx: N/A

MoD: Pheochromocytomas are tumors that secrete catecholamines, including epinephrine and norepinephrine, arising primarily from the chromaffin cells in the adrenal medulla.

Dx:

1. 24-hour urine positive for metanephrines
2. Imaging (CT or MRI) to localize tumor

Tx/Mgmt:

1. Alpha blockers first (phenoxybenzamine)!! (If beta blockers were given first, it would cause unopposed alpha action causing a hypertensive crisis. Treat the crisis with nitroprusside)
2. Beta blockers (propranolol) for two weeks
3. Surgical resection is first line treatment

Endocrine Diseases Which Cause Hypertension

Endocrine diseases that cause hypertension include hyperaldosteronism, pheochromocytoma, Cushing syndrome and disease, hypothyroidism, and primary hyperparathyroidism.

Pituitary Disorders

Pituitary Adenomas

Buzz Words: bitemporal hemianopsia + headache

99 AR

Pheochromocytoma mnemonic and overview

Clinical Presentation: Pituitary adenomas are the most common pituitary pathology. Pituitary adenomas are usually benign and most commonly prolactinomas (see below), but can grow and cause parasellar symptoms, which are symptoms related to the effect of a growing mass within the sellar region (a saddle depression within the skull that houses the pituitary gland). Parasellar symptoms include visual changes caused by compression of the optic chiasm, headache caused by mass effect, and reductions in pituitary hormone release (mostly GH, LH, and FSH) caused by compression of the hypothalamic-pituitary stalk. Other symptoms may also depend on which pituitary hormone is being hypersecreted, including TSH, ACTH, prolactin, and GH (see respective sections for symptoms specific to each hormone).

PPx: N/A

MoD: The pathogenesis of these neoplasms is not fully understood, as the mutations that cause them have not been well documented.

Dx:

1. LH, FSH, prolactin, IGF-1 levels
2. 24-hour urine free cortisol
3. MRI of the brain

Tx/Mgmt: Surgical resection (transsphenoidal approach) of the adenoma is first line, except in the case of prolactinomas (see below).

Acromegaly/Gigantism

Buzz Words: Coarse facial features + increased ring/hat size + large jaw + skin tags + bitemporal hemianopsia (parasellar manifestation; Fig. 13.7).

Clinical Presentation: Patients with acromegaly may present with coarsening of the facial features over time with a particularly large jaw. They may notice that their hats or

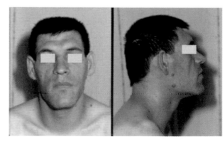

FIG. 13.7 Acromegaly facial coarsening. (From *Orphanet J Rare Dis* 3:17, 2008. http://dx.doi.org/10.1186/1750-1172-3-17. © Chanson and Salenave; licensee BioMed Central Ltd. 2008 Published: 25 June 2008, Figure 2.)

rings are getter tighter. Associated with aortic regurgitation, hypercalcemia, carpal tunnel syndrome. The most common cause of death is from cardiomyopathy. These patients also have gonadotropic depression and sometimes elevated prolactin.

PPx: N/A

MoD: Excess GH released by pituitary adenoma causes excess insulin-like growth factor (IGF)-1, which leads to excessive growth of bone, soft tissues, and organs.

Dx:
- Elevated IGF-1 level
- Inadequate GH suppression with oral glucose suppression test
- MRI of pituitary

Tx/Mgmt: Resection of pituitary adenoma

Diabetes Insipidus

Buzz Words: Frequent urination + very thirsty

Clinical Presentation
- **Central Diabetes Insipidus (DI):** Most common. Causes: idiopathic (most common), head trauma, head/brain surgery.
- **Peripheral DI:** Causes: chronic lithium use (most common), hypercalcemia, hereditary.

MoD:
- **Central DI:** Low ADH secretion
- **Peripheral DI:** Decreased responsiveness of renal tubule receptors to ADH. Normal ADH levels.

Dx:
- Decreased urine osmolality
- High serum osmolality (<300)
- Water deprivation test → no change in urine osmolality
- Low ADH in central DI, normal/high ADH in nephrogenic DI

Tx/Mgmt:
- **Central DI:** Desmopressin; treat underlying cause
- **Peripheral DI:** Sodium restriction and thiazide diuretics

Panhypopituitarism

Buzz Words: Symptoms of ACTH deficiency (postural hypotension, tachycardia, weight loss, hypoglycemia) + symptoms of hypothyroidism (fatigue, cold intolerance, dry skin, bradycardia), + symptoms of gonadotropin deficiency (amenorrhea or infertility in women; decreased libido and infertility in men)

99 AR

SIADH vs diabetes insipidus

MoD:

- Pituitary causes: adenoma, malignancy, hemochromatosis, hemorrhage, infarction
- Hypothalamic causes: mass, radiation therapy, sarcoidosis, trauma, infection

Dx:

- Low ACTH, cortisol, TSH, T4, LH, FSH and testosterone
- Normal aldosterone levels

Tx/Mgmt: Hydrocortisone, levothyroxine, testosterone for men, and estradiol and progestin for women

Pituitary Apoplexy (Sheehan Syndrome)

Buzz Words: Hypotension + postpartum woman + hemorrhage in labor + no lactation

Clinical Presentation: A woman on postpartum day 8 from a vaginal delivery complicated by 1500 cc of postpartum hemorrhage and hypotension during labor complains of extreme fatigue and inability to produce breastmilk for her infant.

PPx: N/A

MoD: An infarction of the pituitary in the setting of postpartum hemorrhage (Sheehan syndrome) or a sudden hemorrhage into the pituitary gland, usually into a pituitary adenoma (pituitary apoplexy), both resulting in hypopituitarism.

99 AR

MRIs of Sheehan Syndrome

Dx:

1. Low ACTH, TSH, LH, and FSH
2. MRI of pituitary

Tx/Mgmt:

1. Treat adrenal insufficiency with corticosteroids
2. Surgical decompression of pituitary in cases with severe neurologic deficits

Growth Hormone Deficiency

Buzz Words: Short stature (commonly seen in children) + decreased bone density (high rate of fractures)

Clinical Presentation: A 20-year-old presents with short stature in the 5th percentile.

PPx: N/A

MoD: See hypopituitarism section (same causes as other pituitary hormone deficiencies)

Dx: Low IGF-1 (low GH can confirm if IGF-1 is borderline)

Tx/Mgmt: GH therapy for childhood onset of disease, follow up IGF-1

SIADH

Buzz Words: Hyponatremia + weakness + seizures + small cell carcinoma (SCLC) of the lung

Clinical Presentation: A patient with a 50 pack-year smoking history presents with seizures. His labs are unremarkable except for a sodium of 105.

PPx: Prep10060vent underlying cause (see below), such as avoiding smoking and maintaining cardiovascular health for stroke prevention.

MoD: Excess ADH causes increased water retention at the level of the collecting ducts in the renal tubules, resulting in volume expansion and hyponatremia. The posterior pituitary or an ectopic source, such as a neoplasm (especially SCLC), central nervous system (CNS) disorder (stroke, infection, trauma), medications (chlorpropamide, carbamazepine, cyclophosphamide, and selective serotonin reuptake inhibitors [SSRIs]) or surgery.

Dx: SIADH is a diagnosis of exclusion, but the following lab values support a diagnosis of SIADH: hyponatremia in the setting of hypoosmolality concentrated urine (>100 mosmol/kg) with reduced urine volume.

Tx/Mgmt: Treat underlying cause and water restrict all patients. For symptomatic patients, normal saline may be used.

- Note: Do not correct hyponatremia too quickly or central pontine myelinosis may occur due to rapid flux out of cells into the extracellular fluid space.

Prolactinoma and Hyperprolactinemia

Buzz Words: The combination of bitemporal hemianopsia, headache, and galactorrhea in an older male

Clinical Presentation: A 42-year-old woman presents with decreased peripheral vision, decreased libido, headaches, and unexpected milk production from her breasts (galactorrhea). Men may present with impotence.

PPx: N/A

MoD: Unknown

Dx:
1. Clinical presentation
2. Serum hormone levels (including prolactin)
3. Brain MRI

Tx/Mgmt:
1. Cabergoline or bromocriptine (for pregnant women), both dopamine agonists
2. If symptoms persist or there is not a sufficient reduction in size of the prolactinoma, transsphenoidal surgery may be required

Craniopharyngiomas

Buzz Words: Child falling off the growth curve with headaches or visual changes

Clinical Presentation: Bimodal age distribution (5–14 years old and 50–70 years old), but predominantly in the pediatric population with presenting symptoms of growth failure and/or headaches.

PPx: N/A

MoD: Craniopharyngiomas are suprasellar tumors, arising from epithelial cells.

Dx: Brain MRI

Tx/Mgmt: Surgical resection

Hypogonadism, Primary and Secondary

Buzz Words: Low sperm count + decreased libido + decreased muscle mass + decreased body hair

Clinical Presentation: Common causes of hypogonadism include tumor in or trauma to suprasellar area (most commonly prolactinoma), diabetes mellitus, narcotic pain medication, obesity, exogenous steroid or testosterone use, so look for signs of these other diseases in the question. A typical patient is a man presenting with fertility issues and has evidence of decreased testosterone levels.

PPx: N/A

MoD: In primary hypogonadism, disease primarily involves the testes, characterized by low testosterone and high LH and FSH. Infertility (low sperm count caused by decreased spermatogenesis due to low testosterone) in these cases is harder to treat in comparison to secondary hypogonadism. In secondary hypogonadism, disease primarily involves the pituitary or hypothalamus, characterized by low testosterone, LH, and FSH. Spermatogenesis can be increased (raising sperm count and improving infertility issues) in these patients by increasing LH and FSH.

Dx:
1. Clinical presentation
2. Semen analysis (for sperm count)
3. Serum morning total testosterone. If morning total testosterone is low, repeat it and draw LH and FSH.
4. If secondary hypogonadism is suspected, measure other pituitary hormones too (TSH, etc.)

Tx/Mgmt: Testosterone replacement therapy (via transdermal patch) if patients have demonstrated low morning serum testosterone on three occasions.

Multiple Endocrine Neoplasia (MEN1, MEN2)

Definition

- MEN Type 1: parathyroid hyperplasia, pancreatic islet cell tumor, pituitary tumors; associated with Zollinger-Ellison syndrome (ZES), which produces gastrinomas.
- MEN Type 2A: medullary thyroid carcinoma, pheochromocytoma, hyperparathyroidism
- MEN Type 2B: medullary thyroid carcinoma, marfanoid habitus (tall and thin, large wing span), pheochromocytoma, neuromas

Buzz Words: Personal/family history of endocrine tumors + severe peptic ulcer disease (gastrinomas) + high PTH + high calcium + thyroid nodule + galactorrhea (MEN1)

Clinical Presentation: Patients are typically asymptomatic initially as hyperparathyroidism is the presenting manifestation of MEN1 and 2A syndromes. For MEN2B, presenting symptoms can be a thyroid nodule. Unrelenting peptic ulcer disease can be a hint for ZES.

PPx: Genetic screening prior to symptoms is recommended, as MEN2A and 2B can progress to medullary thyroid carcinoma. For these patients, prophylactic total thyroidectomy is indicated.

MoD: Autosomal dominant disorder.

Dx: Diagnosis is based on the presence of two or more of the tumors specific to one of the MEN syndromes, supported by genetic testing for RET proto-oncogene germ line mutation and labs indicating normal/high PTH and high calcium (MEN1 and 2A).

Tx/Mgmt:

- For patients who are positive for the RET proto-oncogene, total thyroidectomy is indicated to prevent medullary thyroid carcinoma.
- Surgery is also indicated for pheochromocytomas (MEN2A and 2B).
- For symptomatic hyperparathyroidism (bone loss, kidney stones, etc.), surgery is indicated (but watch out for those recurrent laryngeal nerves!).

QUICK TIPS

MEN Type 1 → **PPP** = **p**arathyroid hyperplasia, **p**ancreatic islet cell tumor, **p**ituitary tumors

QUICK TIPS

MEN Type 2A → **MPH** = **m**edullary thyroid carcinoma, **p**heochromocytoma, **h**yperparathyroidism

QUICK TIPS

MEN Type 2B → **MMPN** = **m**edullary thyroid carcinoma, **m**arfanoid habitus, **p**heochromocytoma, **n**euromas

99 AR

MEN syndrome diagram

GUNNER PRACTICE

1 A 34-year-old female presents with altered mental status after a CT contrast study. Her vitals are: HR 115, BP 180/100, T 40.2, RR 22, O₂ sat 95%. Her sister who is accompanying her noted that she had been vomiting and had an episode of diarrhea prior to becoming delirious. The patient has a history of anxiety on lorazepam and hypertension well-controlled on medications. No previous surgeries. The sister also mentioned that the patient is easily irritable and agitated and has been losing weight despite not actively trying to. What should be your next step in management?

A. Propranolol
B. Pain medication
C. Epinephrine
D. Lorazepam

2. A 65-year-old male underwent a thyroidectomy and bilateral neck dissection for thyroid cancer. On postop day one, he began developing perioral numbness, paresthesias in the tips of his fingers and toes, and muscle cramps. He has a history of diabetes and hypertension. He had no previous surgeries and smokes 2–3 packs a day for the past 40 years. Which of the following additional symptoms are LEAST likely to be seen in this patient?

A. Hyperreflexia
B. Brittle nails
C. Prolonged QT interval
D. Wheezing

3. A 40-year-old man presents for surgical consultation for medullary thyroid carcinoma. He is extremely thin and tall. He is being treated for depression by his psychiatrist and has prediabetes. He also complains of episodic headaches, palpitations, and diaphoresis which last for a few seconds and occur every few weeks or so. He has had no previous surgeries. What other neoplasms might this patient have?

A. Pituitary tumors
B. Mucosal neuromas
C. Parathyroid adenomas
D. Pancreatic tumors

Notes

ANSWERS: What Would Gunner Jess/Jim Do?

1 WWGJD? A 34-year-old female presents with altered mental status after a CT contrast study. Her vitals are: HR 115, BP 180/100, T 40.2, RR 22, O$_2$ sat 95%. Her sister who is accompanying her noted that she had been vomiting and had an episode of diarrhea prior to becoming delirious. The patient has a history of anxiety on lorazepam and hypertension well-controlled on medications. No previous surgeries. The sister also mentioned that the patient is easily irritable and agitated and has been losing weight despite not actively trying to. What should be your next step in management?

Answer: A, Propranolol

   This patient is experiencing a thyroid storm and needs emergent antiadrenergic drugs for symptom control, thionamides to correct the hyperthyroid state, and glucocorticoids to decrease peripheral conversion of T4 to T3.

   B. Pain medication → Incorrect. The vitals are inappropriate for a normal pain response.

   C. Epinephrine → Incorrect. This patient is not having an allergic reaction to the contrast dye.

   D. Lorazepam → Incorrect. This patient's presentation is not consistent with a panic attack.

2 WWGJD? A 65-year-old male underwent a thyroidectomy and bilateral neck dissection for thyroid cancer. On postop day one, he began developing perioral numbness, paresthesias in the tips of his fingers and toes, and muscle cramps. He has a history of diabetes and hypertension. He had no previous surgeries and smokes 2-3 packs a day for the past 40 years. Which of the following additional symptoms are LEAST likely to be seen in this patient?

Answer: B, Brittle nails

   This patient is experiencing acute hypocalcemia from damage to the parathyroids during his thyroid surgery. Acute manifestations include perioral numbness, paresthesias in the distal extremities, muscle cramps, hyperreflexia, prolonged QT intervals on EKG, broncho- or laryngospasms, fatigue, and irritability or personality changes. Brittle nails, coarse hair, and dry skin may be signs of chronic rather than acute hypocalcemia.

3 WWGJD? A 40-year-old man presents for surgical consultation for medullary thyroid carcinoma. He is extremely thin and tall. He is being treated for depression

by his psychiatrist and has prediabetes. He also complains of episodic headaches, palpitations, and diaphoresis which last for a few seconds and occur every few weeks or so. He has had no previous surgeries. What other neoplasms might this patient have?

Answer: B, Mucosal neuromas

This patient likely has MEN2B syndrome, which is characterized by medullary thyroid carcinomas, mucosal neuromas, pheochromocytomas, oral or intestinal ganglioneuromatosis, and marfanoid habitus. His episodic headaches and palpitations are from a pheochromocytoma. Like MEN2A, this syndrome is associated with the loss of the tyrosin kinase proto-oncogene called RET.

A. Pituitary tumors → Incorrect. These are associated with MEN1. MEN1 syndrome may present with parathyroid tumors, pituitary tumors, and pancreatic islet cell or endocrine tumors. Patients may complain of gastric ulcers (from a Zollinger-Ellison tumor) or kidney stones (from increased calcium from the increased PTH from parathyroid neoplasms).

C. Parathyroid adenomas → Incorrect. These are associated with MEN1 and EN2A. MEN2A may present with medullary thyroid carcinoma, pheochromocytomas, and parathyroid tumors.

D. Pancreatic tumors → Incorrect. These are associated with MEN1.

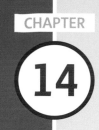

Gunner Jim's Guide to Exam Day Success

Leo Wang and Hao-Hua Wu

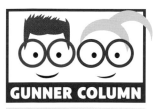

GUNNER COLUMN

Do these three things to perform well on any shelf:

1. Master one review book.
2. Do as many quality questions as you can.
3. Review questions in Excel.

"Master One Review Book"

The internal medicine shelf is notorious for being one of the most difficult shelf exams you will take and requires a lot of knowledge to succeed. The most important thing you can do prior to the start of your rotation is to identify the resource that best covers the material on the medicine shelf and stick with it. This being said, there is a ton of information for the medicine shelf, and you may find yourself wanting other resources. Our augmented reality component provides the depth needed to explore the eclectic multimedia sources that can prep you for the exam.

Most of your learning takes place when you complete questions, so don't be discouraged if you cannot memorize every word of your review book like you did for step 1—this is not possible, even for the most accomplished physicians. Instead, use your review book as a point of reference and annotate the margins.

If you see one topic come up on multiple chapters (or maybe even multiple shelf exams), make sure to write down the page numbers where it appears and flip to those pages every time you review. The more connections you make, the more you will master.

In addition, highlight themes that keep coming up. Any time patients in the question stem have recently changed their medication regimen, suspect the medication change as the cause of their symptoms until proven otherwise. Any time a patient comes in with almost anything, the first two things you should order are a BMP and CBC. Any suspicion for infection should lead you to get blood cultures. These organizing principles transcend individual topics and can help you do well on any shelf exam test question.

"Do as Many Quality Questions as You Can"

The key to success is practicing in an environment that simulates the pressure of test day. And nothing simulates that pressure better than taking practice questions under stringent time constraints.

After you identify your review book, select as many authoritative question banks as you can. We recommend Gunner Practice, UWorld, and NBME Clinical Science practice exams. Do at least 10 questions a day under timed conditions (1.5 minutes a question), starting on the first day of your rotation.

Remember, you can complete the same question multiple times in the course of study! In fact, it is recommended that you retry the questions you got wrong in the first place, just so that you know you would get it right on the test.

It is also important that the questions you complete are of high quality. This means that the length and content of the question stems reflect what you would actually see on test day. Many question bank resources are too easy (giving you a false sense of confidence) or ask about material that will not show up on the exam (wasting your time).

Once you have selected your question bank resources, count the total number of questions and divide it by the number of days you have available to study. Then make sure you set a study plan where you can make at least two passes through your questions. The first pass is completion of all available questions. The second pass is completion of all the questions you got wrong or made a lucky guess on during your first pass. Seeing how many of the second pass questions you get correct should be a nice confidence boost leading into exam day.

"Review Questions in Excel"

How you take notes for the questions you complete is imperative to success.

The most effective strategy is to pick **one** take-home point for every question you complete and record it on an Excel sheet specific for your clinical rotation.

For instance, if you got a question about the treatment of sickle cell wrong, write "Tx of sickle cell" in column A of your Excel sheet and then "hydroxyurea" in column B of your Excel sheet. This will allow you to create an immediate pseudo flashcard. When you review this material the following week, you can put your cursor over column A, say the answer out loud, and check your answer by shifting your cursor to column B. This will save you a lot of time and jump directly to what the most important takeaway is for each question. You can also make your own flashcards on the Gunner Goggles iOS app.

If you understand everything in the question and answer choices, don't record it in the Excel sheet.

If you don't understand multiple things in the question and answer choices, record the most important takeaway point and move on. For test day, it is better to be confident in what you know well than to undermine your confidence by fixating on what you are weak at.

By test day, you should have one Excel sheet that contains one important take-home point from every question you were unsure about. The tabs on the bottom should be organized by question bank resource. This Excel spread would ideally only take 3–4 hours to review, and is something you would go over the day before the exam.

Last but not least, **trust the process**. Philadelphia 76ers fans endured years of painful basketball losses while Sam Hinkie rebuilt the team, but were instructed to "trust the process." Students often enter test day anxious and overwhelmed, which can cause them to second-guess their answer choices. Trust the process—trust that you will have covered everything leading up to the medicine shelf exam and have some faith in your answer selections. After all, you were on this rotation for at least 8 weeks. For these reasons, don't second-guess yourself. Your first instinct is usually right.

In summary: Read, Apply, Review. And Trust the Process.

Index

Page numbers followed by *f* indicate figures, *t* indicate tables, and *b* indicate boxes.